Notes and Observations on the Ionian Islands and Malta

With Some Remarks on Constantinople and Turkey, and on the System of Quarantine as at Present Conducted

VOLUME 2

JOHN DAVY

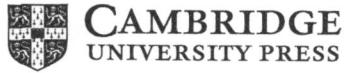
CAMBRIDGE
UNIVERSITY PRESS

CAMBRIDGE UNIVERSITY PRESS

Cambridge, New York, Melbourne, Madrid, Cape Town,
Singapore, São Paolo, Delhi, Tokyo, Mexico City

Published in the United States of America by Cambridge University Press, New York

www.cambridge.org
Information on this title: www.cambridge.org/9781108042369

© in this compilation Cambridge University Press 2012

This edition first published 1842
This digitally printed version 2012

ISBN 978-1-108-04236-9 Paperback

CAMBRIDGE LIBRARY COLLECTION

Books of enduring scholarly value

Travel and Exploration

The history of travel writing dates back to the Bible, Caesar, the Vikings and the Crusaders, and its many themes include war, trade, science and recreation. Explorers from Columbus to Cook charted lands not previously visited by Western travellers, and were followed by merchants, missionaries, and colonists, who wrote accounts of their experiences. The development of steam power in the nineteenth century provided opportunities for increasing numbers of 'ordinary' people to travel further, more economically, and more safely, and resulted in great enthusiasm for travel writing among the reading public. Works included in this series range from first-hand descriptions of previously unrecorded places, to literary accounts of the strange habits of foreigners, to examples of the burgeoning numbers of guidebooks produced to satisfy the needs of a new kind of traveller - the tourist.

Notes and Observations on the Ionian Islands and Malta

The English doctor John Davy (1790–1868) was the younger brother of the chemist Sir Humphry Davy, of whom he wrote a memoir, also reissued in this series. After graduating from Edinburgh University, he entered the Army as a surgeon and was posted overseas. From 1824 to 1835 he was stationed in the Mediterranean, and later at Constantinople. Davy took detailed notes of the places he visited and the people he met, and turned some of these writings into books; his scientific observations led to him being made a Fellow of the Royal Society in 1834. Davy's account of his time in the Mediterranean was published in two volumes in 1842. Volume 2 continues the description of the Ionian islands and their people. Later chapters focus on health issues, such as malaria and other diseases, with the final chapters discussing Constantinople and examining the problems faced by Turkish army hospitals.

Cambridge University Press has long been a pioneer in the reissuing of out-of-print titles from its own backlist, producing digital reprints of books that are still sought after by scholars and students but could not be reprinted economically using traditional technology. The Cambridge Library Collection extends this activity to a wider range of books which are still of importance to researchers and professionals, either for the source material they contain, or as landmarks in the history of their academic discipline.

Drawing from the world-renowned collections in the Cambridge University Library, and guided by the advice of experts in each subject area, Cambridge University Press is using state-of-the-art scanning machines in its own Printing House to capture the content of each book selected for inclusion. The files are processed to give a consistently clear, crisp image, and the books finished to the high quality standard for which the Press is recognised around the world. The latest print-on-demand technology ensures that the books will remain available indefinitely, and that orders for single or multiple copies can quickly be supplied.

The Cambridge Library Collection brings back to life books of enduring scholarly value (including out-of-copyright works originally issued by other publishers) across a wide range of disciplines in the humanities and social sciences and in science and technology.

NOTES AND OBSERVATIONS

ON

THE IONIAN ISLANDS AND MALTA.

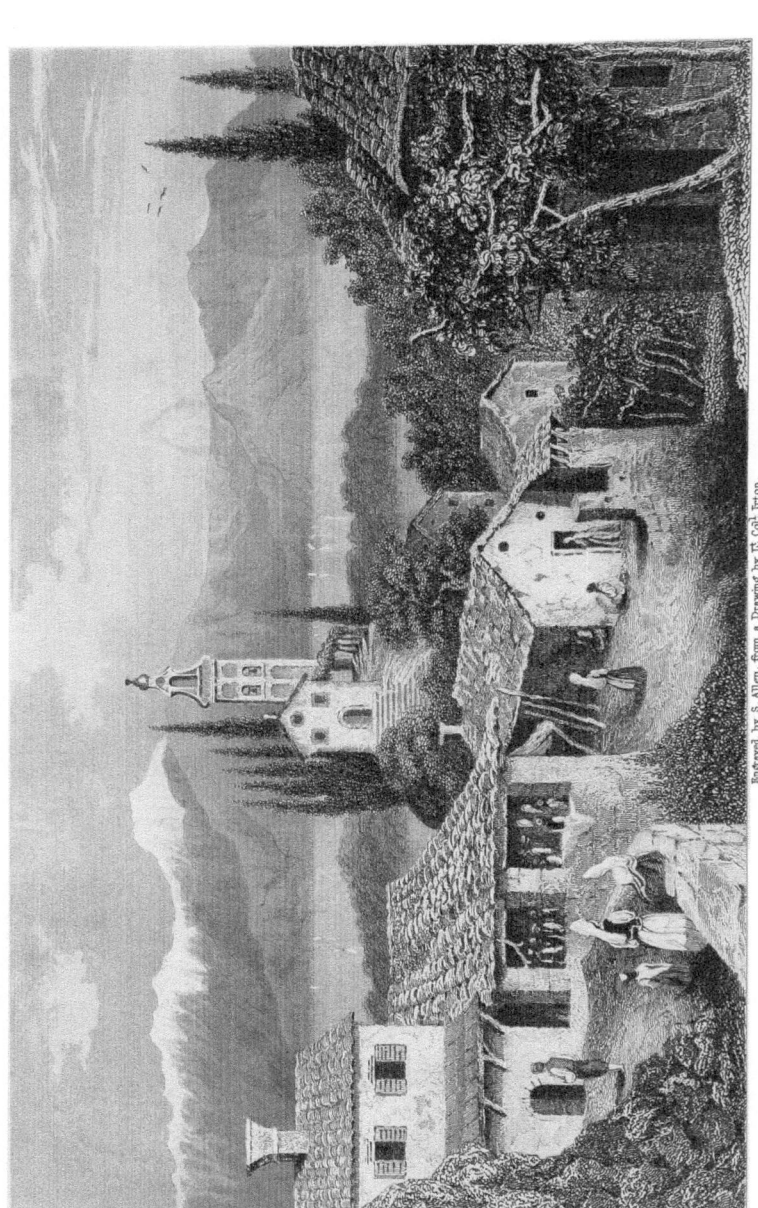

Engraved by S. Allen, from a Drawing by D. Col. Irton.

VILLAGE OF CALAFATIONES.

CORFU.

Published by Smith, Elder & C? Cornhill, London.

NOTES AND OBSERVATIONS

ON THE

IONIAN ISLANDS AND MALTA:

WITH SOME REMARKS ON

CONSTANTINOPLE AND TURKEY,

AND ON

THE SYSTEM OF QUARANTINE AS AT PRESENT CONDUCTED.

BY

JOHN DAVY, M.D., F.R.SS., L. & E.

INSPECTOR-GENERAL OF ARMY-HOSPITALS, L. R.

IN TWO VOLUMES.

VOL. II.

LONDON:

SMITH, ELDER & CO., 65, CORNHILL.

MDCCCXLII.

CONTENTS.

Page

CHAPTER I.

SKETCH OF THE PRESENT GOVERNMENT OF THE IONIAN ISLANDS.

Form of the Ionian Government as established by Charter in 1817.
The Senate, how Constituted. Its Duties. The Legislative As-
sembly. Mode of its Election. Its Functions. The Parliament.
The Local Governments of the different Islands, and their Compo-
sition. How Subordinate to the General Government. Form and
Administration of Legal Power. Composition of the Courts of Jus-
tice. Supreme and Local Church Establishment. Civil List.
Character of the Government. Remarks on the same. Acts of
Parliament illustrative of the Forms of Government, . . 1

CHAPTER II.

ON THE STATE OF THE ARTS IN THE IONIAN ISLANDS.

Statistical Returns illustrating the State of the Arts. Remarks on
these. Trades followed, chiefly those concerned with Common
Wants. How carried on. Examples in illustration of the low
degree of Skill with which they are conducted. The Fine Arts
little advanced. Comparison of the different Islands. Remarks
on the rude State of the Arts in Cerigo, and on the Ignorance of
the People. Small Communities unfavourable to Progress in the
Arts. Retarding Circumstances, ... 32

Page

CHAPTER III.

MISCELLANEOUS NOTICES OF SOME OF THE UTENSILS, IMPLEMENTS, AND
PROCESSES IN USE IN THE IONIAN ISLANDS.

Mills. A very primitive Corn-Mill described. Oven in common use.
Kitchen Fire-places. Lamps. Still. Water-lever. Different
Modes in use of watering Gardens. Manner of washing Clothes.
Bleaching. Dyeing. The Sandal. Remarks on its usefulness.
Boats of peculiar Construction. Modes of taking Fish. Of snar-
ing Birds, ... 43

CHAPTER IV.

ON THE COMMERCE OF THE IONIAN ISLANDS.

Great Capabilities of these Islands for Commerce. Tables illustrative
of their present Commercial Condition. Peculiar Mode of Conducting the Trade in Grain. Currant and Oil Trade. Disadvantages under which they labour. Remarks on the Commercial Resources of the Islands, and the Improvement of certain
Productions and Manufactures. Exertions of Government in
behalf of Improvement. Establishment of an Ionian Bank—an
Agricultural Society. Great Improvement and Extension of the
Roads. Other Improvements in Progress. Tables in illustration
of the Commercial Relations between the Ionian Islands and Great
Britain. Tables illustrating the Currant-trade, . . 57

CHAPTER V.

ON THE STATE OF KNOWLEDGE IN THE IONIAN ISLANDS, AND ON THE MEANS
OF EDUCATION.

Remarkable deficiency of useful Scientific Knowledge. Circumstances
to which owing. Illustrations drawn from the Liberal Professions
and the Superstitions of the People. Outline of the System of
Education in use, instituted by the Government. Medals for the
Encouragement of Learning. Seminary for the Instruction of
Students of Divinity. Brief Sketch of the Progress of Public
Education. Remarks on the Tendencies to Abuse. Example of
Success in Cerigo. Dangers to which a University is exposed in a
Small Community illustrated, ... 96

CHAPTER VI.

ON THE CHARITABLE INSTITUTIONS OF THE IONIAN ISLANDS.

Smallness of their Number. Monti di Pietà. Civil Hospitals. Lunatic Asylum. Desiderata in regard to Medical Institutions. Foundling-Hospital. Remarks relative to its former Abuses. Observations on the Condition of the Indigent Poor. Remarks on the Population, ...   117

CHAPTER VII.

ON THE CHARACTER AND GENERAL CONDITION OF THE PEOPLE OF THE IONIAN ISLANDS.

General Resemblance of the People of the different Islands. Points of Difference. Habits and Manners of the Inhabitants divided into Classes. Notice of the Principal Towns ; of the Houses of the Upper Class ; their Furniture and Household Economy. Amusements and Recreations. Dress of the Peasantry. Other particulars respecting them. Numerous Holidays. Neglect of the Sabbath. Condition of the Women. Marriage Rites. Funerals. Neglected State of Grave-yards, and Want of Respect to the Dead. Remarks on the Character of the People. Extracts from Authors, relative to the same, contrasted, ...   124

CHAPTER VIII.

NOTICE OF A JOURNEY THROUGH THE MOUNTAINOUS DISTRICT OF ZANTE, IN 1824.

This District hitherto imperfectly known. Particulars of Catastari. Monastery of Spelliotissa. Character of the adjoining Hilly Country. Volimes. Pitiable Condition of the Sick. Total Destitution of Medical Aid. Free, independent Life of the Inhabitants. Monastery of St Georgio. Bay of Vromi. Prospects from the Heights of Vrachiona. Village of Maries. Houses and Habits of the Villagers. Cisterns of Oxicora and its basin-like Valley. St Leo. Instances of remarkable Longevity. Large Apiary. Basin-like Valley of Luca. Coldness of its Climate. Monastery of Madonna Paragato. Woodcock Shooting. Gilliamano. Village School. Neglected Grave-Yard. House of the Priest. Farther Particulars

Page

respecting the Occupations of the People. Comparative Severity
of the Winter Season. Villages of Ambelo and Chieri. Malaria
of the former. Manner of Snaring Doves. Diglidani's Leap.
Cultivation and Peculiarities of the Currant-Vine in the Valley of
the Pitch-Springs. Appearance and Dress of the People in the
Mountain Villages, ...   155

CHAPTER IX.

MISCELLANEOUS REMARKS ; WITH EXTRACTS FROM JOURNALS, IN FARTHER
ILLUSTRATION OF THE STATE OF THE PEOPLE IN THE IONIAN ISLANDS.

Notice of a Visit to the Monastery of Taffeo, in Cephalonia, and how
entertained there. A Medical Consultation in the same Island.
Excursions from Cephalonia and Santa Maura to Ithaca. Primitive Reception and Hospitality. Particulars respecting the Island
of Meganisi. Notice of the desert Islet of Tiglia. Particulars of
Leftimo, a district of Corfu. Excursion to Sidari, on the north
coast of Corfu. Particulars of Fano, and other Islets, off the north-
west coast of Corfu. Notice of the Island of Paxo. Its Cisterns.
Bishop of Paxo. Manners of the Inhabitants,   .   .   194

CHAPTER X.

ON MALARIA AND THE FEVERS OF THE IONIAN ISLANDS.

General Healthiness of the Ionian Islands, independent of Fevers of
Malaria-Origin. Tables in Illustration. Different Types of Fever
described. Summer Fever of the Mediterranean. Remittent Fever.
Illustrative Tables. Remarks on the Nature and Treatment of
Remittent Fever. Intermittent Fevers. Malaria. Conjectures
respecting its Nature. Negative Evidence. Facts in illustration
of its Mysterious Origin. Circumstances favouring its Agency.
Cautions against it, ...   218

CHAPTER XI.

ON THE FEVERS OF MALTA.

Kinds of Fever to which Malta is subject. Tables in illustration. Remarks on the Nomenclature of Fevers. Notice of the different kinds
affecting the British Troops and the Inhabitants. Further Observations and Reflections on Malaria, ...   262

Page

CHAPTER XII.

ON THE CLIMATE OF THE MEDITERRANEAN, IN RELATION TO PULMONARY
CONSUMPTION.

Popular Opinion that the Climate of the Mediterranean is less productive of Pulmonary Disease than that of Great Britain. Opposite
results of recent Statistical Inquiries. These results scrutinized.
Comparison of Cavalry and Infantry Soldier as regards circumstances affecting Health. Evidence derived from the Troops serving at home and in the Mediterranean. Proportional prevalency of
Phthisis amongst the native Maltese. Tables in illustration. De-
duction in favour of the Climate of Malta. Problem of the greater
Liability of British Troops to Phthisis in Malta than in the Ionian
Islands. Returns of Fatal Cases in illustration. Circumstances
likely to conduce to the greater Liability in Malta. Remarks on its
Climate, with Suggestions for Invalids proposing to winter there.
Reflections on the Formation of Tubercle in the Lung, and on the
Means of Prevention, ... 280

CHAPTER XIII.

OBSERVATIONS ON QUARANTINE.

Supposed Importance and Object of Quarantine. Notice of the Effects
of the Measures which have been considered necessary for its
Inforcement. Reflections on the existing System. Farther inquiries necessary to decide on many important Points. Foundations of existing System of doubtful Soundness. Question of the
Contagion of Plague. Considerations for and against the Doctrine.
Recent Facts seemingly Demonstrative of Contagion. Remarks
on the time the Disease may be latent. On the questionable Propriety of the Classification of Substances into Susceptible and Non-
Susceptible. Reasons for considering all Substances susceptible,
excepting those which have the Power of destroying Contagion.
Other Objections to the present System of Quarantine. Desiderata
in Relation to farther Inquiry. Prospects of a successful Termination, and of a Revision of the Quarantine Laws. Facts in favour
of both. Advantages likely to result from the adoption of a Milder
and more Efficient System, ... 323

Page

CHAPTER XIV.

ON THE SMALL-POX OF 1830-31, IN MALTA.

How introduced. Progress of the Disease, its Extent and Mortality.
Tables in illustration. Remarks founded on the Numerical Re-
sults. Conjecture that Warm Air freely circulating in the Apartments may be beneficial in the Treatment of the Disease. Influence of Sex, Age, Vaccination. Tables in illustration. Return of
Small-Pox amongst the Men, Wives, and Children of the British
Troops. Remarks on the Results, in Proof of the Protecting
Power of Vaccination. Some Peculiarities of the Disease noticed.
Remarks on Chicken-Pox, in relation to the question of its identity with Small-Pox. Observations on the Degree of Credit due to
the Tables illustrating the Disease, and on the Manner of Forming
them, ...   368

CHAPTER XV.

ON THE CLIMATE OF CONSTANTINOPLE, AND ON SOME OF THE HABITS OF
THE PEOPLE IN CONNEXION WITH CLIMATE AND HEALTH.

Climate of Constantinople different from what might be expected
à priori. Its chief Peculiarities. Observations in illustration.
Some Errors and Exaggerations pointed out. Meteorological
Tables for the Years 1839 and 1840 kept in Pera. Comments on
them. Observations and Remarks in Connexion with Climate.
On the Temperature of the Bosphorus and Black Sea at different
Seasons. A Peculiarity in the Temperature of the Bosphorus
pointed out. Brief Notices of the Dress, Dwelling-Houses, Manner
of Living, &c., of the Turks, in Connexion with Climate and
Health. Notices of the Principal Diseases to which they are sub-
ject in the Capital, and of those to which they are either little Liable,
or are Exempt from. Remarks on the Climate in Relation to the
Inquiries of Invalids and Travellers, ...   393

Page

CHAPTER XVI.

NOTICE OF SOME OF THE PUBLIC INSTITUTIONS IN CONSTANTINOPLE, IN
CONNEXION WITH THE PRESENT STATE OF TURKEY.

Opposite Hypotheses respecting the Present Condition of the Turkish
Empire. Opinion of their Futility. Military Hospitals in Con-
stantinople and its Neighbourhood, Described. Naval Academy.
Military College. Medical School. How defective. Notice of
the great Barracks belonging to the Capital. Of the Quarantine
Establishment. Of some of the Government Manufactories. Contrast between them and the Native Work-Shops—between the
New and the Old Schools—as demonstrative of different Periods.
Prospect of Improvement, founded on the Capacity of the Turkish
Youth. Observations on the Vices of the Government, connected
with the Training of Official Men. Conjectures respecting Reform,
and Revival of Power, on the Supposition that the People are little
changed, and that existing Abuses may be Swept away by a Master-
mind. Farther Conjectures on the same Subject. Remarks on
the Rayah-Christian Population, ... 427

NOTES AND OBSERVATIONS

THE IONIAN ISLANDS AND MALTA.

CHAPTER I.

SKETCH OF THE PRESENT GOVERNMENT OF THE IONIAN ISLANDS.

Form of the Ionian Government as established by Charter, in 1817. The Senate, how Constituted. Its Duties. The Legislative Assembly. Mode of its Election. Its Functions. The Parliament. The Local Governments of the different Islands, and their Composition. How Subordinate to the General Government. Form and Administration of Legal Power. Composition of the Courts of Justice. Supreme and Local Church Establishment. Civil List. Character of the Government. Remarks on the same. Acts of Parliament illustrative of the Forms of Government.

IN accordance with the Treaty of Paris of 1815, these states are under the immediate and exclusive protection of the sovereign of Great Britain. A representative of the protecting power, appointed by the crown, and responsible to her Majesty's government, resides in the islands, with the title of Lord High Commissioner.

The established government of the Ionian Islands is framed on the charter of 1817, to which I would refer the reader who may be desirous of becoming

minutely acquainted with the formula of its constitution, and the details of its forms, which are somewhat complicated.

Including the Lord High Commissioner, it is considered as consisting of three parts, namely, a Senate,
a Legislative Assembly, and a Judicial Power.

The senate is elected out of and by the legislative
assembly; and the latter [after a trial of the ballot],
by the open votes of the " Sincliti ;" that is, such of
the people of the Ionian States as possess a certain amount of property,* or the equivalent (as has

---

* The qualifications of the Sincliti, or noble electors, were not
defined in the charter of 1817. In the eighteenth article of that document, reference is made to the constitution of the Septinsular Republic, bearing date the 24th November 1803, and setting forth that
the organization of the electors, as then laid down, shall be maintained
till " changed or ameliorated" by act of Parliament. The conditions
are contained in the sixth article, and are the following:—" Sono
Nobili attivi e constituzionali, e possono divenirlo successivamente
e indefinitamente per se, e per i loro legittimi discendenti, tanto celibi
come maritati ed uniti in famiglia con altri membri della Medesima
pur maritati, tutti quelli, che sono, o fossero per essere descritti nel
Registro Civico dell' Isola cui appartengono, ed hanno o fossero per
avere, e conservassero complessivamente i seguenti requisiti:—

1. Di essere originari delle Sette Isole.

2. Di essere nati per legittimo matrimonio o legittimati per sus-
sequente, da padre cristiano, e professare la Religiona cristiana.

3. Di possedere un annua rendita liquida fondiale, o usufrutturia,
o reale, o resultante da un' industria assicurata, o da una florida casa
di commercio, fissata, per i conscrivibile alla nobilità attiva delle
rispettive isole, in ducati nostri correnti a lire sei l'uno nelle misure
seguenti :

Per Corfù Ducato mille ottocento (L. 69) ; per Cephalonia sei cento
settanta cinque (L.33, 15s.); per Zante mille trecento cenquanta,
(L.67, 10s.) ; per Santa Maura cinque cento quaranta (L.27) ; per

lately been liberally enacted), of a university degree. *

The Senate, constituting the nominal executive
part of the government, is composed of four members and a president, the latter named by the Lord
High Commissioner, and the former approved by
him. It is divided into three departments, each of
which has a secretary; namely, a general, a finan-
cial, and a political department.

The Legislative Assembly, the functions of which,
independent of electing senators, are nominally analogous to those of our House of Commons, is com-

Cerigo, due cento venti cinque (L.9, 4s. 6d.); per Itaca trecento
quindici (L.15, 15s.); per Paxo cinque cento quaranta (L. 27.)

4. Di non esercitare personalemente alcun arte o mestiere meccanico.†

5. Di non tenere personalmente bottega aperta.†

6. Di avere sempre condotto un vita civile, e saper legere e scrivere
in una delle lingue usati dal Governo.

7. Di non essere stati mai dichiariti colpevoli di delitti puniti con
pene efflittive e infamanti.

8. Di non essere falliti fraudolenti ne detentori gratuiti dell' eredità
di un fallito.

9. Di non essere debitore al publico Erario."

It is curious to observe the great differences in the qualifying rates
of incomes in the different islands, and especially the very high rate
in Corfu, compared with that in Cephalonia, which is little more than
that of Paxo. At that time the olive crop was far the most profitable,
and it probably was made the foundation for the estimate. The produce of the currant-vineyards, on the contrary, was then of so little
value, the English market being closed, that the vines were not worth
cultivating. In Zante, I have been assured, many of the vineyards
at that time were rooted up, and the ground subjected to the plough.

* In 1837: see act of Parliament on the subject, at the end of this
chapter.

† Since abrogated.

posed of forty members.   Twenty-nine of these are
furnished at each election from the several islands, in
the following proportion, viz., Corfu, seven; Cephalonia, seven; Zante, seven; Santa Maura, four;
Ithaca, one; Cerigo, one; Paxo, one;—each of the
three last in rotation electing a second.   The other
eleven are not elected as such at the time: they consist of the members of the preceding senate, of the
last regents of the four principal islands, and one of
the regents of the three smaller islands in rotation;
and they together constitute what has been denomi-
nated the Primary Council.*   Both the legislative
assembly and its primary council, are presided over
by one of its members, and each has its secretaries.

The Senate and Legislative Assembly, constitute
the parliament of the Ionian States, the sessions of
which are regulated,† and the duration of which is

* " A certain time previous to the regular dissolution of parliament, the primary council is required to prepare double lists of the
individuals from whom the members of the new legislative assembly
are to be elected; which lists are to be transmitted to each island, at
least fourteen days before the " death of the parliament." The qualification for the legislative assembly is the same as that for the elec-
tive franchise.   Out of the double list, nominated by the primary
council (fourteen for instance for the larger islands), half the number
are elected by the Sincliti, by a majority of votes; which election, or
rather selection, is final.   The Sincliti are, in the first instance, regis-
tered by the regents of the respective islands, and a return of them is
annually made to the senate.

† The session of parliament is biennial, commencing the 1st of
March, and lasting at least three months; it may take place, however,
at other times, on emergency, by order of the Lord High Commissioner, in whom also is vested the power of proroguing parliament.

for five years, liable to be dissolved, however, by the protecting sovereign, by an order in council.

Besides the general government exerting control over all the islands, there are local governments, one for each island, consisting of a Resident appointed by and acting immediately under the Lord High Commissioner, and a regent assisted by a municipal council of five, and by an advocate-fiscal, archivist, secretary, and treasurer. The regent and advocate-fiscal are appointed by the Senate, with the approval of the Lord High Commissioner; the archivist and secretary by the regent, with the approval of the senate; and the treasurer by the treasurer of the general government, with the sanction of both the Lord High Commissioner and the Senate. The municipal body are selected and appointed by the joint agency of the Sincliti, and of the resident and regent; the former, by a majority of votes, returning ten of them; the regent, with the approval of the resident, selecting five. The municipal council, acting under the regent, is required to attend, according to the charter, to the following subjects, each member having one for his special care, viz. :—

1. Agriculture, Public Instruction, and objects of National Industry.
2. Commerce and Navigation.
3. Subsistence of the People.
4. Civil Police and Charitable Establishments.
5. Religion, Morals, and Public Economy.

Each island is divided into districts, determined by

the municipal council, to which particular officers are assigned, constituting a municipal and an executive police; the former appointed by the respective regents and the municipal council; the latter by the Lord High Commissioner, with the consent of the Senate. The agents of the municipal police are inspectors of districts, primates (primati communali), and messengers. The agents of the executive police are lieutenants (luogotenenti di distretto), and their constables; capi di decima, and their cernide. The number of these officers are proportioned to the extent of the districts and the size of the villages and their wants, for the purpose of keeping the peace and enforcing the laws.

The legal power, which, according to charter, forms a part of the civil government, is exercised by a supreme court of justice (or court of appeal) at the seat of government, and by local courts in the different islands. The former is composed of four members, one of whom acts as a president; two of them are appointed by the Crown, by the Lord High Commissioner's warrant; and two by the Senate. The Lord High Commissioner, and the President of the Senate also form a part of the court, as extraordinary members, acting in particular cases, and especially in instances in which the ordinary members are equally divided in opinion, the Lord High Commissioner having a casting vote, should he and the president differ in judgment.

The local courts in each of the islands are three in

number, viz., the civil, the criminal, and one of commerce, independent of the minor offices of justices of peace, for the trial of petty offences. In each court there are commonly several judges. In Paxo, in 1837, there were two and a president: in Cephalonia, including a president, there were ten. The legal officers derive their appointments from the senate.*

* The judicial establishments maintained in these islands are very expensive, and the payment of them absorbs a considerable proportion of the revenue. The yearly salary of each officer was determined by a law of 24th July 1834, according to which the total amount is L.19,422. As examples, may be inserted the salaries of the respective officers of the courts, in one of the large islands, and also in one of the small, as Cephalonia and Paxo.

CEPHALONIA.

One president, . .	L.425
Four judges, at L. 320 each, . .	1280
Five ditto do., . .	1600
Six registerers, at L.120 each, .	720
Six deputy registerers, at L.78 each, .	468
Four assistant registerers of the first class, at L.65 each, ...	260
Four ditto of second class, L.50 each, .	200
Fourteen ditto of third class, L.35 each,	490
Three messengers at L.30 each, .	90
Four ditto, at L.26 each, . .	104

PAXO.

President, . . .	L.250
Four judges, at L.210 each, . .	840
Two registerers, at L.78 each, . .	156
Two deputy registerers, at L.50 each, .	100
Two assistant registerers, at L.25 each,	50
Two messengers, at L.20 each, .	40

The members of the Supreme Council of Justice in Corfu *were* paid

The principal law-officers are selected from the body of advocates, which is very large. According to a law of 1834, no Ionian subject can practise as an advocate, unless duly enrolled, after election, in the college of his order ; and, according to the same law, in each island such a college should exist, composed of the judicial body, of the advocate-fiscal, and of two advocates elected by those of their order authorized to make the choice. *

at a higher rate; the two Greek judges had L.600 a-year each ; the two English, L.1000; and for some time one of them received L.1900 a-year.

* In future it is required that every advocate shall have studied and graduated at the Ionian university ; be a native ; not under twenty-four years of age ; acquainted with the Greek language ; and professing the christian religion. Before any one can be enrolled on the list of advocates, it is necessary for him to make the following declaration, pledging himself to the same by oath :—" Io A. B. giuro di eseguire le Leggi, statute, ordinanze e Regolamenti, che sono in vigore in questi stati, e che potessero in appresso essere stabiliti. Giuro di non consigliare, o difendere alcuna causa, che sia per mia opinione ingiusta, eccetuate le difese criminali ; di defendere onestamente e diligentemente tutte le cause che mi fossero fidate, e di non arvalorare, e vendere autentico colla mia firma, verun atto che non sia della causa da me stesso patrocinata, o nella quale non fossi consultore. Cosi Iddio mi ajuti."

What effect this new training may have, it is impossible to say. That a great reform is required, appears to be undoubted. From want of principle and integrity, the abuses in the administration of the laws are said to be extreme. " Such things are practised in the courts of law" [says Sir Charles Napier], "which make the people abhor them ;" " where a system of intrigue and of devilry is carried on, that would take volumes to describe." Hitherto bribery and perjury have been carried so far, and so systematically, that in Zante, Sir Charles Napier was informed " there are regular shops for furnishing false witnesses, at so much a-head."

According to charter, the orthodox Greek religion is the established religion of the States; the Roman Catholic is specially protected, and all other denominations are tolerated.

The ecclesiastical establishment consists principally of four metropolitan archbishops, viz., those of Corfu, Cephalonia, Zante, and Santa Maura; and of one archbishop, namely, of Cerigo, who are each independent of the others in their separate jurisdictions; and of two bishops, those of Ithaca and Paxo, acting under the archbishops of Cephalonia and of Corfu. These dignitaries are elected by the clergy of their respective dioceses, by plurality of suffrages and by secret scrutiny, according to the canons and ancient usages of the islands. The election is subject to the *veto* of the executive power.

The highest authority in the Greek Church is exercised by the Exarch, which office in rotation is filled by a metropolitan archbishop, who, whilst he holds it, is required to reside at the seat of government; the period of its tenure is limited to two years and a-half.

The Latin Church is presided over by a vicar-general, who has subordinate to him certain officers, as have also the higher functionaries of the Greek Church.

The Greek bishops owe allegiance to the patriarch of Constantinople, as the vicar-general does to the pope.*

* The clergy of the higher grades, both of the Greek and Latin

The number of officiating priests is very large, not less, it is conjectured, than one to every fifty inhabitants.   Depending on their flock for the means of subsistence, they are commonly very ill paid,* and their condition is often miserable.   Their intellectual deficiencies will be noticed in the sequel, with the measures in progress to educate the order, curtail their number, and increase their respectability and usefulness.

Besides the officers already mentioned belonging to the general and local governments, there are many more connected with the revenue, the customs, public works, ports, the quarantine establishment, and the establishments of public instruction, constituting

Church, are paid by Government, by a law of 1833, according to the following rates:—Each metropolitan of the three larger islands, Corfu, Cephalonia, and Zante, L.312 a-year; that of Santa Maura, L.234; the bishops of Ithaca and Paxo, and the archbishop of Cerigo, each, L.156; the archbishop, the head of the Latin Church in Corfu, L.265; an archdeacon, 380 dollars; three canons, 264 dollars each.

* On an average, they receive from 150 to 180 dollars a-year; that is, from L.32 to L.39, with a house free of rent, which is little better than the wages of a tolerable man-servant in the Ionian Islands, his food provided him.   Some priests, no doubt, receive considerably more, such as are attached to churches, the patron saints of which are popular, and to which many offerings are made, particularly by sailors and the petty traders, before setting sail, or undertaking any thing with which risk is connected.   The church of the Madonna, on the little rocky islet at the entrance of the port of Gaja in Paxo, is of this description: no mariner, I have been informed, thinks of passing it, even though only going to Corfu or Parga, almost within sight, without stopping to say a prayer and make an offering.   On the same rock, according to a story current in Paxo, Antony and Cleopatra, attended by thirty kings, feasted before the battle of Actium.

the civil list; all of whom, including the Lord High Commissioner, the members of the Senate and of the Legislative Assembly, and the staff of the British Force employed in the Ionian Islands, are paid out of the revenue of the States.*

Of the character of the Government, little need be said. It is obvious that it is more free in appearance than in reality; and that it possesses many of the forms of freedom with very little of its substance. Whether this peculiarity, under existing circumstances, be an evil or a good, it is difficult to determine. Taking the most favourable view, it is to be hoped that it may be a preparation for something better: if the people deserve more freedom, they can hardly fail to obtain more; at present it is very questionable whether order could be preserved, and the interests of

* In these islands, no public duty is performed gratuitously. By a law of 1834, L.15,000 are placed at the disposal of the Lord High Commissioner annually, to pay the contingents of his establishment, viz., the residents of the different islands; two members of the Supreme Council of Justice; the secretary of the Senate for the General Department, and the treasurer-general.

The salary of the President of the Senate is L.1350 a-year; of each senator, L.675; and of each member of the Legislative Assembly, L.119, besides payment of expenses whilst in attendance at Corfu during the session of Parliament. Each resident of the larger islands had four dollars a-day, and of the smaller, three; besides army pay as officers, which they invariably are. The pay of the regents, I believe, was similar. Recently, the residents of the larger islands have been allowed L.600 a-year, including their army pay in the amount. The members of the municipal body had each L.5, 8s. 4d. a-month. According to a list of public servants given by Sir Charles Napier, at the time he was resident of Cephalonia, the number employed in that island was 223, at an expense of L.13,385.

the country be tolerably attended to, were the controlling power of the Lord High Commissioner either abrogated or even diminished.*

* A striking example of the good effect of exercising the controlling power, alluded to above, was given by the Lord High Commissioner in 1840, in first proroguing by his own authority, and next dissolving by a mandate from the Queen, the protecting sovereign, the sixth parliament, in consequence of the intemperate and factious proceedings of the Legislative Assembly, on the occasion of discussing the new codes of laws, then submitted to the Parliament,—that branch of the united parliament of the Ionian States, maintaining— in opposition to the law advisers of the crown, in opposition to the Senate and the Lord High Commissioner—that they alone had to exercise the functions of instituting codes of laws, and of making any and all the changes in the Ionian constitution, without the intervention of the Senate, and of proposing them to the protecting power for ratification. In this determination, they considered themselves not as a branch of the Ionian Legislature—not as a part of the parliament—but as an independent constituent assembly, such as they imagined that to have been in the name of which the constitution formed by Sir Thomas Maitland was framed and promulgated. Had the Lord High Commissioner yielded on this occasion, or had he not been supported by her Majesty's Government at home, serious evils might have resulted; for there is reason to believe that, at that time, a design was on foot, abetted by a widely spread party, to create dissension and disturbance in the Ionian Islands, in Greece, and in the Turkish empire, with a view to the formation of a Republican League, under the protection of Russia, preparatory to a prostration under absolute government,—a form in which the nobles might calculate on recovering all their former oppressive power, and see a road opening to them leading to wealth and influence, at Petersburgh, or on the pleasant banks of the Bosphorus. Lord John Russell, in his place in the House of Commons, on the 23d of June of the year referred to, speaking on a motion made by Lord C. Fitzroy respecting the Ionian Islands, expressed his opinion, " that there was good ground to apprehend the existence of a conspiracy to throw off British authority." And, in a despatch to the Lord High Commis-

For a long while, almost from time immemorial, the Ionian people have laboured under great disadvantages, in relation to government.* Bad laws may

sioner, of the 30th of November of the same year, in reply to memorials from some of the inhabitants of Corfu, praying for extension of civil rights, his lordship observed:—" The petitioners do not succeed in their object to show that the great mass of the people of the Ionian Islands desire those changes; and it is my opinion, that if these very changes were immediately adopted, the people themselves would suffer more than all. The people would become the laughing-stock and the prey of a small number of intriguers and ambitious adventurers, and the republic could neither have the protection of a stable government, nor the vigour and energy of a free state.

" The true interests of the Ionian people will be better obtained by the maintenance with a strong hand, and without passion, of a system of order and integrity in the State, and by the encouragement of the people in every enterprise which can elevate their character."

This I have extracted from an article in the *Malta Times*, in which there is much information brought together respecting the Ionian Islands, during the period when Sir Howard Douglas was Lord High Commissioner, and in which his conduct is ably defended from certain attacks made against him, on factious grounds.

* It is rare, indeed, that colonies or dependencies are well governed—that is, with a view to the good of the people, especially their moral and intellectual improvement: if not treated like slaves, they are too often treated like children; and the consequence is, they are more like children than men in their conduct. That the Venetian manner of ruling the Ionian Islands was bad, is commonly admitted; and as Venice degenerated, probably from bad it became worse, till it was atrocious. An author, already quoted, thus speaks of it:—

" Des despotismes, le plus dur, sans contredit, c'est celui des républiques. Celui de Saint-Marc, si pesant pour les provinces de terre firme, l'était bien plus encore pour les iles. Pas d'autres lois là que le bon plaisir des providiteurs, qui pouvaient tout ce que Verrès avait pu en Sicile. Point de frein pour leur cupidité, point de bornes à leur exactions: tout y était pour eux un objet de trafic, tout, à com-

have confirmed or produced bad habits and low
morals; these again, no doubt, have reacted on the

mencer par la justice; tout y était taxé, l'impunité du crime à
commettre comme la remission du crime commis." This is the
opinion of M. Anault, formed on the spot in 1797, when the winged
lion of St Mark had just then given place to the tri-coloured flag,
when the tree of liberty was planted in Corfu, and a municipal body
formed, composed of eighteen Greeks, four Roman Catholics, and
two Jews. An *Ionian citizen*, in a letter lately addressed by him
to Lord John Russell, expresses a similar opinion, and even more
strongly, of the old Venetian Administration, when the Ionian
people were "double slaves," corrupt, and ignorant, under the despotism of the Venetian Government, and the feudal oppression of the
signori of the country; when "religion, life, honour, personal liberty,
the sacred rights of property, were in a state of humiliation; the
people obliged to sell their produce, and particularly oil, in the markets of Venice, at a fixed price; and the Greek Church was subjected
to the supremacy of the Latin." He adds :—" The signori of the
country, to complete the sacrifice of these people, had arbitrarily made
prisons under their houses, for the confinement, at their pleasure, of
not only those who did not pay them, or, in their idea, had offended
them, but also those who, not being of noble degree, dared to wear a
long coat instead of a jacket; who, not being a noble, dared to wear
a hat instead of a cap; who, not being a noble, dared to pass the
coffee-house of the signori with their head covered; or in the middle
of the street or road, when they ought, with uncovered head, in
sign of respect, to hurry on to the footway on the opposite side of
the road; and, if a signore thought that he must wash out an insult
in the blood of a plebeian, it was enough if, before he killed him,
he arranged with the Venetian provveditore how many barrels of oil
he was to pay, in the case of killing him, under the head of fine, to
which the provveditore had the power of commuting every corporal
punishment, even that of death, to which the signore murderer might
be apparently condemned : if they agreed, he killed him ; but if they
did not, he did not kill him : the provveditore, however, would never
give up any barrels of oil offered him, because they did not strike the
bargain."

administration of the laws; and their abuse has had effect on the minds of the people in deepening their degradation. The old Venetian laws are now either abolished, or are on the eve of being so; the new codes of laws, civil, criminal, and commercial, lately completed, have been formed after the best models of modern jurisprudence.* Their influence, honestly

* They were commenced in May 1841. The same writer, just quoted in the preceding note, thus expresses his sentiments on the probable influence of the new laws justly administered, but in language, as regards the class of nobles, I would hope too strong. " The class of nobles will never forgive the English nation for having introduced a form of government into these islands which has destroyed the foundation of their despotic power, which, exercised as it had been for nearly five centuries, obtained in their eyes the character of a legitimate right, of which the British nation had deprived them These nobles having, with very few exceptions, determined to avenge themselves for a loss of such magnitude, formed the plan of erecting themselves into a party apparently liberal, and, under the mask of assumed patriotism, to turn the public spirit of the people into a hatred of the British Government. Their design is clear. If they succeeded, by means of the agitation of the people roused by them, in obtaining absolute freedom in the exercise of the rights of voting for the electoral body, then will the Legislative Assembly be formed of persons of their party hostile to the English name, ready, with the concurrence of the Senate, already chosen from amongst their body, to paralyze the fundamental laws of the new regime,—then would they regain in the Senate, composed of themselves, their ancient despotism, and oblige the Lord High Commissioner to desist from exercising his controlling power as much in legislative as administrative affairs, or to exercise it in a declaration of open war, and in continued opposition to the powers of the State, in which the people naturally taking part, a total dissolution of the political connexion between the protected and protecting power must ensue. But her Majesty's Government, in order to disconcert the plans of the nobles, had recourse to the most efficacious means to destroy their whole

administered under a strong, and just, and enlightened controlling power, ought to have the best effect

influence on the people. Perceiving that the present form of government has destroyed the material and direct baronial oppression in
these States, but there has remained that indirect influence over the
people which, in an arbitrary legislation, the powerful exercise over
the weak in the administration of justice, her Majesty's Government
hastens the introduction of a new law, by means of which the administration of justice is raised to such a moral level as to be capable
of producing in the people the intimate conviction,—that, in the eye
of the law, the person and property of each individual is placed
beyond the control or caprice of the judge and the oppression of the
powerful, and thus every possible influence of the nobles on the mass
of the people would be at once destroyed. The nobles in a body are
furious at this. This class, which forms a corrupt judicial body,
expects to see the effects of the new legislative system frustrated,
and have placed their only hopes in the recall of the present Lord
High Commissioner (then, Sir Howard Douglas) and the arrival of a
new one, who, knowing little or nothing of the people, may probably fall into the error of nominating for the new judicial organization, when it comes into operation, men corrupt, ignorant, and
inimical to the new legislative system, who are capable of reviling
and robbing it of its salutary effects; and, in truth, my lord, this
would be fatal,—the nature of the new judicial system is such, that
its first impression must be strong and favourable. It will depend
upon the moral executive use of these laws, to impress upon the
minds of the public the idea of their impartiality, in order to force
them into the conviction, ' that in the eye of the new law all men
are equal.' My lord, when once the people are sure that under these
new laws their lives, honour, and their personal safety are secure from
the caprice of the judge and from the oppression of those in power,—
that they have no need of feudal protection, and need not stand in
awe of the higher classes,—the feudal proprietors (nobili) will then
have lost all their influence over them; and the people of these States
enjoying, for the first time in five centuries, a state of perfect security, cannot but become positively attached to her Majesty's government and throne. The turbulent class of the gentry, having lost

in developing the good qualities of the public mind and in checking the bad,—and in the formation of good principles and habits, the foundation of character.*

their influence over the populace, will remain impotent, and her Majesty's government may tranquilly await the time for the greater civilization of this people, by allowing them gradually such greater latitude of political liberties as their civilization advances, and as the actual institutions for public instruction may render them capable of acting up to."

* The subjoined passage, from an able and eloquent writer, is worthy of the deepest consideration of the Ionian people, especially at the present time, when, probably, very sanguine expectation is indulged in of an improved order of things to result from their new laws :— " It is the general spirit and habits of thinking in a community that are all in all: that charters, and statutes, and judges, and courts of law, are all of no avail for perpetuating a constitution, or even for securing the regular administration of its blessings from time to time —are all of no avail, if a vital principle does not animate the mass, and if there be not sufficient intelligence and spirit in the community to be anxious about its own happiness and dignity, its laws and government, and those provisions and forms in both, which are favourable to its liberties."—(*Lectures on Modern History, by Wm. Smyth,* vol. i., p. 163.) And hardly less deserving of attention from the same people are the following reflections of a profound writer on the mere forms of freedom, *i. e.,* viewing them merely as the scaffolding of the building :—" I am curious," says Niebuhr, the distinguished author alluded to, " about the Norwegian constitution ; it will probably, like the Spanish, be a misshapen failure. This constitution-making seems likely to come into full work, but the manufacturers furnish as wretched wares as some years ago, when they brought themselves into such discredit. The first vital point is, that a nation should be manly, unselfish, and honourable. If it is this, it will of itself develope free institutions, and they will be lasting. Constitutional forms will do nothing for a weak or foolish nation. What is the advantage of selecting representatives, if men of ability are wanting to represent the people? That is the root, not the fruit. Can a man gather ripe and

Whether the constitution on which the existing government is founded is a judicious one, fitted for the condition of the people, and likely to improve them, it may be difficult to decide. It may be objected that, under it, the Ionian Islands have neither the advantages belonging to free states nor to colonies. Were they free, with an army and navy of their own—with diplomatic and consular agents of their own—a field of honourable and profitable exertion, now closed, would be open to them;—talent might be brought into activity—merit rewarded. Were they a colony, with the rights of British subjects, independent of the advantages resulting to them as such, they would not have to contribute a large proportion of their revenue for military protection.* The late Lord High Commissioner, Sir Howard Douglas, has, it is understood, reported fully to her Majesty's government on the condition of those islands in connexion with their peculiar political state. It is to be hoped these reports will be printed; and that some of his recommendations will be followed, made with a view to lighten their burdens† and encourage amongst

good fruit from a tree which has no root? Let every individual then, and every government, first labour to make itself and the people truly vigorous, masculine, single-sighted, and unselfishly virtuous. To attempt to effect this by forms is to put the horse behind the cart, and think it will draw just as well."—*Account of the Life of B. G. Niebuhr, from his own Letters, &c. ; Quarterly Review, September* 1840.

* About L.35,000 a-year.

† Lord John Russell, in the House of Commons, on the 22d of April 1841, is reported to have said,—" Sir Howard Douglas frequently urged on the government, attacked as he was by those who

them intelligence, enterprise, and industry—the moving powers of national prosperity—by supplying improved and increased means of education, happily begun; by giving the preference for civil appointments to qualified, deserving natives—and by diminishing or totally repealing the export duties, now so high, on the staple produce of the country.

In alluding to the disadvantages which may be supposed to result to those islands from their peculiar connexion with Great Britain, the benefits they certainly owe to British protection should be kept in grateful remembrance by the people,—for they are neither few nor inconsiderable—comprised in the fullest protection at home and abroad, at comparatively small expense; in their shipping being privileged, and enjoying the exemptions belonging to British subjects in our ports,*—and in a political training and educa-

said he was hostile to giving free institutions to the Ionian Islands, strong representations in favour of a diminution of their burdens—a fact so highly creditable to him, that I cannot refrain from mentioning it on this occasion."—*Hansard's Debates*, vol. lvii., pp. 1013-14.

* The Ionian subject abroad looks with confidence to the British ambassador or consul for protection. Since the Ionian Islands have been under the protection of Great Britain, not even a piratical inroad has been attempted, from which formerly the people suffered severely. Wisely disarmed, the population now is comparatively peaceable; the crime of murder is becoming rare, and security of person and property increasing. Under the new laws, well administered, further and great improvement in this respect may be expected, and will be required, to enable the country to exert its energies and to flourish. The following remarks on this subject, written in 1835 by the well-informed individual whom I have more than once already quoted, are deserving of consideration, both as regards the past and the future.

tion which they are receiving under the surveillance
of the government of a free country.

" We certainly afford them protection against external enemies;
but a people so demoralized " (he is speaking principally of the people
of Santa Maura) " require to be protected against themselves ; or
rather, the *few* industrious *good* against the *many* unprincipled *bad.* If
this kind of protection cannot be afforded, it were better to resign the
prominent part we now take in the administration, and allow them to
work out their own reform.   I am but too well convinced that, in the
absence of a wise and vigorous head, that British protection, when the
power it gives is resigned to unprincipled natives, may be made, not
only to sanction much injustice, but actually exerted as an engine of
oppression, and a means of stifling just indignation.

" I believe some statesmen have thought that the Ionians are at
length able to govern themselves; my humble but firm opinion is,
that they are wholly incompetent to the charge.   True, they have
been between twenty and thirty years under the tuition of a great,
and enlightened, and a just nation ; but there were many difficulties
to contend with in the first years of our protection, which that able
statesman, Sir T. Maitland, had not time to overcome, and which Sir
F. Adam struggled against during the greater part of his administration."   He adds,—" In the Ionian Islands feudal influence still exists
to an extraordinary extent ; and the oppression and frauds which
were once exercised by open force, are now practised through the
agency of the laws, by means of intrigue and chicane, of which the
mere theorist, or even practised statesman, of any other country, can
have but a slight conception.   That a truly conscientious man is
hourly exposed to certain destruction ; that, feeling this, all men are
tempted to ally themselves to powerful individuals, whose will for
them is law, and who can, by the command of testimony, or other
means of corruption, prove or disprove, to an extraordinary extent,
whatever they undertake, is but too certain.   The man who should
dare to set up for independence of a party would be surely hunted
down.   Self-preservation imperiously dictates a close union with the
bad and powerful.   I have seen many fearful instances of this ; and
while society is so constituted, common honesty, and much less patriotism, sufficient for self-government, cannot exist.   If left wholly

By way of illustration of the manner in which the civil government conducts the public business, a few

to themselves, and the British garrison were withdrawn, the first measure would inevitably be the instant massacre of the nobles by the goaded peasantry. I can speak with certainty of Cerigo and Santa Maura, and it is the firm opinion of both these classes. This I conceive (though it would deliver the islands from many atrocious characters) is not the kind of self-government contemplated by the theoretical statesman I have alluded to. But it is a contingency which may be relied on; and the nobles tremble, and the peasants exult, when they contemplate the probability of being abandoned by England, as they were by the Russians in 1803. The same horrible effects would surely follow.

" Many years under a directing government must elapse before they can advantageously or rationally govern themselves; but very little (though something) has hitherto been done, and there is much to do. A Lord High Commissioner, who, like Sir T. Maitland, possessed head and heart sufficient to oppose the powerful oppressor and protect the injured and weak, would, like that good man and able statesman, be shamefully calumniated; but he would have with him the hearts of those whose voice is never heard by a British public, that of the Ionian peasant-proprietors, who, vitiated as they are, yet monopolize the patriotism which a statesman would gladly appeal to—who, with all their barbarism and ignorance, are heirs to many of the noble points of the Greek character. They have all the quickness of intellect that distinguished their ancestors, with frames fitted for toil, and minds singularly alive to emulation, and hungry for instruction. If a statesman were determined to act the Napoleon principle with them, that is, to proportion reward to merit, he could renew the magical effects of ancient legislation; but at present the honours and rewards are confined to the courtiers; while the love and pride of country, and readiness to make sacrifices for its improvement, are chiefly to be found among the peasantry. Yet the intriguing and selfish noble continues to engross the attention of the government; and, though the legislator and supposed interpreter of the peasant, too often sacrifices his dearest interests for the attainment of his own grovelling objects. Among the evils to be avoided I might advert to the danger of conceding too much power to the senate, and creating an oligarchy

instances may be brought forward of acts of Parlialiament, in themselves not uninteresting or unimportant.

Fourth Session of the United States of the Ionian Islands, held in virtue of the Constitution of 1817.

No. LVIII.

Title.—Act of Parliament respecting the Reading-boards and Books to be used in the Schools of Mutual Instruction.

Preamble.—In order that primary instruction, by means of the established Lancasterian schools, may answer the sole end for which the system was introduced into these islands, by the authority of his highness the President, and the most excellent the Senate, with the vote and assent of the most noble the Legislative Assembly of the

---

odious to the people, and which the constitution has wisely guarded against by giving the *veto* to the Lord High Commissioner.

" I might point out the evils attending the undue interference of intriguing individuals at Corfu, whose insidious operations, if permitted, would effectually paralyze every attempt to advance the interests of the people; but these subjects are beyond my limits.

" The Ionian government, to accomplish its purpose, must still, as prescribed by the treaty of Paris, be directed by a Lord High Commissioner; and he, if supported at home, and the clamour of a few bad men can be disregarded, may carry *any reform*, if he rely on the co-operation of the people, and be aided by capable English agents as his residents. Such a line of policy would excite the unbounded gratitude of the patriotic—would enable the islands to enjoy the advantages which nature has almost in vain hitherto showered upon them. They are growing into importance from the march of events connected with Russia and Turkey, and our intercourse with each by means of the Mediterranean. By favouring the development of their resources, mental and physical, we should rapidly recover the ground we have of late been losing, and combine our glory with their happiness." This, it should be remembered, was written in 1835.

United States of the Ionian Islands, in this fourth meeting of the fifth Parliament, and with the approbation of his excellency the Lord High Commissioner of his Majesty the Protecting Sovereign, it is decreed and enacted as follows :—

Art. I. In none of the above-mentioned schools, whether central or auxiliary, shall any reading-board or book be used without the written license of the Exarch of these states, all the Prelates of the several islands being consulted, and the majority of them in favour thereof.

Art. II. The books and reading-boards, previously to their being submitted to the Exarch and Prelates for the license mentioned in the preceding article, are to be examined by the Professors of Theology in the Ionian University, who will certify whether they do, or do not, contain any thing contrary, or in any manner prejudicial to the dogmas, canons, doctrines, or customs of the dominant orthodox religion of these states.

Art. III. The license is to be printed on the title-page of the book, or at the head of the reading-board.

Art. IV. In the month of August next the reading-boards or books at present in use in the Schools of Mutual Instruction are to be submitted to the examination prescribed by Arts. I. and II.; and from the 1st of September 1837 they cannot be used without the license of the Exarch, as ordered by the said articles.

Art. V. Any director, master, or monitor, who may be guilty of any infraction of the foregoing articles, or may order, authorize, or suffer any such infraction, shall be immediately dismissed from his situation.

Art. VI. The present act to be printed, published, and transmitted to the proper authorities for due execution.

Corfu, 13-25, 1837.

Fourth Session of the Fifth Parliament, &c. &c. &c.

No. LIX.

Title.—Act of Parliament to guard against a scarcity of Wheat.

Preamble.—Experience having shown that the restriction on trade in the article of wheat in Corfu, as it was fixed by act No. 30 of the present Parliament, is of the greatest benefit to the population of this island, whilst it insures also the supply of wheat throughout the state ; considering that the measures adopted on this important subject should be directed to any possible reduction on the price of this article of necessity, even more than to the forming of a branch of public revenue : therefore, by the authority of his highness the President, and the most excellent the Senate, with the most noble the Legislative Assembly of the United States of the Ionian Islands, in the fourth meeting of the fifth Parliament, and with the approval of his excellency the Lord High Commissioner of the Protecting Sovereign, it is decreed and enacted as follows :—

Art. I. Speculations of individuals with respect to wheat in Corfu are prohibited, excepting in mere *transitu ;* but trade in any other kind of grain is perfectly free ; well understood that this prohibition does not extend to wheat, the produce of this island.

Art. II. There is to be in Corfu a depôt of wheat, in sufficient quantity for the usual consumption of the island, and for supplying any accidental and momentaneous wants of the other islands of the state.

Art. III. This depôt is to be under the direction of the municipal council of Corfu as a branch of the public revenue.

Art. IV. A special commission will regulate the details of the depôt ; it is to be composed of two public functionaries and three heads of families, to be chosen every six months by the municipal council.

The two public functionaries forming part of the said commission are to be the municipal officer for matters of trade and navigation, who is to be the president, and the collector of public revenue, who will have charge of the depôt and its accounts.

Art. V. The persons employed in the grain department are to be proposed by the municipal council, and they will be nominated, and their salaries fixed, by the Senate.

Art. VI. The commission will sit when any cargo or cargoes of wheat are announced in port ; also, whenever the president may think it necessary, and at all events once a-week.

Art. VII. The issuing-stores of the department will be kept open on the days, and for the hours, that the stores of private speculators in the other kinds of grain are usually open.

Art. VIII. A member of the commission, in turn, will daily inspect the issuing stores.

Art. IX. The measurers and porters for the deposits in Port

Franco are to be appointed by the collector, and paid by the depositors at the same rate as those of the grain department.

Art. X. At the end of every six months the municipal council will publish in the Ionian Gazette a statement of the purchases and sales of wheat—the prices—the gain or loss upon the same—and the remains in store.

Art. XI. The Senate, on the proposition of the municipal council, will fix the sums to be placed at the disposition of the latter for the purchase of wheat.

Art. XII. The price of sale will be fixed monthly by the municipal council on the report of the special commission. In fixing the price they will be guided by the following points :—

1. The cost of the wheat.
2. The casual surplus or deficiency.
3. The expenses of the administration.
4. The interest on the capital employed, at the rate of four per cent. per annum.

Art. XIII. All surplus in the chest, not sufficient at the time it occurs to effect a reduction of one obolo in the price of bread, is to be applied to that object as soon as an increased surplus may render the same practicable.

Art. XIV. The accounts of the grain department in Corfu are to be examined and passed in the same manner as all the other public accounts.

Art. XV. The present act is to be printed and published, and will continue in force up to the termination of the first ensuing ordinary session of Parliament.

Corfu, 29th *March* (10th *April*) 1837.

Fourth Session of the Fifth Parliament, &c. &c. &c.

No. LXXIV.

Title.—Act of Parliament for granting certain privileges to the study of Literature and the Sciences in the Ionian University, and to the useful and industrious classes of the people.

Preamble.—Agreeably to Art. XVIII. sect. 2. chap. iii. of the constitution of 1817, and in order to remove certain restrictions that lie heavy upon the useful and industrious classes of the people, as well as to encourage the study of literature and the sciences in the university of this state; by the authority of his highness the President and the most excellent the Senate, with the assent of the most noble the Legislative Assembly of the United States of the Ionian Islands, in this fourth session of the fifth Parliament, and with the approval of his excellency the Lord High Commissioner of the protecting Sovereign, it is decreed and enacted as follows :—

Art. I. It shall be lawful for artists, mechanics, and shopkeepers, to offer themselves for inscription in the list of " *Sincliti.*"

Art. II. Laureation shall be equivalent to the income that constitutes the qualification, as follows :—

1. Degrees taken in the Ionian University, or in the universities of Great Britain.
2. Conferred in foreign universities before the publication of the present act.
3. Conferred in foreign universities upon young Ionians, who may be studying there at the time the present act is published.
4. Taken in foreign universities for branches of science not laureated in the Ionian University, except the law.

Art. III. The present shall be printed, published, and transmitted to the proper authorities, in order to be carried into effect.

Corfu, 5th June, 1837.

No. LXXXII.

Title.—Act of Parliament for promoting and effecting the Draining of the Marshes and Low Lands in the Ionian Islands, and the good condition and cultivation of lands, with consideration also of the public health.

Preamble.—Whereas, in several islands of these States, there are many and extensive tracts of land which, owing to their being covered with stagnant water, are unproductive as well as prejudicial to the public health, greatly impeding the progress of agriculture and industry, and the increase of population,—as the expense required for the draining and subsequent continued cultivation of such lands ought not to fall upon the government, and at the same time there is reason to believe that not all the proprietors, individually, are in a situation to meet it;—considering the urgent necessity for the intervention of government to remove so many evils, by encouraging and protecting the enterprises of joint stock companies and every other tending to the internal improvement of the country;—by the authority of his highness the President, and the most excellent the Senate, with the vote and assent of the most noble the Legislative Assembly of the United States of the Ionian Islands in this fourth session of the fifth Parliament, and with the approval of his excellency the Lord High Commissioner of his majesty the protecting Sovereign, it is decreed and enacted as follows:—

Art. I. The municipal councils shall draw up without delay, detailed statements of all the lands in their respective islands that are covered with stagnant water, absolutely barren, or producing scarcely anything, owing to their being thus inundated, and that are therefore prejudicial to the public health; with the understanding that, in these statements, fisheries that have an opening to the sea are not to be included.

Art. II. The above statements are to specify the extent of the land, —its boundaries; the number and names of the proprietors, *coloni*, or *livellatarj*; of what part each is owner; the evils arising from the actual condition of such lands; the kind of work required upon them; the time necessary for draining them and rendering them permanently productive; the probable expense of so doing; and what advantages are to be expected from their draining and cultivation.

Art. III. To facilitate their operations, they will be assisted by the agricultural committees,—by the executive police,—by the civil engineer, the inspector of roads, and the public land-surveyor, in the islands where there is one.

Art. IV. The municipal council will first direct their attention to the lands more immediately contiguous to the towns, to those that are situated in the most populous places or near them, and to those that require immediate remedy.

Art. V. When a plan has been decided upon, the municipal council are to communicate it to the parties concerned, who are to be requested to forward any remarks they may wish to make thereon, within a reasonable time, to the local government, who will transmit the same to the Senate, together with the plan, a regular report and proposition, and such other elucidations as it may think necessary.

Art. VI. When the above-mentioned proprietors, *coloni*, or *livella-*

tarj, are willing to undertake the performance of the work specified, but declare themselves, and are found to be, without the necessary means, the executive power will advance them, by way of loan, the sums required for executing such work, upon the security of the land about to be improved, taking interest at four per cent. per annum, until the repayment of the principal. The Senate may take every precautionary measure it thinks proper, according to circumstances, in order to ensure the application of the money exclusively to the object for which it was granted.

Art. VII. The proprietors, *coloni*, or *livellatarj* may, in the case pointed out, claim the assistance of the agricultural committee in the direction of the work, with the means in the power of the latter, and without affecting their capital.

Art. VIII. If any, or all the proprietors, *coloni*, or *livellatarj*, who may be called upon as by Article V., to effect the projected work refuse to do so, the Senate, when it thinks the work necessary for the public health, will offer to take in exchange for other landed property, or to purchase the part or parts belonging to the dissentients, or to take the work into its own hands, at the option of the parties interested; and in this last case for the parts taken the executive government may treat with third persons, or with joint-stock companies, and raise sums upon loans, on its own security, with previous notice to the original proprietors; and the parts so cultivated by the public are to remain under mortgage until the complete repayment of the capital laid out, and the interest thereon, which is not to exceed six per cent. per annum.

The above lands being drained, improved, and brought into cultivation, the sale of them is to be held good until the repayment as above, deducting from the annual income the interest, *a scaletta*. Only that part of the land thus taken by the government is to be liable for the expense, all other property of the owner being free from such charge.

The owner may at any time redeem the land taken by the government, by paying the expense and interest, as before stated.

Art. IX. Land belonging to the public is to be drained with the sanction of the Senate, which may contract for the purpose with third persons, or with joint stock companies, on the principles established by act No. 78 of this Parliament.

With regard, however, to the draining of such land as would require an outlay in great disproportion to the advantage likely to be derived from its cultivation, on which account the work could only be desired for the sake of the public health, the Parliament will decide whether it shall be performed, and how the means are to be provided, whether by the alienation of some other public property, or by allotting a sum from the treasury.

Art. X. Over-marshy land, which having remained without tillage for many years, has been drained and improved, if it be kept under mortgage by the public, in virtue of Art. 8, no claims of former creditors of the owner, nor rights of feudal tithes, can be admitted until either the creditors or the owners have paid the expense incurred for the draining, in proportion to the part affected. If the land has been taken by the public in exchange, such claims shall be asserted over the property given instead of it. In the case of alienation by sale, if the debtor has no other property, the creditors have the right, as long as the land in cultivation may remain in the hands of government, to claim from said land, after deducting the purchase-money, and the expenses of cultivation and draining.

Art. XI. Land originally the property of government, or afterwards become so, and drained, shall be put up to sale, and the proceeds shall be applied to the draining and cultivation of other lands belonging to the public in the same island.

Art. XII. The executive government also, upon information and plans received from the respective municipal councils, will establish express regulations for giving due effect to the principles of the present law.

Such regulations are not to alter the existing laws, and are to be laid before the Legislative Assembly, at its next meeting.

Art. XIII. The present is to be printed, published, and transmitted to the proper authorities for execution.

Corfu, 19*th June*, 1837.

Second Session (extraordinary) of the Seventh Parliament of the United States of the Ionian Islands, held in virtue of the constitution of 1817.

No. XXI.

Title.—Act of Parliament for fixing a duty on the Grain imported into the States.

Preamble.—Whereas the stability and permanency of every government require that the resources of the State should be placed on a sure foundation, and as little as possible affected by casualties.

Whereas, every sound principle of political economy, and the experience of ages have shown that those imposts which affect all the subjects in general of any State, whilst they are least burdensome, constitute a certain resource.

Whereas, a moderate and well calculated duty upon the importation of grain, falling equally upon Ionians and foreigners residing within the State, not only is scarcely felt, but affords a certain branch of public revenue, and at the same time encourages the cultivation of this most essential article.   Whereas, lastly, the repeal of this duty, without substituting any other in its room, has occasioned a deficiency in the public revenue, and the exigencies of the State call for a speedy and effectual remedy.   Therefore, by the authority of his highness the President, and the most excellent Senate, with the opinion and assent of the most noble the Legislative Assembly in this (extraordinary) second session of the seventh Parliament, and with the approval of his excellency the Lord High Commissioner of the protecting Sovereign, it is decreed and enacted as follows :—

Art. I. Upon all kinds of grain imported for consumption into the United States of the Ionian Islands, the respective custom-houses will exact a duty as follows:—

On wheat, for every *kilò*,* pence 5.

On all other kinds of grain and pulse, except such as are already comprised in the existing tariffs, for every *kilò*, pence 3.

Art. II. To facilitate trade, the collectors of public revenue are authorized to permit the landing of any cargo of wheat, or other grain, without requiring the duty to be paid in advance, on condition that said cargo be deposited in proper stores, at the choice and expense of the owner of the grain, which must be secured by two locks, different from each other, of one of which the key is to remain with the collector, and that of the other with the owner, in order that, in case of sale for consumption, the duty fixed by the present law be, first of all, paid into the public chest.

Whenever the owner may think it necessary to air his grain so deposited, the collector is to allow him to do so.

---

* The kilo is the English bushel, or eighty imperial gallons.

Art. III. The disposition of the present act not interfering in any way with the provisions of act No. V. of the present Parliament, is to take effect from the 1st April next, N.S.

Art. IV. The present is to be printed, published and transmitted to the proper authorities for due execution.

Corfu, 11th March, 1841.

CHAPTER II.

ON THE STATE OF THE ARTS IN THE IONIAN ISLANDS.

Statistical Returns illustrating the State of the Arts. Remarks on
these. Trades followed, chiefly those concerned with Common
Wants. How carried on. Examples in illustration of the low
degree of Skill with which they are conducted. The Fine Arts
little advanced. Comparison of the different Islands. Remarks
on the rude State of the Arts in Cerigo, and on the Ignorance of
the People. Small Communities unfavourable to Progress in the
Arts. Retarding circumstances.

As tending to mark the stage of society and its condition, the state of the arts in a country is necessarily
a subject of interest, and deserving of consideration.

Conte Paolo Mercati, in a valuable little work,
published in 1811, entitled, "Saggio Storico Statis-
tico della Citta et Isola di Zante," has given some
details relative to the occupations and trades followed
in his native island and city, which may be usefully
applied to the topic in question.

At that time, the population of the island, according to this author, amounted to 33,353, of each sex,
and of all ages, in the town and the country,* as
shown in the following Table :—

* In 1836 it was estimated at 35,348.

	Males under sixteen.	Ditto to sixty.	Old Men.	Females under sixteen.	Ditto to fifty.	Old Women.	Jews.	Absentees.	Total.
City,	2460	3863	665	2035	3319	1125	274	383	14,124
Country,	3917	5761	891	2811	4539	1083	...	227	19,229
Total,	6377	9624	1558	4846	7858	2208	274	610	33,353

The whole population he considered as divided into three classes, viz., the nobili, cittadini, and plebeii, —of the first of which there were then no less than ninety families. The occupations, too, he classed in three divisions, as shown in detail in the following list, distinguishing between those who followed them, whether they resided in the town or country, the latter including the country villages.

	City.	Country.
Priests, ...	90	153
Deacons, ...	2	4
Clerks, ...	46	70
Monks, ...	63	52
Lay Brothers and Novices, . . .	6	0
Nuns, ...	5	14
Advocates, ...	41	0
Notaries, ...	25	41
Physicians and Surgeons, . . .	16	0
Blood-letters, ...	14	62
Druggists, ...	18	0
Masons, Stonecutters, Quarriers, . .	95	242
Blacksmiths, ...	61	6
Carpenters, Turners, Carvers, Spindlemakers,	137	15
Tanners, ...	35	0
Ship and Boat-builders, . . .	49	0
Mill-wrights and Millstone-cutters, .	19	20

	City.	Country.
Coopers,	59	0
Musical Instrument-makers,	3	0
Rope-makers,	13	0
Shoemakers,	256	0
Carpet-weavers,	8	0
Silk-weavers,	55	0
Dyers,	41	7
Tailors,	149	0
Capote-makers,	29	0
Hatters,	5	0
Spinners of fine cotton thread,	750	0
Gold and Silver smiths,	110	0
Watchmakers,	6	0
Coppersmiths,	8	0
Tinsmiths,	11	0
Potters,	34	17
Armourers,	18	0
Gilders, Varnishers, and House Painters,	14	0
Butchers,	65	0
Fishermen,	189	95
Bakers,	75	0
Confectioners,	15	0
Distillers,	17	0
Soapmakers,	19	0
Wax-chandlers,	9	0
Glaziers,	11	0
Printers,	2	0
Coffeehouse-keepers,	19	0
Mercers,	188	0
Grocers, and the Sellers of Provisions of different kinds,	168	0

In the above enumeration farmers and farm-labourers are not included; these constituted the chief portion of the residue of the population, and resided in the country, with the exception of 478, who lived in the town.

Zante, at the time that Conte Marcati wrote, was the richest and most flourishing of all the Ionian Islands ; and as I believe it still maintains this character, and that since that time it has undergone little change, the state of the arts there may be viewed as a favourable example, and rather in advance of their condition in the other islands.

In casting the eye over the list, one is struck with the absence of certain trades which administer to the intellectual wants and to the refinements of a highly civilized and well-educated people—such as, in relation to the first, printers, stationers, and booksellers, and the auxiliary callings of paper-makers, type-founders, engravers, &c.; and in relation to the second, such as coachmakers, wheelwrights, cabinet-makers, upholsterers, &c. &c. As late as 1824, when I was in Zante, there was not a single bookseller's shop in the city ; and the little stationery that was to be procured was to be met with here and there—at the druggist's, perhaps, or the mercer's.

The next impression received from the list is the very limited number of manufacturers, comprised chiefly in eight carpet-weavers, fifty-five silk-weavers, fifty-one potters, and nineteen soap-makers. Soap, carpeting, and silk, are the only articles expressly made for exportation, and these, with the exception of soap, chiefly to the adjoining islands, and in small quantities.

Another peculiarity, in referring to the list, which is obvious, is the absence of merchants—an omission which is not strictly correct, at least at the present time, for Zante is not without merchants; but they are few in number, and chiefly foreigners, belonging to English houses, and are engaged chiefly in selling and purchasing by commission.

Considering the list generally, the conclusion one must draw is, that the trades of Zante are principally those essential to the common wants of life ; and the same is applicable to all the other islands, with the exception, perhaps, of the seat of government, Corfu, where, probably, by this time, a bookseller's shop may exist, and other shops may be opened, to meet the demands of the garrison.*

As regards workmanship, the trades which are

---

* The only printing press in the Ionian Islands is one in Corfu, the property of the government, which is under a censorship, and is chiefly employed in printing the Ionian Gazette, acts of Parliament, and other official documents. Were the censorship removed, and perfect freedom given to the press, it is not probable that any enterprising individual would come forward to attempt a printing establishment ; or, if attempted, that it would succeed, excepting conducted on a small scale, and limited in its operations to ephemeral publications, likely to do more harm than good. Very recently a serious riot took place in the seat of government, and the military were attacked by a mob that threatened to murder a missionary, whose offence was the distribution merely of religious tracts. A free press has been given to Malta, and, as might be expected, it has been abused in the manner just alluded to; but it is to be hoped that good will ultimately come of it ; that it will tend to call forth the intellectual powers of the people ; and that, witnessing its evil effects, they will become guarded in its use, and learn to control their bad feelings and passions. Freedom of the press, like freedom of speech, requires manly control to be useful or even tolerated, and its exercise is a discipline of the mind of the most valuable kind.

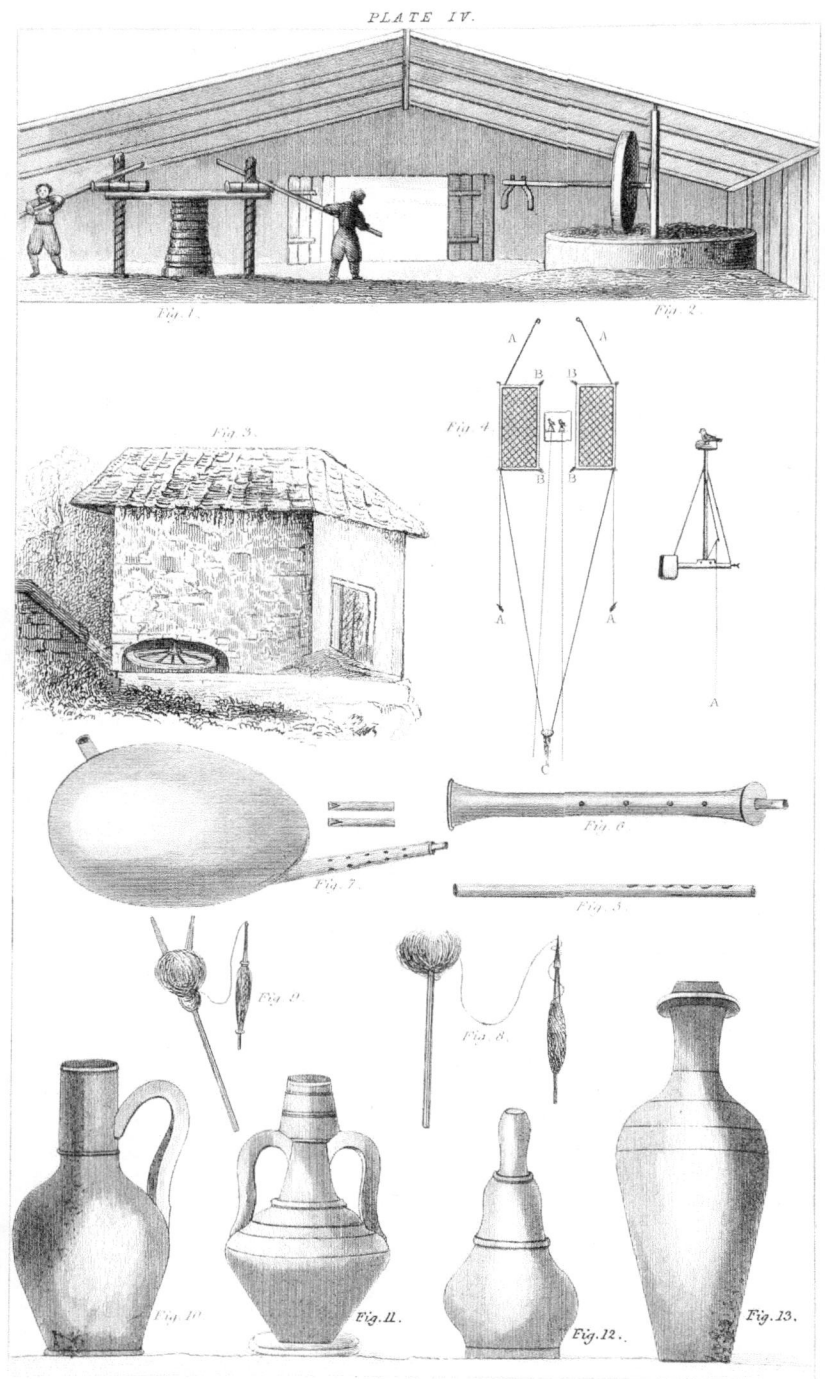

PLATE IV.

Fig. 1.   Fig. 2.

Fig. 3.   Fig. 4.

Fig. 6.

Fig. 7.   Fig. 5.

Fig. 9.   Fig. 8.

Fig. 10.   Fig. 11.   Fig. 12.   Fig. 13.

OLIVE PRESS & CORN MILL, &c. IN USE IN THE IONIAN ISLANDS.

followed are in a low stage of art. The execution is commonly coarse, displaying little skill or dexterity, and extremely little knowledge, and, consequently, the value of the materials forming the articles made is but little enhanced by the labour bestowed. Take, for example, the pottery or the carpeting. The former is made of the gray clay of the island; and, whether glazed or unglazed, is of the coarsest quality. The forms, however, are commonly graceful, particularly of the jars—whether of small size and porous for holding and cooling water, or of large dimensions for holding wine and oil. They much resemble in shape ancient vases;* and it can hardly be doubted that the art has been perpetuated from ancient times, but, excepting in the forms of the vessels, retaining nothing of that excellence which distinguished the earthenware of ancient Greece. The carpeting, made principally of goats' hair, has no pretensions to beauty; it is coarse and strong, of the rudest manufacture, indicating the merest infancy of the art. The same remark is applicable to the silk camlet manufacture, which, though a good article (excepting that it is ill dyed), and well adapted for the purpose to which it is chiefly applied, viz., the making of coats and jackets for use during the summer season, is wove in a primitive loom, the same, probably, that has been employed in the east for thousands of years. The soap of Zante is another instance of rude art;

---

* In Plate IV. some of the forms of the common earthenware at present in use in the Mediterranean are represented.

though formed of good materials, and always of olive-oil, it is of indifferent quality, from the careless manner in which it is made, being commonly gritty, from the alkali not having been properly prepared, and always of an unpleasant smell. The natives of these islands, in brief, have not yet received the stimulus necessary to induce them to apply with energy to any manual occupation or manufacture, and seem to bring to them as little capital as possible, to exercise them with the smallest possible degree of knowledge and skill, to be contented with earning a mere subsistence, and to be unambitious of improvement. These remarks even apply to the gold and silver smiths, who often, in a comparatively rude state of society, acquire skill and execute works of distinguished beauty; but the articles of plate made in the Ionian Islands are without pretensions to beauty; whether for the use of the table, as spoons and forks, or for the ornament of the person, as ear-rings and buckles, the workmanship is coarse, and the forms inelegant. Nor is cheapness a common recommendation. The prices of most articles made in the islands are comparatively high, and the demand made for any work at all unusual is exorbitant.*

When the common and the ornamental arts are so

* When I was in Zante, in the summer of 1824, I paid at the rate of thirty oboli, about fifteen-pence a pair, for coarse cotton socks of homespun thread, knit in the island; for sewing together, so as to make a note-book, with plain paper cover, a quire of paper, which cost twelve oboli, thirty-eight oboli; for putting a horn handle to a tea-pot that cost in England when new about two dollars, one dollar.

little advanced, it would be unreasonable to expect
to find the fine arts cultivated. The Greek Church
has always been unfavourable to painting and sculp-
ture, and this may be one of the causes of the almost
utter neglect of them in these islands. I doubt much
whether, amongst their whole population, there is an
individual capable of painting a portrait; or now,
that the Cavalier Prosoleny is dead, who studied at
Rome, and justly acquired some reputation as a sculptor, whether there is another who could model a bust
or give the design of a monument.*

If the different islands are compared, one with another, some marked differences may be perceived in
relation to the means of art which they possess. As
Zante may be considered the least deficient, Cerigo
probably may be pointed out as most so; nor is it
surprising, keeping in mind its detached situation, its
peculiar position, the poverty of its population, and
the manner in which, for centuries, they have been
cut off from intercourse with any civilized people.

In 1826, when the total population of this island
was 13,020, it appears, from an official return, that
there were only 25 employed in what were designated
manufactures, as dyers, potters, and tanners; and
only 177 individuals in arts of the first necessity, as
masons, carpenters, smiths, shoemakers; whilst 475

---

* The son of this artist, reported to be a young man of talent, is
now at Rome, prosecuting his studies in the same line of art at the
expense of the government. The school of design, which was continued many years under the direction of Prosoleny, is now closed.

were engaged in petty traffic, and 2650 in hus-
bandry.

Whilst Major Macphail was resident of Cerigo, he
exerted himself strenuously to improve the island.
He has assured me that the rudeness of the people
and their ignorance were almost beyond belief; and
that in carrying on ordinary works connected with
road-making, the natives could contribute little more
than bodily labour; if a rock was to be blasted, or
an arch turned, he had to direct it, and a cyclopædia
was the source of his information. The mason who,
under his directions, constructed the first bridge that
was ever seen in Cerigo, had not the least confidence
in the strength of the arch, being ignorant of the
principle, unacquainted even with the form: shortly
after it was completed a violent storm occurred by
night; the following morning early the mason was
found on his knees, looking despondently at the
bridge, and praying to the Virgin to defend it, and
save it from destruction from the torrent.

The preceding slight details are sufficiently characteristic of a very backward stage of the arts and of
society; and others might be given tending to the
same point, and illustrative also of the little tendency
to improvement which is commonly found to exist in
small communities.

The demand for provisions being very limited, the
supplies are furnished by a few dealers, who can easily
combine to raise prices. To prevent this, the local
government considered it necessary to fix the market

prices even of the necessaries of life, as bread, butcher-
meat, &c.—the necessary consequence of which has
been, that little attention has been paid to quality,
and the people have become accustomed to, and contented with, inferior articles of food, some of which
it is not improbable may have an injurious effect on
the constitution, and it is possible may have affected
their mental qualities as well as their bodily.

Again, perhaps, owing to the small number of artificers, and the high price of work, a habit appears to
have been formed of having no more done than is
absolutely necessary—of leaving things in an un-
finished state, and of neglecting repairs, especially in
the country. The consequences have been sloven-
liness, discomfort, and ultimate loss.* In the country
it is very unusual indeed to see any of the wooden
work of buildings, not even the doors and window-
frames, protected by paint; the majority of the
country-houses are out of repair, and very many of
them are in an unsafe and ruinous condition. And
this, moreover, it hardly need be pointed out, is not
without its consequences; living in the country is, to

---

* In illustration equally of carelessness and want of skill, mention
may be made of what has happened to a mud-boat employed in Zante
for the purpose of deepening the port there, which, for many years,
has been becoming shallower, from mud brought by an adjoining
stream and deposited on its bottom. Whilst in use, some of the cogs
of the wheels of the machine got broken. No Zantiote artist was
competent to repair them; in Corfu one might be found; but he was
not sent. The damage increased till the wheels were irreparably
useless. For six months the mud-boat has not been employed, and
must remain so till new wheels can be procured from England.

a proverb, disagreeable, there being so little comfort there and ordinary enjoyment; and though in scenery often of surpassing beauty, delighting the traveller, it is avoided by the landed proprietors, and allowed to remain neglected, to the great detriment of their own interests and of those of the public.

Another circumstance may be mentioned, which probably has some influence in checking improvement in art, and even in conducing to its deterioration; it is the absence of the apprenticeship system—in consequence of which it is seldom that any trade is well learnt. Most young men start in life on their own account with the smallest possible amount of skill in their particular business; and having but little encouragement, it is not surprising that few, if any, of them ever become accomplished workmen. In Greece, in Malta, and in Turkey, the usage in this respect is the same; and in all these countries most of the arts, as in the Ionian Islands, are in a rude and almost primitive state.

CHAPTER III.

MISCELLANEOUS NOTICES OF SOME OF THE UTENSILS, IM-
PLEMENTS, AND PROCESSES IN USE IN THE IONIAN
ISLANDS.

Mills. A very primitive Corn-Mill described. Oven in common use.
Kitchen Fire-places. Lamps. Still. Water-lever. Different
Modes in use of watering Gardens. Manner of washing Clothes.
Bleaching. Dyeing. The Sandal. Remarks on its usefulness.
Boats of peculiar construction. Modes of taking Fish. Of snar-
ing Birds.

I ENTER on these notices, partly for the sake of illustrating further the state of the arts in the Ionian
Islands, and through them the condition of the
people; and partly with the hope that some of the
simple implements and processes which will be described, may be found available and useful in our
colonies, in their early stage,—recommended at least
by their requiring little outlay of money, and little
skill of construction or execution.

Several kinds of mills are employed for the grinding of corn and other grain,—as the hand-mill,—the
mill worked by horses and sometimes by women,—
the wind-mill, and the water-mill; of these, the wind-
mill is least in use; the others of more simple struc-

ture are commonly preferred; one or other of them is to be met with in every village.

The water-mill is the only one I shall now particularly mention. It is of the same kind as that seen by Sir Walter Scott in the Shetland Islands, only perhaps a little larger, and so amusingly described by him in his Diary, published in his Life,—consisting of a horizontal wheel, supported by a perpendicular beam, and moving the upper on the nether mill-stone, and moved by a stream of water descending with considerable velocity from a certain height, at an acute angle.*—(Plate IV., fig. 3.)

This form of water-mill, with its hopper, as it is quite elementary, is probably of great antiquity, and may be considered the representative of the first invented. In support of this idea, I may mention that its use is very widely spread in countries far apart, and in remote or secluded regions, to which modern art hitherto has hardly penetrated. I have myself witnessed it in daily use, not only in the Ionian Islands, but also in the higher alpine country of Savoy,—in the neighbourhood of Constantinople, and in Asia Minor, near Penteraclea;† and I have heard

* Sir Walter Scott describes the mill-stone of the *Cleik-him-in* mills as "a stone quern of the old-fashioned construction."—*Life of Sir Walter Scott*, vol. iii., p. 145.

† Penteraclea, the ancient Heraclea, on the southern shore of the Black Sea, brings to my recollection the coal-mines, or rather coal-seams, which I visited in the neighbourhood of that town, along the sea-coast, admirably situated for working, and, from the size of the beds at the surface, and the good quality of the coal, not inferior to some of the best bituminous kind of England,

of it as still employed in the hilly parts of Syria,—in ancient Assyria, the country of the Nestorian Christians,*—in some of the mountainous parts of Spain, and even in the wilder parts of Ireland;—the late lamented Sir David Wilkie assured me that he had seen it in Conamara.

The oven commonly employed in these islands is also of the simplest construction, and very easily made. It consists of a dome of clay, or of brickwork, with an opening closed by a stone, by which the fuel is introduced to heat it. The figure of the cross may be often seen on the stone door, and above it: that represented in Plate VI., fig. 3, was in the kitchen of the headman or primate of Santa Matia, a village in Corfu.

of very great promise. I have said, they hardly deserve the name of mines, and that is, because they are so inartificially and unprofitably worked, rather quarried than mined, in a manner very characteristic of the low state of-mining art in Turkey. The rock formations in which they occur, are those commonly associated with this mineral,—sandstone, shale, and limestone.

In the same district in which I saw the primitive mill, I witnessed the people of the country—Turks, men, and women—occupied in reaping,—the women, however, in a company, a little apart from the men;—they used the sickle, and, what was peculiar, they had the little and ring finger of the left hand, with which they grasped the corn in cutting, armed each with a wooden projecting sheath, by which the tips of these fingers were defended and the grasp enlarged. They are put on and off as easily as a thimble.

* Dr Grant, in his interesting account of the Nestorians, or the lost Tribes, recently published, in a note, p. 211, says:—" They have also water-mills for grinding, made in the most simple manner. These have but a single wheel, and the revolving stone and wheel are attached to the same perpendicular shaft."

The kitchen fire-place of the houses in Corfu, of all but the poorest, is well adapted for the purposes for which it is wanted, and for economizing fuel,—wood, and charcoal, the fuel invariably used in these islands. The structure of which it consists is of brick-work,—a standing-out platform with a funnel above for receiving and carrying off the smoke, through a chimney with which it communicates, as represented in Plate VI., fig. 5.*

The lamps in use amongst the natives are principally of old fashion; some of them are of antique form. The figures given in Plate VI. are of the most common kinds. Fig. 9 is made either of brass or silver; fed with good oil (it is olive-oil that is always used) it is an excellent lamp, giving a good steady light, and it is easily kept in order and managed; indeed, for its management there is an ample provision in the many adjuncts appended, as snuffers, picker, and tongues, besides an extinguisher. It consists of a body, the reservoir of the oil, and a cover; has sometimes three, sometimes four burners, and may be raised or depressed at pleasure. Figs. 7 and 8 represent lamps of earthen-ware used by the lower class of people; and are probably precisely the same as were used by people of the same class in these countries, two and three thousand years ago.

---

* The part A (fig. 5), is for a wood-fire; B, for a charcoal-fire; the two small stoves marked B, in front, communicate with air-holes, C; the two behind these have no flues; live coal is put into them, and they are used for keeping things hot.

Figs. 10 and 11 are of night lamps of a very simple kind : one is such as, I believe, is sometimes employed in this country in a sick chamber,—merely a little cotton, moulded in a conical form, put on a plate or saucer with a little oil. The other is a small floating lamp,—a thread of cotton, supported by wire passed through pieces of cork, by which it is floated on the oil. It is frequently to be seen before shrines in churches, and before pictures of the Virgin and of favourite saints in private dwellings ;—the madonna and certain saints being too frequently the objects of superstitious worship, and each person having a patron protecting saint, to whom he is considered in a manner dedicated.*

The still employed—and it is almost exclusively used for preparing a coarse spirit, well called aqua ardente—is of very rude construction; that represented in Plate VI., fig 2, is to be met with in some parts of Santa Maura and Corfu. The refrigeratory is sometimes of wood, sometimes an earthen vessel; through which two straight metallic tubes pass, communicating with a single large pipe from the head, which is very small and luted on, and, as well as the body, is generally of copper.

The lever-apparatus† for raising well-water, is in

---

* Determined by the accident of birth; every day of the year in the Greek calendar having its saint.

† *Vide* Plate VI., fig. 6. It consists of a long pole supported by a cross stick resting on a forked upright; a stone is commonly tied to one end as a counterpoise to the bucket when filled with water. The

common use in the Ionian Islands, as well as in most parts of the east, and, there is reason to believe, from time immemorial. It is recommended by its simplicity of structure, its cheapness, and the facility with which it is used. Here it may be remarked, that although irrigation is not practised to the extent that it might be, with advantage, in these islands, yet that the use of watering their grounds is in principle fully understood by the natives. Not to recur to the more extensive operations of watering the currant-plantations and the olive-trees, it may be mentioned that where there is garden cultivation, as in the neighbourhood of the towns of Zante and Corfu, two methods of watering are employed, viz., by the hand and by gutters. The gardener carries a jar with a large mouth under one arm, and pouring the water from it on the other hand, he scatters it over the thirsty plants. The gutters are little channels made in the soil, closed at one end, and supplied with water from a well by means of the lever and bucket, till the ground is thoroughly saturated. The time of watering is the evening, usually after sunset. In the process the foot is often employed—the naked foot—for the purpose of closing one channel, or breaking down a little embankment to turn the

chief labour is in letting down the empty bucket (B), as it is opposed to the weight (A). The bucket having a cross bar, is suspended by a hook, which is sometimes a piece of stick, and then it is tied to the slender pole (D); when of iron, it is fastened permanently.

course of the water into the different beds,—bringing to recollection the scriptural expression of watering the seed "with the foot, as in a garden of herbs."*

By the villagers, who are fond of flowers—and it is a prevalent taste, particularly in Corfu, where they pride themselves on their fine carnations—another method of watering is used, which probably has been found by experience to have a better effect. The florist takes the water into his mouth and spurts it on his plants. The slightly raised temperature of the water may be beneficial, and also the small quantity of saliva mixed with it which may act as a manure.

In the Ionian Islands and in the Levant generally, the business of washing clothes is commonly conducted in the following manner, the particulars of which I collected in Zante. The linen is moistened with salt, brackish, or fresh-water (the two former are preferred). They are heaped one upon another in a basket or tub, with a hole in its bottom. A quantity of wood-ashes is thrown upon the top; lukewarm water is poured upon the ashes, and then hot water. A drop of oil is occasionally added to the water that leaks through, to ascertain the presence of the alkali of the ashes; when the oil mixes with the water, no more warm water is added. The clothes are allowed to remain a few hours saturated with the ley, and are then washed. Very little soap

* Deuteronomy xi. 10.

is required. It should have been mentioned that lemon-peel and laurel-leaves are often added to the wood-ashes, to impart an agreeable fragrance. Most commonly in washing, the linen is not rubbed with the hands, but is beaten with a wooden mallet. Preparatory to the bleaching of linen, it is dipt in salt-water. This was mentioned to me by a physician of Zante, who supposed that the salt-water aided in the bleaching effect by the chlorine which its salts contain, and flattered himself that his countrywomen practically had been in advance of modern chemistry: but, I apprehend, the salt-water is chiefly useful in keeping the linen moist, moisture being a great help in bleaching; and that as no chlorine is rendered free, this substance cannot operate. Many prejudices prevail amongst the people of the Ionian Islands respecting the influence of the moon;—one of these is, that linen exposed to it in bleaching is rendered rotten.*

Dyeing in the Ionian Islands is little more than a domestic art. Most of the home-spun webs are dyed at home by the wives and daughters of the villagers. Blue, red, and yellow, are the favourite colours. The first is imparted by woad (*Isatis tinctoria*), which is found wild, and is also cultivated for the

---

* They dread more the new moon than the moon at its full. On a new moon they abstain from sowing seed, or grafting fruit-trees, or cutting timber, with the belief that the two first cannot succeed, and that wood then felled will suddenly decay. They consider, too, the new moon equally unfavourable to the making of wine and the bleaching of linen.

purpose. Madder is employed to give a red colour, and saffron to give a yellow, both which are grown in the islands. The process of dyeing with woad is briefly the following :—The green leaves, after having been bruised with a mallet, by being beaten on a stone, are exposed on the ground to dry, with an admixture of the leaves of the mastic, as a defence, it is said, from " the evil eye," that widely spread Eastern superstition, the imaginary cause of so many evils.* Thoroughly dried, the woad will keep twelve months, without losing its virtue. When used, hot water is poured on it in a wooden trough, the bottom of which is full of small holes to allow the excess of water to drain off. In a short time fermentation commences, and very offensive effluvia are emitted ; now a lexivium of wood-ashes is added, and the woollen cloths to be dyed are immersed in the mixture. In summer, the time of steeping is about eight days ; in winter, about ten. The colour received is dark blue, and is permanent.

The sandal commonly worn by the Ionian peasantry is so useful an article, so cheap, so easily made, and so good a substitute for the shoe, that it may be deserving of being better known, especially in the army, the providing of shoes for which in the field is often difficult, and sometimes impracticable.† In

---

* Greek and Turk has the same belief in the evil eye, and wear charms to avert its influence. The death of a child, the lameness or sickness of a horse, all sorts of accidents or misfortunes, are attributed by both people to its operation, in defiance of religion and fatalism.

† In Ceylon, during the rebellion in 1818–19, I witnessed an in-

Plate VI. fig. 12, the form of sandal most generally used in these islands, is represented. The strongest sandals are made of bullock's hide, preserved by salting, immediately after taking it from the animal. It is of one piece, with one seam only, from the point towards the instep. It is secured from slipping from the foot by a thong passed through loops, and wound round the leg above the ankle. A pair of sandals in constant use will last two or three months. So much are they approved by our soldiers, that when detached, employed on the roads, where their military appearance is little attended to, they commonly adopt them.

Neither as boatmen nor fishermen are the people of the Ionian Islands in any repute. The circumstances of situation, so favourable, and their natural wants, if not interfered with, would probably have induced them to exert themselves in both capacities, and with success. The principal check exists in the

stance of the evil above alluded to. For months, not only the men, but also the majority of the officers employed in the remote and wild districts, had to march bare-footed, and over very difficult ground, their shoes and boots having been worn out, and a fresh supply not having been attainable. Had the sandal been brought into use in this emergency, much suffering might have been prevented, and probably some lives saved; for the sores arising from injuries received by the unprotected feet, in some instances, had serious consequences. A sandal of the fresh hide of a bullock or goat, affording good protection, may be made in a few minutes, by cutting out a piece of the hide, the form of the foot, but a little larger than the sole, and fastening it by a strip of hide passed through holes in the overlapping margin, to the ankle.

PLATE VI.

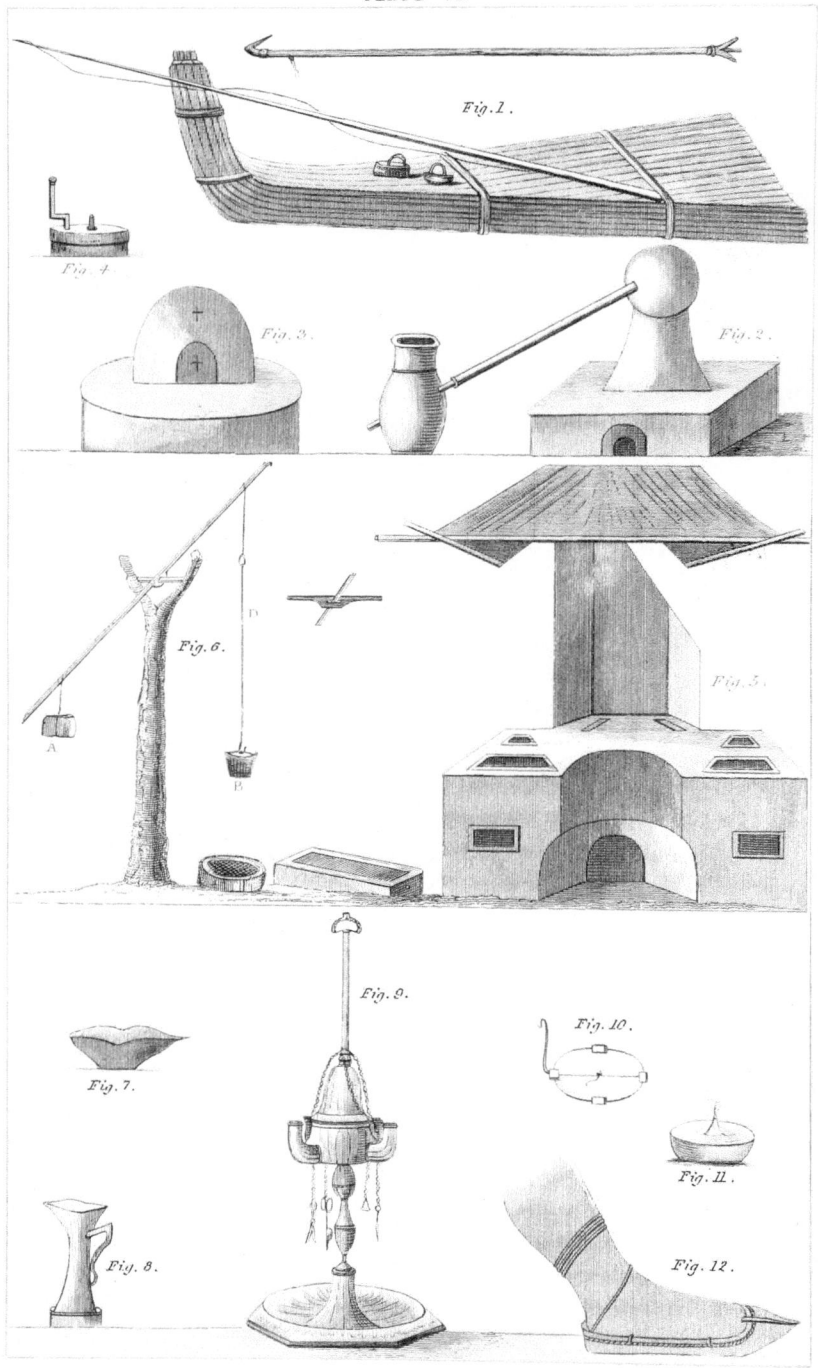

Fig. 1.

Fig. 4.

Fig. 3.

Fig. 2.

Fig. 6.

Fig. 5.

Fig. 9.

Fig. 7.

Fig. 10.

Fig. 11.

Fig. 8.

Fig. 12.

DOMESTIC IMPLEMENTS &c. IN USE IN THE IONIAN ISLANDS.

sanatory regulations connected with the quarantine system, which, as at present established, are a great impediment to all minor sea enterprises. Some of the boats in use are sufficiently characteristic, as the very primitive monoxolon, a canoe formed by hollowing the trunk of a tree, employed in the shallow waters of the lagoon of Santa Maura, and of the lake Corissia, in Corfu; and the paterella or bullrush boat, of which a sketch is given in Plate VI., sometimes employed by the fishermen of Corfu, and which is so light that it is easily carried by one man.*

Of the modes of taking fish, deserving perhaps of notice on account of their singularity, I shall make mention of two—one practised in Zante—the other

---

* The paterella, from which the sketch above alluded to was taken, was in use near Sinarades, on the western coast of Corfu, and was made of dried bullrushes from the Val di Roppa. It was about four feet long, not including the prow, about three feet wide at the stern, and was capable of carrying one man well, but barely two. The boatman sits on it cross-legged, and manages it with a long light reed, at one end terminating in a hook, at the other in a prong—the latter is used as a paddle. The other articles of equipment were a cane fishing-rod, a basket to hold fish, a pot with a paste made of rotten cheese, flour, and water, and a wallet containing bread. The fisherman paddled himself to the rock of singular form, called " The Bride," off the shore, about two miles from Pelica; and when we passed, about an hour after, he was throwing some of the paste into the water, to entice the fish and bring them together, before he commenced fishing, using the same for bait. The paterella, I may remark, may be deserving of the attention of travellers engaged in exploring new regions, on account of its facility of construction. Reeds may serve as well as rushes, or indeed any light, spongy, tough plants admitting of being bound together in a suitable form.

on the south-western coast of Corfu, and probably elsewhere in the islands. The method in use in Zante is for catching mullet : the fisherman uses a mullet as a decoy, which is attached by the gills to a line tied to a rod stuck in the sand, and is allowed to swim about. The fisherman stands near the rod on the look-out; and when a fish appears allured sufficiently near by the decoy, he flings a casting-net with which he is prepared, and, if dexterous, commonly encloses the fish. The decoy, it is said, should be a female. In Corfu the fowling-piece is applied to the business of fishing—constituting the reverse of that aërial species of angling for swallows, already mentioned. The sportsman, besides his gun, is provided with a little jar of oil, for the purpose of rendering smooth the water when ruffled, to enable him to see the fish. Shot is used about the size of duck-shot; and one individual of whom I inquired, who appeared to be well practised in the art, said the fish he shot were from half-a-pound in weight to three pounds. A rocky coast, with rather deep water along-shore, is best fitted for this kind of sport.

The people of these islands are passionately fond of field-sports, as are the Greeks generally,* and

* A marked difference in this respect exists between the Greeks and their neighbours the Turks—and indeed, it may be said, the oriental people generally. The Turk may be seen coursing on horse-back, following his greyhounds at full speed in pursuit of the hare with the keenest impetuosity, but I believe he never goes out for the quieter and less exciting amusement of fowling, in which the Greeks of Constantinople indulge as much as those of the islands.

shooting is their favourite amusement, but in the ignoble manner of taking advantage of the birds at rest; indeed I am not aware of any southern people or inhabitants of a hot climate who practise shooting on the wing. They are also addicted to the snaring of birds, especially doves; and in the island of Cerigo to the hunting of quail, which they run down. Another method of taking doves is by decoy with nets,* which a priest, whom I saw using it in Malta, called his " land-fishing." In Plate IV., fig. 4, is a sketch of the whole apparatus, an explanation of which will be found in the note below.† The following of this amusement requires

* My knowledge of the above method was got in Malta, and I may be in error in describing it as practised in the Ionian Islands. What induces me to have a doubt on its being followed there, is the degree of quiet patience which it demands, and for which these people are nowise distinguished.

† The apparatus consists of two parts : two nets, each about seven feet long and about three wide ; and two perches for the decoy doves. The nets are, as it were, anchored at AA by cords, allowing of lateral movement; at B two corresponding corners of each are fastened by tying the wooden stretchers of the nets to stakes driven into the ground. From the other end of the near stretchers two strong cords proceed, which meet at C, from which one strong cord is continued to the fowler's seat, masked by a wall; by pulling this cord he raises and turns over the nets. The perch consists of a small circular leaden stand, at the extremity of a wooden rod, which is fixed to a support of wood, attached by two small hinges to a horizontal piece of wood, which is placed on the ground and fixed by a heavy stone on one end of it. From the rod close to the hinge-piece a perpendicular rod proceeds ; the other three lines aaa are to add to the strength of the rods. The long line A is held by the fowler, who pulls it when he wishes to raise the dove to attract the attention of passing birds, which it does the more, as, in the act of being raised, it flaps its

great devotion to it and extraordinary patience, as the doves pass in flights, and are birds of passage. Sometimes, after watching from early dawn to nightfall, not a bird will appear; occasionally, large numbers in succession. Seventy are sometimes caught in one day.

wings. The decoy-birds are hooded, and are tied to the stand, which is slightly raised by being placed on a stone. The nets having only end-stretching rods, are easily and quickly turned over on the alighting of a bird between them.

CHAPTER IV.

ON THE COMMERCE OF THE IONIAN ISLANDS.

Great Capabilities of these Islands for Commerce.   Tables illustrative
of their present Commercial Condition.   Peculiar Mode of Conducting the Trade in Grain.   Currant and Oil Trade.   Disadvantages under which they labour.   Remarks on the Commercial Resources of the Islands—and the Improvement of certain
Productions and Manufactures.   Exertions of Government in
behalf of Improvement.   Establishment of an Ionian Bank—an
Agricultural Society.   Great Improvement and Extension of the
Roads.   Other Improvements in Progress.   Tables in illustration
of the Commercial Relations between the Ionian Islands and Great
Britain.   Tables illustrating the Currant-trade.

WHETHER the productions of the Ionian Islands are
considered, or their geographical situation, it cannot
be questioned that they possess great natural advantages well fitting them for the purposes of commerce.
Their position, close to the coast of Greece—at one
extremity, at the entrance of the Adriatic ; at the
other, at the entrance of the Archipelago—does not
require to be dwelt on in relation to their commercial
capacity.   The productions of the soil—oil, fruit, and
wine—are peculiarly commercial articles; olive-oil
and the currant have been long staple commodities :
and the olive-tree and currant-vine have been cultivated chiefly with a view to the exports of their produce.   Yet it must be confessed that the Ionian

people generally are not a commercial people. The following return shows, in conjunction with other particulars, the proportion of the whole population so engaged, chiefly, it should be remembered, however, in petty trade.

RETURN OF THE POPULATION, AND OF THE BIRTHS, MARRIAGES, AND DEATHS IN THE IONIAN STATES, FOR THE YEAR 1836.

States.	Square Miles.	Males.	Females.	Aliens and Resident Strangers.	Population to the Sq. Mile.	Agriculture.	Manufactures.	Commerce.	Births.	Marriages.	Deaths.
						Persons employed in					
Corfu, . .	227	35,221	29,886	9,806	287	15,077	1,621	1,443	2,208	473	1,580
Cephalonia,	348	34,864	28,333	936	182	12,689	1,471	835	1,694	550	931
Zante, . .	156	19,675	15,673	4,127	226	7,672	1,947	421	1,329	370	1,115
Santa Maura,	180	9,097	8.098	190	95	2,458	132	470	521	119	370
Ithaca, . .	44	4,942	4,702	108	219	1,407	196	931	197	90	119
Cerigo, . .	116	4,156	4,551	37	75	1,522	264	198	283	89	157
Paxo, . .	26	2,561	2,503	223	195	217	198	65	116	32	113
Total, .	1097	110,516	93,746	12,427	186	41,042	5,829	4,363	6,384	1,723	4,385

The other returns, which follow, throw further light on this subject. They are extracted from a work compiled from official documents.*

SHIPPING, 1833.

Flag.	Ships Inwards.	Ships Outwards.
	Tons.	Tons.
Ionian, ...	130,797	137,013
British, ...	25,941	24,449
Austrian, ...	40,463	39,678
Russian, ...	6,886	6,059
French, ...	546	451
Neapolitan, ...	6,764	5,419
Papal, ...	2,313	1,975
Sardinian, ...	932	1,483
Turkish, ...	2,988	3,060
Greek, ...	35,570	34,083
All other, ...	1,709	2,162
Total, ...	254,909	255,832

* Tables of the Revenue, Population, Commerce, &c., of the United Kingdom and its Dependencies.

IMPORTS INTO THE IONIAN ISLANDS, 1833.

Articles Imported.		Quantities.	Value in Sterling Money.
PRODUCE.			£
Sugar, ...	lbs.,	917,953	16,079
Coffee, ...	...	357,215	8,250
Drugs, Gums, Medicines, Dyeing Materials, &c., . . .	...	...	9,954
MANUFACTURES.			
Cotton, ...		...	58,709
Hemp and Flax (exclusive of cordage),		...	5,655
Woollen, ...		...	22,002
Silk, ...		...	5,263
Earthenware, ...		...	2,446
Furniture, ...		...	2,052
Hardware, ...		...	7,780
Nails, ...		...	2,847
Cordage, ...	lbs.,	173,246	2,561
Glass, ...		...	2,471
All other articles, . . .		...	38,761
Raw silk, ...	lbs ,	1,718	682
... cotton, . . .	...	63,453	1,906
Wool, ...	...	8,760	139
Hemp and flax, . .	...	104,217	2,476
For large casks, . .	{ Staves, No.,	420,363 }	7,003
	{ Hoops, ...	561,594 }	
Iron, ...	lbs.,	232,722	1,601
Timber, ...		...	13,817
Firewood, . . .	passi,	15,032	6,291
Wheat, . . .	bushels,	769,579	147,882
Indian Corn, . . .	...	223,437	21,876
Barley and Oats, . .	...	178,074	13,491
Beans and other Legumes,	...	34,639	3,846
Potatoes, . . .	lbs.,	939,013	2,588
Rice, ...	...	755,713	6,609
Maccaroni, . . .	...	223,439	2,351
Flour, ...	...	146,874	961
Biscuits, ...	...	120,178	737
Cheese, ...	...	1,056,846	11,929
Butter, ...	...	72,847	2,610
Salt Meat, . . .	...	25,070	592
Stockfish and Baccala, .	...	1,287,609	10,933
Bottargo and Caviare, .	...	99,577	4,434
Sardinias, Anchovies, &c.,	...	2,070,185	23,268
Onions and Garlic, . .	migliaris,	9,655	2,065
Dried Fruits, . . .	...	...	5,134
Poultry, ...	heads,	26,180	1,083
Carry forward,			

Articles Imported.		Quantities.	Value in Sterling Money.
			£
Brought forward, . .			
Foreign wines, . .	barrels,	667	3,360
... spirits, . .	...	834	2,136
Cattle, ...	heads,	8,483	29,182
Horses, Mules, and Asses, . . .		791	4,641
Sheep, Goats, and Pigs, . . .		66,604	26,360
Tobacco, . . .	lbs.,	88,083	1,621
All other articles, ...		...	15,177
Total, . . .		...	563,611
Transit, . . .		...	83,654

EXPORTS FROM THE IONIAN ISLANDS, 1833.

Articles Exported.		Quantities.	Value in Sterling Money.
PRODUCE.			£
Olive oil, ...	barrels,	62,663	102,275
Currants, ...	lbs.,	17,131,371	89,885
Wine, ...	barrels,	19,717	5,441
Spirits, ...	...	1,013	1,144
Valonia, ...	lbs.,	104,796	240
Salt, ...	bushels,	37,555	469
Wheat, ...	...	...	...
Indian corn, . . .	...	130	11
All other produce, . . .		...	2,412
MANUFACTURES.			
Cotton, ...		...	954
Silk, ...		...	49
Woollen and Goat hair, . . .		...	82
Earthenware, ...		...	517
Articles of coarse Clothing, . .		...	269
Shoes, ...		...	61
Hides, ...	No.,	1,950	399
Cordage, ...	lbs.	552	20
Hardware, ...		...	413
Casks for Currants, . .	No.	6,543	4,138
Barrels for Oil and Wine, . . .		4,658	474
Soap, ...	lbs.,	3,080,374	33,861
All other Articles, ...		...	1,400
Foreign Manufactures, . . .		...	6,155
Total, . . .		...	250,669
Transit, . . .		...	129,665

In comparing the amount of imports and exports in 1833, as given in these Tables, it should be remembered that in this year there was no olive crop in Corfu. It also requires to be kept in recollection that a large sum is annually paid by Great Britain to our troops stationed in these islands; in the year mentioned it was L.113,481.

Of the different islands, the people of Cephalonia and of Ithaca are most enterprising and most disposed to engage in foreign trade, especially the former. This is indicated by the number of ships belonging to Cephalonia, manned, navigated, and employed by natives. In 1828, I was informed by an English merchant belonging to a house of commission established at Argostoli, that whilst Corfu possessed only about twelve vessels, besides boats, and Zante only four, Cephalonia had three hundred vessels, square-rigged, each with a crew of from twenty to thirty men.* But the trade in which they were occupied was not that of carrying fruit or oil from their own shores to foreign ports, but of carrying grain from one foreign port to another—that commerce which, for many

* According to the Statistical Tables of Cephalonia there were, in 1823, belonging to this island, 119 ships ; 107 sailing vessels, or boats ; 49 vessels for passage or small boats ; and 69 fishing-boats. Which statement is correct I do not know. If it is supposed to be for the interest of a people to give false information, official returns may be utterly worthless. Sir Charles Napier mentions an instance in point, when speaking of these tables, how the currant-proprietors concealed half the produce, having the idea that the currants were to be subjected to increased taxation. The deception was detected by the Custom-house books.

years during the revolutionary war, was engaged in
with so much success by many of the Greeks, and to
which Hydra, and Spezia, and Ipsara, when most
flourishing, almost entirely owed their wealth.

As not uncharacteristic of the present stage and
condition of the people, I shall give the few particulars which I have collected respecting the manner in
which this branch of trade is carried on, and of the
habits of those engaged in it.

The manner in which it is conducted is every way
rude and primitive.   Each ship employed commonly
belongs to its captain and two or three other proprietors ; and as the purchases of grain are chiefly made
with ready money, seldom by barter, and never on
account or credit, they have to advance the sums
requisite, with the understanding that the profits are
to be divided between the owners and sailors in certain proportions ; so many shares to each owner ; so
many to the captain ; so many to the mate ; and to
the sailors individually so many, according to their
respective merit.   The sailors receive no pay nor
wages ; but they are allowed to take small invest-
ments of their own, to the amount of from fifteen to
twenty dollars' worth, with which they trade on their
own account.   Many of the shipowners and merchants
are said to be quite illiterate, unable either to read
or write.   As a substitute for written accounts, an
individual having six vessels, or shares in so many,
provides himself with six chests, in which he deposits
his share of the profits of each voyage, with an addi-

tional chest for the capital. He is able to recollect the amount he advances for each venture—the sum he withdraws from the principal chest. To ascertain whether he is a winner or loser, he compares the contents of his chests, or transfers the contents of the six into one. The profit calculated on is at least twenty-five per cent. of the money laid out : four voyages to the Black Sea are expected to afford profit sufficient to cover the original cost of the vessel. The sailors are frugal and economical in the extreme ; at sea they live chiefly on stockfish, Sardinias, bread and garlic, with some oil and wine. These are the provisions they lay in, in Cephalonia ; in the Black Sea, they live chiefly on the fish which they catch there, drying the surplus ; so that, when there, they have occasion to purchase little else than bread. Their cargoes of grain are commonly freighted for Leghorn, where they are sure to find a good market, if they are not able before to effect an advantageous sale amongst the islands. It is said that, in many instances, the proprietors, especially in the case of boats, being too poor to advance the sum requisite to purchase a cargo of corn, hire themselves out in the Levant, carrying from port to port till they have gradually realized the funds necessary to make the great purchase, the staple of their enterprise.

The oil and currant-trade, from the export duty on which, the revenue of the government is, in large proportion, derived,* is principally conducted by

* The gross revenue of these islands, from 1834 to 1840, varied

foreign merchants, and the latter principally in foreign bottoms.   The greater part of the oil is sent to Venice, in island vessels, and the greater part of the currants in English vessels to the ports of Great Britain.

Even the trade in currants and oil is considered on the decline, or precarious.   Very much less oil than formerly is now made and exported, and at a reduced price; and though the quantity of currants grown is not yet diminished (in Cephalonia, indeed, it is much increased*), nor their value materially lowered, yet it is expected that it will fall, as the culture of the currant-vine is extended in the Morea, its native place, where, during the late war, especially after the invasion of the country by the Egyptian army, it suffered greatly, and was much reduced.   There the soil is considered better; labour is cheaper; the export-duties somewhat less;—in brief, provided the country

from L.200,846 to L.139,771.   During the same period, the amount derived from the three principal branches, namely, export-duties on currants and oil, and customs, fluctuated as follows :—Currants, from L.54,306, to L.29,921 ; oil, from L.62,901, to L.3665 ; customs, from L.36,693, to L.23,907.

* When the Morea was devastated by war during the period of the Greek revolution, and its currant-vineyards were mostly destroyed, a sudden and great impulse was given to extend the cultivation of this vine in the Ionian Islands.   In a memorial of the Cephalonians, in 1829, praying for a diminution of duty on currants, then amounting to about 600 per cent. on the price paid to the growers of the fruit, exclusive of about 56 per cent. paid to the Ionian government, it is stated that the produce of currants, from five millions of pounds weight in 1820, was increased, in nine years, to ten millions.

remain tranquil and is tolerably governed, all the circumstances are in favour of its successful competition.

Both these important branches of commerce and of native industry labour under disadvantages, in the heavy duties imposed on them ; they are both subject to a double duty ; one of export from the islands, at a very high rate ; the other of import, also at a high rate.*

* In 1841, the quantities of currants grown in the Ionian Islands, and in the Morea, were estimated as follows:—

		Lbs.	Tons.
Zante,	. .	8,521,000 or	3850
Cephalonia,	.	14,561,000	6500
Ithaca,	. .	0,478,000	210
		23,560,000	10,560
Morea,	. .	9,300,000	4,600
		33,360,000	15,160

The duty exacted by the Greek government on currants exported from the Morea, is about seventeen per cent. *ad valorem.*

The duty on the exports of currants and oil from the Ionian Islands is eighteen per cent. *ad valorem;* on wine of the islands the same; on soap eight per cent. The same duty is exacted on export, whether from island to island or to a foreign port, according to the regulations of government, of May 1833.

The import duty in this country is the same on the currants of the Ionian Islands and of the Morea, viz., about 3d. a-pound (22½ per cwt., and 5 p. ÷ additional), reduced from 6d.; that on olive-oil is L.4, and four scudi the ton.

It is believed that, were the duty on currants (now upwards of 130 per cent. on the prime cost of the article in the islands), reduced to the same as that on raisins (imported chiefly from Spain and Turkey), namely, about 15s. per cwt., the consumption soon would be greatly augmented, to the benefit of the revenue.

The price of currants is liable to great fluctuation from the precariousness of the crop, and the perishable nature of the fruit. Last

The impolicy of the export-duty has been often argued, especially by the late enlightened Lord High Commissioner. So long as, owing to peculiar circumstances, there was little competition, the effect of it was comparatively slightly felt; but it may be otherwise soon, now that that competition is coming into activity. The difficulty is to find other sources of revenue; this is the problem—and so it is likely to continue, until enterprise, and industry, and intelligence are stimulated farther, and the resources of the people and the country are profitably developed.

Were the best modes of agriculture introduced, and all the soils capable of cultivation brought under culture, it can hardly be doubted that sufficient, and more than sufficient, grain might be grown for the supply of the inhabitants, instead of about three months' consumption, as at present.*

Were the best vines planted, and the requisite capital and skill expended and applied to them, and

year it was from sixty-two to seventy dollars per 1000 lbs.; this year forty-two dollars. The currant-grounds in the Ionian Islands and the Morea are so near that they may be considered in regard to climate, almost as one vineyard; the season that is favourable to the one is favourable to the other, and *vice versa;* and, in consequence, a bad crop in Zante is rarely if ever compensated by a good one in Cephalonia, or a good crop in the islands enhanced in value by a bad one in the Morea.

* The fixed duty laid on foreign wheat, at the rate of 3s. 4d. the quarter, *i. e.* of 5d. the kilo (equal to the English bushel, or eight imperial gallons), by act of Parliament, March 1841 (*vide* p. 29), is advocated, on the ground of improving the revenue (to the amount of about L.18,600 per annum), and of encouraging the island culture of grain.

the best methods of making wine employed, it hardly admits of doubt, as has already been pointed out, that excellent wines might be made, not inferior to the best of Spain and Portugal, and Madeira, perfectly fitted for exportation and for the English market, and that thus a new and lucrative branch of commerce might be established.*

Were the olive-plantations not neglected—were the oil prepared in the most approved manner,—it is equally certain that the produce of oil would be far larger, and of very superior quality. This country might be supplied with oil for the table from the Ionian Islands equal in fineness to that of Lucca or of Provence; and with olives, in their green state, not inferior to those imported from France and from Italy. Compare the selling price of the latter with that of the common salted olives in use in the Ionian Islands, and we have a striking example of the increased value of an article, in consequence of the application of skill in its preparation. In these islands the people do not seem to reflect that, without high excellence in art, there can be no very profitable remuneration of labour. It would be well for them

* Formerly, it would appear that Greek wines were in considerable estimation. Thus, in some aphorisms for cider, communicated to the Royal Society in 1662, the writer commences with remarking,—" He that would treat correctly of cider and perry must lay his foundation so deep as to begin with the soil. For as no culture or graffes will exalt French wines to compare with the wines of Greece, Canaries, and Montefiasco, so neither will the cider of Bromyard and Ledbury equal that of Allen-more, Horn-Lacy, and King's-Chapel, in the same county of Hereford."—*Birch's History of Royal Society*, vol. i., p. 144.

to consider the effects of art in imparting value to materials—whether they be canvas and marble, or glass, or iron, or clay—under the almost creative power of the painter and sculptor, or of the optician, chronometer-maker, and porcelain manufacturer. Examples even more instructive might be pointed out to them in many of the humbler walks of art—requiring no capital, no machinery—only patient industry, and the skill which can hardly fail to result from the exercise of it; such, for instance, as the hosiery-knitting carried on by the women of the Shetland Islands at their leisure hours, and straw-plaiting in the adjoining Orkney Islands. Articles of Shetland hosiery, made by the home fireside, of wool of the island, homespun, are now for sale in Edinburgh, of higher price than similar articles of silk; I have seen a pair of stockings which were valued at L.5; and I have heard of an Orkney straw bonnet that was sold for L.17 sterling.

The soil and climate of the Ionian Islands are perfectly fitted for all the fruit-bearing trees and plants of the south of Europe, especially the orange, the lemon, the citron, the pomegranate, the melon, the fig, and the grape.* Were the best varieties of each

* Some years ago, before Parga was crushed by the tyranny of Ali Pasha of Janina, the citron was cultivated there extensively, for exportation to Germany and Poland, almost exclusively for the use of the Jews, who employ the fruit in one of their religious ceremonies, and who, as they require it to be without blemish, willingly pay a high price for it in its perfect state. After the destruction of the citron groves of Parga with the town, a gentleman, a foreigner, residing

kind carefully cultivated, it can hardly be doubted that the fruit would be excellent (of which there is proof already in several instances). It is probable that they might become profitable articles of export, especially now that steam-navigation is affording increased facilities of intercourse, and is shortening so much the time of transit, and, moreover, since the inland communication between the villages and towns, by means of the new roads, has been so much improved.* By the Adriatic, Germany might be supplied from these islands, and by the Gulf of Lepanto a good part of northern Greece.†

in Corfu, began the cultivation of the tree in a favourable sheltered spot near Benitza, in that island, and with perfect success. Whilst oranges and lemons were allowed to drop from the trees neglected, not being considered worth the trouble of gathering and sending to market on account of their cheapness, the choice citrons had great attention paid to them, and were most carefully exported, repaying amply.

* When I was in the Ionian Islands I heard of many instances, besides the one mentioned in the preceding note, of oranges and lemons being allowed to drop from the trees, not being considered worth the gathering, owing to the difficulty of sending them to market, though only a few miles distant from town, where there were no good roads, and at a time when the fruit, owing to the little demand for it, would not repay any expensive mode of conveying it.

† From the Statistical Tables of Cephalonia, composed by the municipal officers in 1823, it appears that the quantity of almonds and walnuts grown in that island then amounted to 465 barrels a-year. Both are of excellent quality, and might be grown to almost any amount. The almond, with a soft shell, admitting of being crushed between the fingers, is particularly good, and deserving of more extensive cultivation. Even for its wood, the walnut-tree would be valuable.

The principal islands are well adapted for the mulberry-tree, and the climate is excellent for the silkworm, as has been proved by trial on a small scale. The growing of silk, therefore, might become a source of much profit, and may be particularly deserving of attention, as it promotes habits of care and of forethought, requires no hard labour, and may profitably occupy the idle time of women and children.

In the preceding chapter allusion has been made to the inferior quality of the soap manufactured at Zante; it cannot be doubted that the article might be greatly improved, and that, so improved, the demand for it would increase, and that it might become a lucrative concern. The same remark is applicable to the silk manufacture of the same island, and to its carpet manufacture. Until there is an increase of skill, and a greater outlay of capital in machinery, these and the other arts can never thrive—can never be sources of profit ; and now, considering the facility of communication, they must either improve or be extinguished : in their present state they cannot long stand the competition to which they are exposed.

At present only a trifling quantity of sea-salt is exported from these islands: whether their dry summer climate is considered, or the purity and strength of the salt-water of the sea which washes their shores, or the fitness of many parts of their shores for the formation of salines, it is highly probable that, were intelligent enterprise directed to the increased production of this important article, it might become a source of considerable profit. The wealth and greatness of Venice, looking to their origin, have been ingeniously traced to the trade of the republic in salt, which was long the staple commodity of its commerce: it cost little in preparing; it sold for much; the trade in all its branches afforded advantages of various kinds; and there appears no reason why some of these advantages, at least, may not be again experienced, were the example to be followed.*

Whether the pottery of the Ionian Islands admits of any material improvement, is questionable. The kind of clay at present used is only fitted for making porous vessels for holding and cooling water, coarse jars when glazed for holding oil, and a few other articles of the rudest and cheapest description for home use. The finer earthenware of the ancients was made of a red clay, free from calcareous matter, and glazed and ornamented with a black varnish,

* The management of a saline is of the simplest kind: all that is required is a flat surface on which to admit sea-water, and some slight embankments and sluices to confine it: the separation of the water from the salt is effected by the sun and air. It has been imagined by some that salines are unwholesome: of this I cannot find any satisfactory proof. Their neighbourhood sometimes is unwholesome. This is remarkably the case in the instance of the salines of Santa Maura; and it is also remarkable that the spot itself has often been exempt from malaria, when the adjoining garrison has been suffering severely from its effects, and that at a time when the effluvia arising from the water in process of evaporation have been very offensive. It may be mentioned incidentally as a curious circumstance, that the heaped salt, collected after the evaporation is finished, emits a very grateful perfume, very similar to that of the violet, the cause of which remains to be ascertained.

which is now lost to the arts. If any improvement
should be attempted in the earthenware manufactory,
it is probable that it would be advisable to keep the
ancient in view as a pattern; the material, in some
parts of Corfu, is abundant, and were diligent inquiry
made, the composition of the ancient varnish could
hardly fail of being discovered.* In Constantinople,
large numbers of men and boys are profitably employed in the making of pipes, of the kind of clay just
alluded to: the labour is easy, the art nowise diffi-

* Since the above was written, I have made some experiments on
the black varnish or glazing of ancient pottery, from the results of
which it appears to be glass, coloured by black oxide of iron, perhaps mixed with particles of metallic iron, to which its high lustre
may be owing. It is of the hardness of glass, brittle, and translu-
cent, as is proved by the colour of the earthenware appearing through
it where it is very thin. It is powerfully attracted by the magnet.
Before the blow-pipe, it is fusible: its colour remains unchanged,
however powerfully it is urged by the flame. It is insoluble, and
retains its colour in nitric and muriatic, and nitro-muriatic acid; but
when fused with boracic acid, and then acted on by muriatic acid, its
colouring matter is dissolved, silicious matter remaining; and the
solution is slightly precipitated by ammonia.

Considering this glazing as a compound of silica and alkali, coloured
in the manner mentioned, it may be inferred that it was applied to
the earthenware in the form of a paste, and that the vessels were
afterwards subjected to a temperature sufficiently elevated to melt
the paste and convert it into glass, but not high enough to fuse the
substance of the pottery, which I find is fusible at a very high temperature. Probably the ancient vases of superior quality, in which
the red colour of the clay is so finely contrasted with the shining
black of the varnish, were subjected to heat in close vessels,—equally
defended from the fumes of the charcoal-fire and the oxidating influence of common air; and, I believe, there is a passage in Pliny,
which I cannot now find, in accordance with this idea.

cult. Were there any spirit of enterprise, it might very readily be introduced into these islands, and it might become a source of profitable industry.*

The attention of government, in these islands, is now most laudably directed to ameliorations of various kinds, from a growing sense not only of their advantage, but also of their necessity, to prevent further degradation and increase of difficulties connected with revenue, and of distress amongst the people.

Up almost to the present time, the Ionian Islands had been without a banking system; this the government, during the last year, has wisely attempted to introduce, and has been able to effect, by means of British capital; and now, I am informed, an Ionian bank is in full and satisfactory operation in Corfu, and branch banks in Zante and Cephalonia. The consequences of a deficiency of a banking system had been most unfavourable to the public credit, to enterprise, and improvement; and, it may be added, to the morals of the natives and to their national character, conducing to usurious interest,† to unfair

* By means of a very simple kind of mould, the Turkish pipe-bowls are made with great ease and rapidity. To preserve the fine red colour of the clay in the baking (a colour the same as that of the ancient pottery, the material being the same), they are heated in the manner in which I have supposed the ancient pottery was baked, in a dome of clay from which the air is excluded, the fire being heaped up around.

† The legal interest has been ten per cent., and so scarce has money been, that there has been no difficulty in obtaining good security at

dealing, to gambling, and to hoarding and miserly habits. The new bank, conducted on the principle of a joint-stock company, will tend mainly to correct these evils, by affording accommodation at a moderate rate of interest, and offering the means of secure investment. It is likely to be, of all things, most instrumental in promoting those ameliorations, which the condition of the country so much requires.*

this rate. Usurious interest of thirty, forty, fifty per cent., hitherto has not been uncommon.

The money tariff of the Ionian Islands—that authorized in May 1828—is peculiar, in the very small value of the lowest denomination of coin : it is as follows :—

SILVER COIN.

			s.	d.
Crown,	= 600 oboli,	=	5	0
Half-crown,	= 300 ...	=	2	6
Shilling,	= 120 ...	=	1	0
Sixpence,	= 60 ...	=	0	6
Threepence,	= 30 ...	=	0	3

COPPER COIN.

Penny,	= 10 oboli,	=	0	1
Halfpenny,	= 5 ...	=	0	$0\frac{1}{2}$
Farthing,	= $2\frac{1}{2}$ ...	=	0	$0\frac{1}{4}$
Obolo,	= 1 ...	=	0	$0\frac{1}{10}$

* Notwithstanding the obvious advantages of the banking system, noticed above, it has not been received in the Ionian Islands without opposition ; it has found enemies there as well as supporters. Its enemies belong to that party which is hostile to British protection. They, it is said, point to the bank as a thing pregnant with evil,— "a horse of Troy" (this is their word of alarm), hiding speciously mischief incalculable, utter ruin. The British government, they say, by means of this bank, meditate a transfer of the landed property of the islands to British subjects, by the cunning process of taking

To which also it may be expected other measures lately introduced by the government will contribute, particularly the formation of an agricultural society, to institute inquiries, propose improvements, and make trial of new methods, in all the branches of rural industry.* For these purposes, it is to have

advantage of the distress and necessities of Ionian proprietors, making pecuniary advances to them on mortgage, and then (after some changes made in the law relative to real property) taking possession of the property by foreclosing! Never, perhaps, was a *mala mens* in a party more preposterously exhibited, or in a manner more insulting to the common sense of the people whose fears they wish to excite. The government of Great Britain—of that country which paid twenty millions sterling to abolish slavery in its West Indian possessions—giving support to a bank to ruin Ionian proprietors! Absurd as the notion is and deserving of contempt, the designs of those who bruit it abroad ought not to be overlooked. Though they may not be able to overthrow the bank, they may for a time, a short time, impede its operations and its influence, to the detriment of all concerned. From the latest accounts, it is satisfactory to find that, notwithstanding the suspected latent designs against it, its state is prosperous—that a dividend of six per cent. has been made to the shareholders—and that its capital is about to be increased, for the purpose of extending its operations. In the *Morning Herald* of the 17th of March of the present year, a detailed statement is to be found of the condition and prospects of this bank, laid before the proprietors at their first general meeting in London, on the 13th of the same month, in accordance with what has just been mentioned of its improving prospects.

* Before Sir Frederick Adam left the Ionian Islands, an attempt was made at his request, by Mr Falconar, to cultivate the Indigo plant, and, it is said, with a very promising result, the soil and climate appearing to be both equally favourable to it. This I learn from Mr Robert Jameson's paper on the island of Cerigo, already referred to. As this species of cultivation may be of very great importance to the islands, I shall add a few particulars relative to the

pecuniary aid from the government; and branch societies, with certain funds at their disposal for the objects of the institution, are to be formed in the different islands. Of the same beneficial character is the system of road-making, which was commenced some years ago, and is already considerably advanced; when finished, it will afford every facility to inland communication.* The new roads, where completed, as in Corfu, appear to vast advantage, com-

manner of conducting it, derived from the same source. "The ground (for indigo) should be slightly tilled, and the seed sown somewhere between March and the middle of April, and the weeding ought to take place when the plant is a month old. By the middle or end of July the plant is matured, and the manufacture of the indigo commenced. In India, the greatest expense at first is the erection of a manufactory, on account of the expense of the materials, which is not so here. Towards maturity, a steadiness of temperature seems to be favourable to the plant, which is said not to be the case in India; but here, from Tables kept for two years, it would appear that the difference of temperature between six P.M. and midnight, averages in July and August scarcely 6° Fahrenheit, and between midnight and sunrise, which is the coolest part of the twenty-four hours, it is about 12°. Perhaps this may be assigned as the cause of the experimental crops here yielding much more matter, even under the disadvantageous mode of manufacture followed, than is obtained in Bengal. Further trial of the manufacture of this substance is worthy of the serious attention of the Ionians."

* The new system of roads, on the Macadamized plan, was commenced little more than twenty years ago in Corfu, and even later in some of the other islands, particularly Zante. They were first made chiefly by statute labour, under in some respects severe regulations: discontent and murmuring were the natural result. A road-fund was next formed (the statute labour being discontinued) by an additional tax on oil and currants exported, already highly taxed, and on some other articles. This fund proved inadequate; it was hardly sufficient,

pared with the old : they are, in brief, excellent
carriage-roads, made of the best materials; whilst
the old ones were mere bridle-paths, or, if regularly constructed, paved,—the pavement generally
out of order, and in many places broken up, totally
impracticable for wheels ; indeed, until the new
roads were opened, there was not a single carriage or even cart in use in all the islands. Other
undertakings may be mentioned, either in progress
or proposed, conducive to the same useful ends; as
the establishment of savings-banks ;* the improving

I am informed, to keep the roads completed in order, much less to
defray the expense of their extension. The last measure adopted,
effected by the late Lord High Commissioner, Sir Howard Douglas, is
a return to statute labour, but so modified as to be agreeable to the
people, not oppressive, being restricted to branch-roads, and limited
as to seasons and distance, as well as amount,—no peasant being liable
to be called on to work more than four miles from his dwelling, or in
the sowing-season or that of harvest, or of labour in the vineyard ; and
being restricted also to the mere road;—bridges, when required, having
to be constructed at the public expense, working tools provided, and
the land purchased through which the roads are to pass. The result
of this method is said to be very prosperous, and the extension of the
roads, by means of it, rapid and great. In Corfu, where most progress has been made, the use of carts has become common. A cart
drawn by one horse, and managed by one man, carries the load of
five horses or mules, conducted by five men! Probably the camel
might be introduced into these islands with advantage. Of all beasts
of burden, in relation to the expense of its keep and its powers, it is
the most economical; and the climate, there is reason to believe,
would prove very suitable to it. It would be easy for the local government to make a trial of it. Three or four pair might suffice,
which could be procured from Greece or from Italy.

* Savings-banks were established by the late Lord High Commissioner, Sir Howard Douglas, in all the islands; with a rate of interest

of ports and moles;* the forming of docks and building-slips; the draining and cultivation of marshes;

of six per cent. on all deposits; and I am informed that, with a view of drawing attention to them, and especially that of the rising generation, and of affording encouragement, at the same time, to merit and foresight, he made from his own funds small purses of four dollars, and presented them to each central school in the different islands, to be invested in the Island Savings-bank, for boys as well as girls. The following return of the state of the savings-banks in the different islands, is copied from the Corfu Government Gazette:—

QUADRO DIMOSTRATIVO DELLO STATO DEI BANCHI DI RISPARMIO DELLE ISOLE JONIE AL 31 LUGLIO 1841, ESTRATTO DAI CONTI DELLE RISPETTIVE TESORERIE LOCALI.

Isole.	Bilancio al 30 Aprile 1841.	Secondo Tremestre del 1841.		Bilancio al 31 Luglio 1841.	Osservazioni.
		Somme . Depositate.	Somme Ritirate.		
	L. S. D.	L. S. D.	L. S. D.	L. S. D.	
Corfu',	1647 18 10 7/0	109 0 6 4/0	72 8 1 8/0	1684 11 3 3/0	
Cefalonia,	152 5 7 8/0	43 7 5	15 0 0	180 13 0 8/0	
Zante,	34 .2 11	.. .. ..	11 7 0	22 15 11	
Santa Maura, }	32 15 2 5/0	.. .. ..	7 7 3 2/0	25 7 11 3/0	
Itaca,	.. .. ..	.. .. ..	.. .. ..	.. .. ..	
Cerigo,	6 10 1 3/0	.. .. ..	.. .. ..	6 10 1 3/0	{ Al 30 Gi-ugno 1841.
Paxo',	1 6 3 3/0	.. .. ..	0 14 1	0 12 2 3/0	
Totale, L.	1874 19 0 6/0	152 7 11 4/0	106 16 9	1920 10 6	

The great difference of amount of deposits in Corfu, and the other islands, is remarkable. It is owing to the larger number of English and Maltese resident there, by whom alone hitherto use has been made of these banks. The neglect of them by the natives is a strong proof both of ignorance and aversion to change; but no more than might be expected, considering their past condition, in connexion with a long continued system of misrule. Much perseverance undoubtedly will be required on the part of the government—on the part of the Lord High Commissioner—to bring these savings-banks, or any other good institution, into useful operation.

* The new mole at Lixuri, in Cephalonia, on account of its importance, is deserving of special mention. It has converted an open beach into a good port, and rendered Lixuri independent of Argos-

and, what is most important of all, the establishment
of schools and of a college and university, for the
culture of the mind and the acquiring of useful knowledge, without which all other attempts at improvement must be of little avail.

In illustration of the commercial relations existing
between the Ionian Islands and this country, I shall
insert some valuable Tables, for the use of which I
am indebted to Mr Porter, of the Board of Trade:
they form part of the Statistical Tables annually laid
before Parliament, prepared by this gentleman. They
show how limited the transactions of trade are between the two countries, both as regards the number
of articles and the amount of their value, with a very
few exceptions as regards the latter. I shall insert
also a detailed statement of the produce, for many
years past, of the currant-vineyards of the Ionian
Islands and of the Morea, drawn up by Mr Han-
cock, a merchant largely engaged in the fruit-trade,
the accuracy of which may be depended on; followed

toli, affording every facility of commerce for imports and exports to
the richest part of the island, ships now coming where before boats
only could approach. And in conjunction with the mole, a custom-
house has been opened and a sanita establishment, in a handsome building previously erected.

Amongst the new works at present contemplated, and for which
estimates have been made, I am informed, are the following:—a
breakwater at Samos, in Cephalonia, for the purpose of forming a
port there; the prolongation of the mole at Pronos; and the construction of one at St Euphemia, in the same island; and in Ithaca,
the supplying of the town of Vathi with water from the Paganò
wells.

by some remarks, by the same gentleman, on the fluctuations in the price of the article, the circumstances connected therewith, and the losses which the producers of the fruit are likely to sustain, unless the duty on it is still further reduced.

TABLE I.—FOREIGN AND COLONIAL MERCHANDIZE IMPORTED INTO THE UNITED KINGDOM FROM THE IONIAN ISLANDS.

Articles.	1831.	1832.	1833.	1834.	1835.
Brimstone, . Cwts.,	...	...	...	16	...
Cheese, ...	...	...	...	1	...
Corn, Wheat, . Qrs.,	249	1062	...	...	...
Cotton Manufactures, entered at value, £	...	...	8	3	...
Currants, . Cwts.,	162,363	108,079	97,912	153,404	127,571
Dye and Hard Woods, viz., Fustic,. Tons.,	22	148	187	276	120
Figs, . . . Cwts.,	...	...	...	...	...
Furs, Marten, . No.,	...	...	...	21	...
... Otter, ...	...	...	...	2	...
Hats, Straw, . .	...	...	...	...	...
Indigo, . Lbs.,	188	...	...	...	...
Leather Gloves, Pairs,	...	24	...	...	...
Lemons and Oranges, in Packages, viz.—					
Not exceeding 5000 cubic inches, Pack.	...	...	...	...	...
Exceeding 5000 and not exceeding 7300 cubic inches, ...	1	9	72	...	...
Exceeding 7300 and not exceeding 14,000 cubic inches, ...	...	...	...	2	...
Liquorice Juice, Cwts.,	...	...	...	...	2
Oil, Olive, . Galls.,	100,242	12,336	58,138	311,704	68,800
Opium, . . Lbs.,	...	...	...	...	...
Pepper, ...	...	...	...	...	...
Raisins, . . Cwts.,	...	...	...	...	...
Seeds, Flaxseed, and Linseed, Bushels,	...	...	...	1	...
... Tares, ...	148	82	...	...	...
Shumac, . . Cwts.,	...	...	99	...	...
Silk, Raw & Waste, Lbs.,	...	...	1,350	...	...
Silk Manufactures of Europe, &c. entered by Weight, ...	...	5	...	...	...

TABLE I.—FOREIGN AND COLONIAL MERCHANDIZE IMPORTED—
(*continued.*)

Articles.	1831.	1832.	1833.	1834.	1835.
Skins,Kid,Undressed,No.	312	...	...	...	...
... Lamb, ditto, .	265	..	...	...	...
Spirits,Rum, Proof, Gal.,	6	...	...	...	...
... Brandy, ...	...	...	...	996	...
... Geneva, ...	...	...	...	...	...
Sugar, Unrefined, Cwts.	1	...	...	...	...
Tallow, ...	...	...	...	...	...
Tea, . . Lbs.,	...	...	...	...	...
Timber, Masts, Yards, and Bowsprits, under 12 inches diameter, No.	1	1	...	...	..
... Staves, Great hunds.	...	...	8	...	...
Tobacco, Unmanufactured, . Lbs.	...	...	471	...	
... Manufactured and Snuff, .	5	8	...	4	11
Valonia, . Cwts.,	7,461	8,563	31,495	7,001	3,150
Wool, Cotton, Lbs.,	...	...	...	...	...
... Sheep's, ...	...	...	...	...	...
Wine, viz. :—					
French, . Galls.,	28	2	54	...	...
Portugal, ...	315	...	...	...	...
Spanish, ...	171	...	56	71	23
Madeira, ...	80	...	...	...	...
Other sorts, ...	304	380	637	849	393
Wine of all Sorts,	898	382	747	920	416

IMPORTS—(*continued.*)

Articles.	1836.	1837.	1838.	1839.	1840.
Brimstone, . Cwts.,	...	...	...	...	...
Cheese, ...	...	1	...	...	...
Corn, Wheat, Qrs.,	...	...	5,370	13,928	1,960
Cotton, Manufactures, entered at Value, £	...	...	1	13	...
Currants, . . Cwts.	136,773	156,043	94,440	133,374	133,343
Dye and Hard Woods, viz. Fustic; Tons,	72	120	46	53	62
Figs, . . Cwts.,	811	804	123	684	432
Furs, Marten, No.,	...	...	...	...	...
... Otter, ...	...	...	...	...	...
Hats, Straw, ...	...	...	4	4	...
Indigo, . Lbs.,	...	...	...	...	...
Leather Gloves, Pairs,	...	3	...	...	...

TABLE I.—IMPORTS—*(continued.)*

Articles.	1836.	1837.	1838.	1839.	1840.
Lemon and Oranges, in Packages, viz. :—					
Not exceeding 5000 cubic inches, Pack.,	3	...	...	...	...
Exceeding 5000 and not exceeding 7,300 cubic inches, ...		...	...	...	...
Exceeding 7,300 and not exceeding 14,000 cubic inches. ...	...	...	...	...	...
Liquorice Juice, Cwts.,	...	...	...	..	...
Oil, Olive, . Galls.,	40,808	80,076	47,300	56,750	56,319
Opium, . Lbs.,	...	...	...	4	...
Pepper, ...	...	...	...	...	2
Raisins, . Cwts.,	2	745	...	...	76
Seeds, Flaxseed and Linseed, . Bushels,	484	...	...	...	...
... Tares, . .	...	...	...	...	...
Shumac, . Cwts.	...	...	...	...	...
Silk, Raw & Waste, Lbs.,	...	14	143	...	...
Silk Manufactures of Europe, &c. entered by Weight, ...	...	5	...	...	...
Skins, Kid, Undressed, No.	...	. .	...	...	...
... Lamb, ditto, ...	...	...	...	...	...
Spirits, Rum, Proof Gals.,	...	...	...	...	...
... Brandy, ...	19	...	...	...	7
... Geneva, ...	...	...	...	230	...
Sugar, Unrefined, Cwts.,	...	...	...	...	...
Tallow, ...	...	...	...	87	20
Tea, . . Lbs.,	...	...	4,230	...	...
Timber, Masts, Yards, and Bowsprits, under 12 inches diameter, No.	1	...	...	...	...
... Staves, Great hunds.,	...	...	...	...	...
Tobacco, Unmanufactured, . Lbs.,	...	...	55	...	8
... Manufactured, and Snuff, ...	...	3	...	9	8
Valonia, . Cwts.,	2,215	1,868	4,646	1,633	2,000
Wool, Cotton, Lbs.,	20	...	...	...	...
... Sheep's, ...	45,799	...	...	...	121,110
Wine, viz. :—					
French, . Galls.,	16	30	2	132	67
Portugal, ...	3	67	14	...	4
Spanish, ...	142	...	25	...	135
Madeira, ...	...	...	...	...	...
Other Sorts, ...	571	932	220	741	1,177
Wine of all Sorts,	732	1,029	261	873	1,383

TABLE II.—BRITISH AND IRISH PRODUCE AND MANUFACTURES EXPORTED FROM THE UNITED KINGDOM TO THE IONIAN ISLANDS.

Articles.		1831.		1832.	
		Quantities.	Declared Value.	Quantities.	Declared Value.
			£		£
Apparel, Slops, and Haberdashery, £		...	1,980	...	2,298
Arms and Ammunition, ...		...	559	...	392
Bacon and Hams, . . . Cwts.,		1	2	4	13
Beef and Pork, . . . Barrels,		...	...	...	...
Beer and Ale, . . . Tuns,		62	1,057	17	326
Books, Printed, . . . Cwts.,		22	562	21	468
Brass and Copper Manufactures, ...		4	22	28	180
Butter and Cheese, ...		235	1,067	198	831
Coals, Culm, and Cinders, . Tons,		2,398	1,082	1,180	519
Cordage, ... Cwts.,		12	30	...	...
Cotton Manufactures, entered by the Yard, . . Yards,		216,159	5,210	758,007	16,261
... Hosiery, Lace, and Small Wares, . . . £		...	615	...	682
... Twist and Yarn, . . Lbs.,		62,450	3,643	55,665	3,048
Earthen-ware, of all Sorts, . Pieces,		48,700	512	75,156	757
Fish, Herrings, . . . Barrels,		60	60	63	70
Glass, entered by weight, . . Cwts.,		876	1,059	178	542
... Ditto at value, . . £		...	...	...	132
Hardware and Cutlery, . . Cwts.,		116	762	213	1,155
Hats, Beaver and Felt, . . Dozens,		127	492	55	375
Iron and Steel, Wrought and Unwrought, . . . Tons,		1,452	11,019	208	1,977
Lead and Shot, ...		42	565	1	16
Leather, Wrought & Unwrought, Lbs.,		252	96	60	16
... Saddlery and Harness, . £		...	106	...	170
Linen Manufactures, entered by the yard, . . Yards,		5,841	302	12,962	819
... Thread, Tapes, and Small Wares, . . . £		...	...	...	...
Machinery and Mill Work, ...		...	45	...	750
Painters' Colours, ...		...	135	...	208
Plate, Plated Ware, Jewellery, and Watches, ...		...	200	...	560
Salt, ... Bushels,		186	13	...	...
Silk Manufactures, . . . £		...	12	...	61
Soap and Candles, . . . Lbs.,		3,150	138	2,352	73
Stationery, of all sorts, . . £		...	695	...	1,435
Sugar, Refined, . . . Cwts.,		8,186	15,620	6,136	15,987
Tin, Unwrought, ...		32	110	...	...
Tin and Pewter Wares, and Tin Plates, ... £		...	245	...	28
Woollen and Worsted Yarn, . Lbs.,		...	...	...	...
Woollen Manufactures, entered by the Piece, . . Pieces,		175	681	454	1,992
... Ditto by the Yard, . Yards,		1,510	151	3,280	225
... Hosiery and Small Wares, £		...	192	...	105
All other Articles, ...		...	1,844	...	3,254
Total Declared Value,		...	50,883	...	55,725

TABLE II.—BRITISH AND IRISH PRODUCE AND MANUFACTURES EXPORTED—
(*continued.*)

Articles.		1833.		1834.	
		Quantities.	Declared Value.	Quantities.	Declared Value.
			£		£
Apparel, Slops, and Haberdashery,	£	...	2,821	...	2,048
Arms and Ammunition,	...	...	306	...	680
Bacon and Hams, . . .	Cwts.,	2	4	6	15
Beef and Pork, . . .	Barrels,	...	...	...	...
Beer and Ale, . . .	Tuns,	40	825	41	726
Books, Printed, . . .	Cwts.,	14	333	8	188
Brass and Copper Manufactures,	...	5	30	38	237
Butter and Cheese, . . .	...	241	922	214	737
Coals, Culm, and Cinders, .	Tons,	1,049	416	1,250	395
Cordage, ...	Cwts.,	...	...	...	...
Cotton Manufactures, entered by the Yard, . . .	Yards,	233,692	5,504	1,747,855	36,313
... Hosiery, Lace, and Small Wares, . . .	£	...	368	...	958
... Twist and Yarn, .	Lbs.,	54,440	2,955	129,622	8,888
Earthenware, of all Sorts, .	Pieces,	99,156	1,121	111,421	1,395
Fish, Herrings, . . .	Barrels,	200	200	202	290
Glass, entered by weight, .	Cwts.,	334	451	1,122	999
... Ditto at value, . .	£	...	16	...	15
Hardware and Cutlery, . .	Cwts.,	364	1,727	440	2,221
Hats, Beaver and Felt, .	Dozens,	98	662	138	791
Iron and Steel, Wrought and Unwrought, . . .	Tons,	118	952	478	3,655
Lead and Shot, . . .	...	7	103	...	...
Leather, Wrought & Unwrought,	Lbs.,	740	161	148	27
... Saddlery and Harness,	£	...	450	...	108
Linen Manufactures, entered by the yard, . .	Yards,	18,129	911	25,252	1,168
... Thread, Tapes, and Small Wares, . . .	£	...	55	...	47
Machinery and Mill Work, .	...	...	6	...	137
Painters' Colours, . .	...	...	137	...	84
Plate, Plated Ware, Jewellery, and Watches, . .	...	...	493	...	411
Salt, ...	Bushels,	...	...	...	...
Silk Manufactures, . .	£	...	287	...	373
Soap and Candles, . .	Lbs.,	5,996	243	4,430	192
Stationery, of all Sorts, .	£	...	815	...	231
Sugar, Refined, . . .	Cwts.,	4,300	11,101	9,435	24,686
Tin, Unwrought, . .	...	...	...	16	55
Tin and Pewter Wares, and Tin Plates, . . .	£	...	79	...	653
Woollen and Worsted Yarn, .	Lbs.,	...	...	224	32
... Manufactures, entered by the Piece, .	Pieces,	482	2,546	710	3,135
... Ditto by the Yard, .	Yards,	1,689	222	4,035	355
... Hosiery and Small Wares,	£	...	241	...	217
All other Articles, . .	...	...	1,542	...	2,036
Total Declared Value,		...	38,915	...	94,498

TABLE II.—BRITISH AND IRISH PRODUCE AND MANUFACTURES EXPORTED—
(*continued.*)

Articles.		1835.		1836.	
		Quantities.	Declared Value.	Quantities.	Declared Value.
			£		£
Apparel, Slops, and Haberdashery,	£	...	2,151	...	2,309
Arms and Ammunition,	...	...	396	...	456
Bacon and Hams,	Cwts.,	1	3	6	22
Beef and Pork,	Barrels,	..	...	...	...
Beer and Ale,	Tuns,	33	975	29	525
Books, Printed,	Cwts.,	11	199	19	369
Brass and Copper Manufactures,	...	216	2,186	149	1,392
Butter and Cheese,	...	231	927	215	822
Coals, Culm, and Cinders,	Tons,	3,004	1,291	728	423
Cordage,	Cwts.,	...	...	...	...
Cotton Manufactures, entered by the Yard,	Yards,	1,223,334	28,430	1,699,538	40,545
... Hosiery, Lace, and Small Wares,	£	...	962	...	749
... Twist and Yarn,	Lbs.,	131,080	8,382	112,997	6,948
Earthenware, of all Sorts,	Pieces,	135,600	1,766	120,730	1,245
Fish, Herrings,	Barrels,	476	500	409	445
Glass, entered by Weight,	Cwts.,	435	1,081	383	561
... Ditto at Value,	£	...	...	...	...
Hardware and Cutlery,	Cwts.,	670	3,459	401	1,785
Hats, Beaver and Felt,	Dozens,	166	792	151	843
Iron and Steel, Wrought and Unwrought,	Tons,	454	3,585	131	1,578
Lead and Shot,	...	28	526	7	160
Leather, Wrought & Unwrought,	Lbs.,	14,548	1,315	1,810	444
... Saddlery and Harness,	£	...	140	...	141
Linen Manufactures, entered by the Yard,	Yards,	25,857	1,473	22,636	1,307
... Thread, Tapes, and Small Wares,	£	...	167	...	133
Machinery and Mill Work,	...	...	478	...	2,744
Painters' Colours,	...	...	130	...	35
Plate, Plated Ware, Jewellery, and Watches,	...	...	364	...	614
Salt,	Bushels,	20	1	...	...
Silk Manufactures,	£	...	600	.	533
Soap and Candles,	Lbs.,	1,463	49	4,434	226
Stationery, of all Sorts,	£	...	986	...	685
Sugar, Refined,	Cwts.,	13,481	37,719	11,062	33,016
Tin, Unwrought.	...	...	...	...	...
Tin and Pewter Wares, and Tin Plates,	£	...	1,093	...	838
Woollen and Worsted Yarn,	Lbs.,	...	...	...	...
Woollen Manufactures, entered by the Piece,	Pieces,	1,063	2,491	1,081	3,285
... Ditto by the Yard,	Yards,	5,445	378	5,976	472
... Hosiery and Small Wares,	£	...	618	...	558
All other Articles,	...	...	2,591	...	2,915
Total Declared Value,		...	107,804	...	109,123

TABLE II.—BRITISH AND IRISH PRODUCE AND MANUFACTURES EXPORTED—
(continued.)

Articles.		1837.		1838.	
		Quan- tities.	Declared Value.	Quan- tities.	Declared Value.
			£		£
Apparel, Slops, and Haberdashery,	£	...	2,210	...	1,476
Arms and Ammunition, .	...	...	436	...	480
Bacon and Hams, .	Cwts.,	1	5	5	18
Beef and Pork, . .	Barrels,	...	...	...	...
Beer and Ale, . .	Tuns,	34	542	15	262
Books, Printed, . .	Cwts.,	14	290	13	259
Brass and Copper Manufactures,	...	12	77	34	175
Butter and Cheese, .	...	180	903	200	969
Coals, Culm, and Cinders, .	Tons,	2,528	1,094	1,002	445
Cordage, ...	Cwts.,	6	16	...	..
Cotton Manufactures, entered by the Yard, .	Yards,	2,338,946	46,269	1,777,030	32,982
... Hosiery, Lace, and Small Wares, . .	£	...	790	...	541
... Twist and Yarn,	Lbs.,	1,800	100	329,466	19,006
Earthenware, of all Sorts,	Pieces,	138,738	1,513	73,400	882
Fish, Herrings, . .	Barrels,	659	696	290	300
Glass, entered by Weight,	Cwts.,	487	770	271	470
.. Ditto at Value, .	£	...	15	...	18
Hardware and Cutlery, .	Cwts.,	603	3,034	255	1,536
Hats, Beaver and Felt, .	Dozens,	97	535	121	678
Iron and Steel, Wrought and Unwrought, .	Tons,	314	3,486	512	5,058
Lead and Shot, . .	...	3	55	1	21
Leather, Wrought & Unwrought,	Lbs.,	468	90	102	22
... Saddlery and Harness,	£	...	125	...	120
Linen Manufactures, entered by the yard, .	Yards,	24,224	1,445	30,700	1,394
... Thread, Tapes, and Small Wares, . .	£	...	308	...	85
Machinery and Mill Work, .	...	...	568	...	67
Painters' Colours, .	...	...	2	...	25
Plate, Plated Ware, Jewellery, and Watches, .	...	...	865	...	472
Salt, ...	Bushels,	...	...	...	...
Silk Manufactures, .	£	...	219	...	5
Soap and Candles, .	Lbs.,	3,213	168	3,964	215
Stationery, of all Sorts, .	£	...	662	...	1,044
Sugar, Refined, . .	Cwts.,	17,765	35,021	10,787	2,774
Tin, Unwrought, . .	...	88	402	16	67
Tin and Pewter Wares, and Tin Plates, .	£	...	1,261	...	849
Woollen and Worsted Yarn,	Lbs.,	...	...	...	...
... Manufactures, entered by the Piece, .	Pieces,	669	2,255	1,124	2,425
... Ditto by the Yard,	Yards,	4,689	279	5,378	305
... Hosiery and Small Wares,	£	...	629	...	410
All other Articles, . .	...	...	3,127	...	2,217
Total Declared Value,		...	124,465	...	96,100

TABLE II.—BRITISH AND IRISH PRODUCE AND MANUFACTURES EXPORTED—
(*continued.*)

Articles.		1839.		1840.	
		Quantities.	Declared Value.	Quantities.	Declared Value.
			£		£
Apparel, Slops, and Haberdashery,	£	...	3,045	...	2,595
Arms and Ammunition,	.	...	305	...	208
Bacon and Hams, . . .	Cwts.,	13	55	23	75
Beef and Pork, . . .	Barrels,	1	3	1	2
Beer and Ale, . . .	Tuns,	21	425	280	741
Books, Printed, . . .	Cwts.,	18	373	16	303
Brass and Copper Manufactures,	...	9	54	50	259
Butter and Cheese, . .	...	160	724	237	1,168
Coals, Culm, and Cinders, .	Tons,	2,094	934	3,329	1,482
Cordage, ...	Cwts.,	...	...	...	...
Cotton Manufactures, entered by the Yard, .	Yards,	1,480,917	26,218	2,365,857	39,245
... Hosiery, Lace, and Small Wares, . . .	£	...	294	...	618
... Twist and Yarn,	Lbs.,	128,216	6,670	201,620	9,311
Earthenware, of all Sorts,	Pieces,	84,492	974	128,600	1,317
Fish, Herrings, . .	Barrels,	...	...	152	163
Glass, entered by Weight, .	Cwts.,	150	353	411	568
... Ditto at Value, . .	£	...	6	...	...
Hardware and Cutlery, .	Cwts.,	420	2,263	256	1,267
Hats, Beaver and Felt, .	Dozens,	81	371	183	518
Iron and Steel, Wrought and Unwrought, .	Tons,	185	2,067	791	6,705
Lead and Shot, . . .	...	3	71	5	121
Leather, Wrought & Unwrought,	Lbs.,	426	65	264	45
... Saddlery and Harness,	£	...	67	...	42
Linen Manufactures, entered by the Yard,	Yards,	27,490	1,396	16,670	782
... Thread, Tapes, and Small Wares, . . .	£	...	212	...	296
Machinery and Mill Work, .	...	...	25	...	61
Painters' Colours, . .	...	...	108	...	94
Plate, Plated Ware, Jewellery, and Watches, . .	...	...	472	...	533
Salt, ...	Bushels,	180	17	...	...
Silk Manufactures, .	£	...	55	...	417
Soap and Candles, . .	Lbs.,	4,068	194	6,555	307
Stationery, of all Sorts, .	£	...	1,432	...	1,302
Sugar, Refined, . .	Cwts.,	5,400	9,441	7,689	12,717
Tin, Unwrought, . .	...	56	223	12	45
Tin and Pewter Wares, and Tin Plates, . . .	£	...	751	...	347
Woollen and Worsted Yarn, .	Lbs.,	...	...	...	...
... Manufactures, entered by the Piece, .	Pieces,	536	1,397	702	2,414
... Ditto by the Yard, .	Yards,	2,593	176	4,038	367
... Hosiery and Small Wares,	£	...	140	...	371
All other Articles, . . .	...	...	2,634	...	2,398
Total Declared Value,		...	64,010	...	89,204

TABLE III.—FOREIGN AND COLONIAL MERCHANDIZE EXPORTED FROM THE UNITED KINGDOM TO THE IONIAN ISLANDS.

Articles.	1831.	1832.	1833.	1834.	1835.
Cassia Lignea, . . Lbs.,	717	...	2,135	7,525	4,402
Cinnamon, ...	...	...	...	...	...
Cloves, ...	193	1,001	...	3,003	4,813
Cochineal, ...	...	759	361	1,579	2,480
Coffee, ...	30,422	57,526	54,448	33,032	37,881
Corn, Meal, and Flour, viz. :—					
Wheat-meal and Flour, Cwts.,	...	12	...	2	...
Cortex Peruvianus, or Jesuit's					
Bark, . . . Lbs.,	...	...	...	...	50
Cotton Piece Goods of India, Pieces,	780	77	331	4,064	329
... Manufactures, entered					
at value, . . £	...	...	...	...	...
Dyewoods, viz., Logwood, Tons,	...	...	...	...	1
Furs, Otter, . . . No.,	...	...	...	...	...
Ginger, . . . Cwts.,	...	...	...	100	...
Indigo, . . . Lbs.,	2,176	4,539	2,622	9,539	5,083
Iron, in Bars, . . Tons,	...	13	...	10	22
Nutmegs, . . . Lbs.,	...	...	...	35	...
Pepper, ...	3,220	...	7,868	31,543	1,584
Pimento, ...	...	...	...	...	...
Rhubarb, ...	...	...	...	...	...
Rice, . . . Cwts.,	...	...	...	86	...
Silk, Foreign, Thrown, Lbs.,	...	..	...	...	...
Silk Manufactures of India,					
viz. :—					
Bandannoes, Romals, and					
Handkerchiefs, . Pieces,	215	200	174	65	...
Crape Shawls, Scarfs, and					
Handkerchiefs, . No.,	24	...	...	...	...
Spirits, Rum, . Proof Galls.,	12,801	13,644	10,317	9,773	9,110
... Brandy, ...	2,794	2,768	4,994	4,850	4,891
... Geneva, ...	489	1,018	1,417	610	1,623
Sugar, Unrefined, . . Cwts.,	1,225	562	897	2,596	1,422
Tea, ... Lbs.,	1,570	46	2,560	286	14,462
Tin, ... Cwts.,	...	...	...	14	32
Tobacco, Unmanufactured, Lbs.,	...	...	...	34,484	20,570
... Foreign, Manufac-					
tured, and Snuff, ...	...	...	166	476	4,135
Wine, viz. :—					
French, . . . Galls.,	...	37	383	41	594
Portugal, ...	193	210	572	797	529
Spanish, ...	31	242	372	382	345
Madeira, ...	...	115	201	...	...
Canary, ...	...	...	...	...	...
Rhenish, ...	...	...	370	42	24
Other sorts, ...	...	...	...	...	...
Wine of all Sorts,	224	604	1,898	1,262	1,492
Wool, Cotton, . . Lbs.,	...	...	...	...	...

TABLE III.—FOREIGN AND COLONIAL MERCHANDIZE EXPORTED—
(*continued.*)

Articles.		1836.	1837.	1838.	1839.	1840.
Cassia Lignea, . .	Lbs.,	2,623	4,969	5,990	2,398	1,381
Cinnamon, . . .	...	227	...	...	...	...
Cloves, . . .	...	2,717	1,165	968	2,508	1,437
Cochineal, . . .	...	1,181	1,792	4,413	2,187	3,875
Coffee, . . .	...	110,114	24,181	96,007	11,849	109,847
Corn, Meal, and Flour, viz. :—						
Wheat-meal and Flour,	Cwts.,	2	7	7	10	21
Cortex Peruvianus, or Jesuit's						
Bark, . .	Lbs.,	315	...	155	...	...
Cotton Piece Goods of India,	Pieces,	200	200	200	280	420
... Manufactured, entered						
at value, .	£	...	50	...	...	...
Dyewoods, viz., Logwood,	Tons,	2	...	...	...	...
Furs, Otter, . . .	No.,	...	...	6	...	...
Ginger, . . .	Cwts.,	5	4	...	...	...
Indigo, . . .	Lbs.,	1,039	4,894	7,843	3,885	8,025
Iron, in Bars, . .	Tons,	...	...	14	15	63
Nutmegs, . . .	Lbs.,	...	188	...	...	...
Pepper, . . .	...	18,910	32,131	11,939	36,336	30,685
Pimento, . . .	...	2,561	1,125	2,928	844	3,399
Rhubarb, . . .	...	150	169	...	...	49
Rice, ...	...	...	327	...	69	1,135
Silk, Foreign, Thrown, .	...	...	...	...	24	...
Silk Manufactures of India,						
viz. :—						
Bandannoes, Romals, and						
Handkerchiefs, .	Pieces,	347	40	70	74	127
Crape Shawls, Scarfs, and						
Handkerchiefs, .	No.,	216	...	...	...	...
Spirits, Rum, .	Proof Galls.,	14,208	10,306	4,518	5,960	1,922
... Brandy, . .	...	6,398	6,504	4,854	6,817	5,449
... Geneva, . .	...	1,161	3,715	2,106	838	2,085
Sugar, Unrefined, .	Cwts.,	3,143	907	2,253	1,061	1,737
Tea, ...	Lbs.,	5,655	7,845	22,313	4,837	5,011
Tin, ...	Cwts.,	8	16	72	24	...
Tobacco, Unmanufactured,	Lbs.,	5,649	24,144	7,022	...	1,463
... Foreign, Manufac-						
tured, and Snuff,	...	1,486	621	302	115	1,050
Wine, viz. :—						
French, . . .	Galls..	387	247	245	1,083	1,014
Portugal, . . .	...	894	998	915	843	731
Spanish, . . .	...	30	356	194	188	343
Madeira, . . .	...	17	172	215	62	113
Canary, . . .	...	...	...	...	...	97
Rhenish, . . .	...	48	...	...	...	...
Other Sorts, . .	...	...	98	...	24	...
Wine of all Sorts, .		1,376	1,871	1,569	2,200	2,298
Wool, Cotton, . .	Lbs.,	...	112	...	...	...

TABLE IV.—A STATEMENT of the Quantity of Currants, in Tons, shipped from Zante during the Years 1816 to 1841 inclusive; from Cephalonia, from 1820 to 1841; and from the Morea, from 1820 to 1841 inclusive; with Places to whence Exported; also from Ithaca, from 1837 to 1841 inclusive.

Year.	Place of Production.	To Great Britain.	To other Places than Great Britain.	Total Crop each Year.	Remarks.
		Tons.	Tons.	Tons.	During these four years the crop of Cephalonia may be estimated each year at 2,000 tons, and that of the Morea at 4 to 5,000 tons.
1816,	Zante,	1572	645	2,217	
1817,	Zante,	2785 ·	383	3,168	
1818,	Zante,	2120	837	2,957	
1819,	Zante,	2868	641	3,509	
1820,	Zante,	2125	553	4,606	The Morea at 3,000 tons.
...	Cephalonia,	1928			
1821,	Zante,	1790	1215	4,855	From 1821 to 1826 (during the Greek revolution) inclusive, the only currants exported from Greece were those up the Gulf, which ordinarily were smuggled, at great risks, to Trieste and Malta, and the produce never exceeded 2,000 tons annually; and in 1825, certainly not half that quantity was saved.
...	Cephalonia,	1850			
1822,	Zante,	2580 / 38	595	5,355	
...	Cephalonia,	2140			
1823,	Zante,	3520	508	6,563	
...	Cephalonia,	2535			
1824,	Zante,	2943	797	5,627	
...	Cephalonia,	1887			
1825,	Zante,	3023	1021	5,972	
...	Cephalonia,	1928			
1826,	Zante,	1817	2670	6.894	
...	Cephalonia,	2284			From 1827 to 1829 the produce of Greece could be freely exported: the produce may have been 2,000 or 2,500 tons annually. Prices, 1829, 42½ dollars, last, 26.28.
1827,	Zante,	2535	851	6,393	
...	Cephalonia,	3007			
1828,	Zante,	2708	933	6,826	
...	Cephalonia,	3186			
1829,	Zante,	2616	2472	7,495	
...	Cephalonia,	2407			
1830,	Zante,	3292	2007	10,000	
...	Cephalonia,	3376			
...	Morea,	1325			
1831,	Zante,	4037	3767	11,236	
...	Cephalonia,	2209			
...	Morea,	1223			
1832,	Zante,	4517	4795	12,968	
...	Cephalonia,	1689			
...	Morea,	1907			
1833,	Zante,	3479	2611	11,027	
...	Cephalonia,	2848			
...	Morea,	2089			
1834,	Zante,	3070	2176	9,777	
...	Cephalonia,	2783			
...	Morea,	1735			
1835,	Zante,	4262	4196	14,852	
...	Cephalonia,	3260			
...	Morea,	3134			
1836,	Zante.	9211	1663	10,874	
...	Cephalonia,				
...	Morea,				

N.B.—The Ithaca crop is not included, but may be calculated at 200 mills from 1816 to 1825. 260 :: 1826 to 1832. 360 :: 1833 to 1835.

TABLE IV.—(*continued*)

Year.	Place of Production	To Great Britain.	To other Places than Great Britain.	Total Crop each Year	Remarks.
		Tons.	Tons.	Tons.	
1837,	Zante,	2,889			
...	Cephalonia,	3,159	2758	11,962	
...	Ithaca,	...			
...	Morea,	3,156			
1838,	Zante,	1,825			
...	Cephalonia,	3,268	872	8,837	
...	Ithaca,	134			
...	Morea,	2,738			
1839,	Zante,	1,875			
...	Cephalonia,	3,161	2154	10,974	
...	Ithaca,	177			
...	Morea,	3,607			
1840,	Zante,	3,735			
...	Cephalonia,	5,458	3269	14,206	
...	Ithaca,	227			
...	Morea,	4,786			
1841,	Zante,				14,900
...	Cephalonia,	Thus far 11,753	Thus far 3147	estimated.	to
...	Ithaca,				15,000
...	Morea,				

" During the Greek revolution, a great part of the currant-crop was lost by uprooting the plants, and other devastations attendant on the war. And the little that was saved was shipped in irregular ways; so that no better account can be given of it than is to be found in the notes attached to the Table, in the column of remarks.

" The failure of the Greek crops, in consequence of the revolution, led to a great scarcity of currants in 1822 and subsequent years, so that, notwithstanding the enormous import-duty of 44s. 4d. per cwt. into this country, which had remained unaltered since the war (between England and France, &c.), the price in

the islands rose to Spanish dollars 96 per 1000 lbs.,
first cost, or about 58s. per cent. on shipboard,* fluc-
tuating between that and 60 dollars, or 37s., until 1826,
when the island crops, particularly of Cephalonia,
began to augment in consequence of new plantations.
From this time there was a very rapid decline in
prices; and in 1831 and 1832, when the Morea had
again begun to contribute a portion, the island prices
were driven down to 16 dollars, or 10s. 6d. per cwt.,
and even lower—the fall in the English markets
having caused this reduction, since the enormous
duty remained, so that there appeared a probability of
the selling price in London yielding no more than
shipping charges, freight, duty, &c., and leaving
nothing in return for the prime cost.   At this time
very strenuous exertions were made by the Lord
High Commissioner of the Ionian Islands, and the
merchants in London engaged in the trade, to obtain
a reduction of the import-duty in this country, in
which they at last succeeded; and in 1834 it was
made one-half, or 22s. 2d. per cwt.

* " At the time 96 dollars per 1000 lbs. were obtained for currants
in the Ionian Islands (1822), the export-duties were somewhat different
from those now exacted, so that the rendering of the cost *on board*
would really have been somewhat different from what is here given,
but I have not the old rates and calculations at hand, and have, therefore, taken it according to the present duties; the difference, however, is not material.   Throughout, where prices are quoted, I have
taken the Ionian price and cost on shipboard, because, until lately, the
greater part of the government dues was taken in kind in Greece from
the growers; but they have now been united into customs duties,
and very nearly assimilated to the Ionian export-duty."

" By the depression above-mentioned in the price
paid to the growers, the duty-paid price in London
had by this time fallen to little more than half what
it had been for some years subsequent to the general
peace in 1815, so that a comparatively reasonable
price, combined with the demand arising from a constantly augmenting population, caused the consumption to keep pace with the supply, and the prices at
the places of origin recovered from their extreme
depression—the growers, in fact, for a time reaped
all the benefit of the reduced duty in England, the
difference going into their pockets, and the duty-paid
price here remaining much as before the reduction—
indeed, in some years going higher, particularly in
1838, when the crops were very short.

" A cause, however, has been for some years in
operation, tending to lower the prices to the producers, viz., the very great increase of new plantations, particularly in Greece,* after the cessation of

* The old currant-plantations of Greece were situated almost entirely
on the southern shore of the Gulf of Corinth, extending from Patras
to the isthmus.   Recently, I am informed, the cultivation of the currant vine has been extended to Acarnania, on the northern shore of the
Gulf, and has even been commenced on the plain of Argos and about
Pyrgos.   In p. 64, adverting to the competition of the Morea with the
Ionian Islands in the growing of this fruit, the advantage of a better
soil in the former is mentioned, whilst another and more certain favouring circumstance was omitted, viz. the superior means of irrigation
available there, especially in the old tract of currant-ground, and in the
new one on the opposite shore, admitting of being well and easily wa-
tered by the numerous small streams which descend from the hills
and mountains flanking these fertile regions.

the revolutionary war; and in Cephalonia, where currant-plantations have, to a great extent, replaced the
cultivation of the wine-grape. The currant-plant
requires several years to come into full bearing; but
the new plantations are now beginning to yield a
large increase. There was, in 1840, a total crop of
14,200 tons; that of 1841 will amount to 15,000;
and it is probable that the plantations now existing
in the Ionian Islands and Greece together, are capable
of carrying the total production, in fruitful seasons,
up to 18,000, or perhaps 20,000 tons.

" Be this, however, as it may, it is quite clear that
the production is rapidly outstripping the present
consumption. The crop of 1840 was brought to
market at a great loss to the importers, in consequence
of the large supply continually depressing the prices,
which has made them more cautious this season; but
the growers, in consequence, have been compelled to
accept only about half the price they obtained in 1841.
The prices have ranged from 32 dollars to 45, or
20s. 2d. to 28s. per cwt., according to quality; so
that the present import-duty into this country of
22s. 2d. per cwt. comes to be equal to 130 per cent.
on the *prime* cost; and the cultivators of this fruit,
so much used by the middling and lower classes here,
have no other prospect before them than a most
ruinous depression of prices from year to year, unless
the British government should consent to relieve
them by a further reduction of the duty.

" It is true that, since the reduction took place in

1834, the loss of revenue has not been made up to the British government. For this, it would be requisite to have doubled the consumption ; and though such augmentation has been checked by the high prices arising from the short crops of recent years, as above explained, yet the increase of last year exhibits a tendency towards such result. The experiment is only now getting a fair trial, as it has only been during the last and present year that the duty-paid price in London, owing to a large production, has fallen below what it was under the old duty (44s. 4d. per cwt.) The duty on raisins was also reduced in 1834 ; and the revenue derived from that article has already been made up to the British government."

CHAPTER V.

ON THE STATE OF KNOWLEDGE IN THE IONIAN ISLANDS, AND ON THE MEANS OF EDUCATION.

Remarkable deficiency of useful Scientific Knowledge. Circumstances to which owing. Illustrations drawn from the Liberal Professions and the Superstitions of the People. Outline of the System of Education in use, instituted by the Government. Medals for the Encouragement of Learning. Seminary for the Instruction of Students of Divinity. Brief Sketch of the Progress of Public Education. Remarks on the Tendencies to Abuse. Example of Success in Cerigo. Dangers to which a University is exposed in a Small Community illustrated.

IT may be asserted, I believe, without fear of contradiction, that science, constituting that knowledge which is power, the exact sciences, which have so many practical and useful applications, are at present almost unknown in these islands.   It is very doubtful if, amongst the whole population, there is an individual competent to ascertain trigonometrically the height of a mountain, or to determine the latitude and longitude of any particular spot, or to undertake successfully the chemical analysis of a mineral, or soil, or water, or, in brief, one who is qualified to give satisfactory information relative to the many questions which are constantly occurring to inquiring minds, intent on improving a neglected country, where hitherto so little has been done, and where, considering the great capabilities of the country, so much remains to be effected. *

Nor is this surprising, taking into account that, till very lately, the Ionian Islands have been almost destitute of the means of instruction, excepting of an elementary kind, restricted chiefly to reading and writing, to grammar, languages, and arithmetic. †

* The above remark, of course, is intended to apply to the natives of those islands; and soon, it is to be hoped, it will cease to be applicable.

† When Corfu was taken possession of by the French (a detachment of the army of Italy) in 1797, it is stated by M. Arnault, who accompanied the expedition in the capacity of civil commissioner, that it was difficult to find a person who could read. This is mentioned in a letter which he addressed to Buonaparte, then commanding in Italy. His words are:—" La chose la plus rare est de rencontrer ici un homme qui sache lire."—(Souvenirs d'un Sexagènaire; par A. V. Arnault de L'Academie Française, Paris, 1833,) with the motto from Plautus. " Verum amo. Verum volo dici." In the same letter as that just referred to, M. Arnault adds—" Mon rapport sur les arts ne sera ni difficile ni long. Cette ville ne renferme qu'un monument elevé, dans la citadelle, au Marechal Schullembourg, qui la défendit contre les Turcs: c'est sa statue pedestre. Point de statue hors celle-la; point de tableau, point de bibliothèque: une salle de spectacle, et pas d'imprimerie." He continues:—" La peuple est superstitieux et lâche. Le marchand de figues et le garçon boucher sont egalement armés: rien n'etait plus commun que les assassinats; mais la corruption de l' ancien gouvernment porte a croire que leur multiplicité pouvoit être ègalment imputée aux gouvernans et aux gouvernées. On trafiquait égalment de la mort et de la vie d' un homme avec le judge et l'assassin. Saint Spiridion, qui a fait encore un miracle il y a trois semaines, en opère encore, moins souvent toute fois qu' un autre

It may be useful, in relation to this subject, to take a rapid glance at the different liberal professions and classes in society.

The clergy of the Ionian Islands, very few of whom have had the advantages of any literary training in a foreign university, are eminently ignorant.   Mental cultivation hitherto has not been esteemed a necessary qualification for the sacred office.   I am informed that even recently the present head of the Greek church, the patriarch of Constantinople, has put forth a synodical circular, discouraging learning, as dangerous to faith, and likely to lead to heresy.*

saint, devant lequel tout le monde est à genoux ici: ce saint s'appelle *Denaro* (l'argent).

    * This was written about a year and half ago. Since then, the patriarch alluded to has been deposed, and also his successor, by the Turkish government.   That there is a decided hostility to learning in the Greek church, amongst the priesthood, especially of the higher and governing order, and particularly at Constantinople, is notorious. Acts have demonstrated their disposition to keep the people in ignorance, by throwing obstacles in the way of education. If knowledge is considered dangerous in the clergy, how much more must it be so considered amongst the people?

    The following statement is made by a writer, who styles himself " An Ionian Citizen," in a letter bearing the date of Corfu, September 1840, addressed to Lord John Russell.—" The rising generation, in 1817, has scarcely, from that period until this day, enjoyed the light of public instruction. The prejudices of their parents, who thought, and many think so still, that the English government wishes to get the youths into the public schools, to instil into them the principles of the Protestant religion, have rendered public instruction almost nugatory to the present time; and your lordship may rest assured that, whilst the priests of the present generation live, and until the clergy of these states shall be generally educated, most parents will

Law and medicine cannot be practised without
some knowledge; and the best informed men in the
Ionian Islands belong to these professions, many of
whom have studied in the universities of Italy.   But
even their knowledge, it is commonly understood, is
generally superficial and technical, and rarely associated with philosophy and science; which also might
be expected, keeping in view how few competent
judges of high attainments there are amongst the
people; how few opportunities they have to extend
their knowledge, after leaving the schools; and what
little inducement there is to persist in study.

Amongst the higher ranks, too, there is a certain number who have studied abroad, and who, as
gentlemen, are not ill informed, especially in modern Italian, and in ancient Greek literature.   Indeed in this class there are many accomplished in the
knowledge of languages, both ancient and modern,
and well fitted, by these their attainments, to appear
to advantage in mixed society.   But their knowledge is rather glittering than useful, and will hardly
bear the test of true knowledge, already referred to,
namely, that it is power.

If the priesthood is ignorant, how can the mass of
the people be otherwise?   They are ignorant in an

continue to be influenced by such prejudices, and refrain from sending their sons to schools of public instruction." This extreme, and I
would hope greatly exaggerated, view of the influence of the priesthood, he immediately after qualifies, by describing the system of
education as recently perfected by Sir Howard Douglas, " as to have
gone far to undeceive and gain the confidence of the public."

extraordinary degree, and as superstitious.   I find amongst my notes some instances which it may not be amiss to adduce in illustration.

The belief in the evil eye is common, and means are taken as a protection from its influence, or to remove the bad effects attributed to it.   For the former purpose, they attach to the necks of young children relics of saints wrapped in linen, and to the necks of young animals a clove of garlic, or a bit of charcoal or of bread; and, for the latter, they have recourse to some cunning woman who has the reputation of possessing a repellant charm, and who, in exercising her art, uses mysterious words, and with two fingers, whilst uttering the unintelligible words, makes the figure of the cross on the child's head.

They believe in the appearance of ghosts and apparitions, and that ghosts have the power of doing mischief, and that protection is afforded against them by relics and charms.

They believe that an excommunicated person, or an atheist, is under a peculiar influence, which after death brings forth his ghost, and prevents the body from being resolved into its elements, preserving it " unconsumed by the earth," and entire.

They believe that the sudden death of animals is occasioned by ghosts which fly about in the air, and that persons afflicted with erysipelas, palsy, and swellings, owe the diseases to the same imaginary agency; and for a cure they trust to charms.   Thus, for the removal of erysipelas, the patient is taken to a charmer, who uses a formula of mystical words; with a steel and flint strikes sparks on the affected part, then anoints it with melasses, and lastly, makes the sign of the cross on it with the blood of the crest of a black fowl, cut for the express purpose.

They believe that the devil has the power of entering into the bodies of men, and that he can be driven out by certain means; and there are churches which are in repute for cures of this kind, and where the unfortunate beings supposed to be so possessed, are taken and kept for several days without food, and are chained and exorcised. In each church, it is said, there are chains for this special purpose.

So deeply are many of them imbued with superstition, that the non-observance of a fast goes more against their conscience than the perpetration of a murder. It is related that, in the latter time of the Venetian government, when a kind of feudal system was in full force, the head of one of the first families in Zante engaged a dependant to assassinate his enemy, on a particular day and hour. The day was Friday, a fast-day. Whilst waiting the time, the master desired the man to eat his supper; but his request was in vain; there was nothing but fish and olives preserved in oil, which the church has denounced as forbidden articles, and the use of them *péccato gravissimo*.

Of late years exertions have been made by government to improve and enlighten the people by instruction, the beneficial effects of which can hardly fail to become apparent in the rising generation.

The system of education at present in use, consists, 1*st*, Of elementary schools, conducted on the Lancastrian plan, or that of mutual instruction, in which the children of all classes are taught reading, writing, and the first rules of arithmetic, and which are supported partly by government, and partly by the parents of the scholars, the former paying five dollars a-month to each master, and the latter together the same sum.

2*dly*, Of secondary schools, somewhat analogous to our public schools, designed for the children of the middle and higher ranks, in which the following course of education is followed:—

1. Languages—Greek, Latin, Italian, and English.
2. Mathematics.
3. History and Geography.
4. Navigation.
5. Calligraphy.

This course is of five years duration. It is expected that those who enter upon it shall have passed through the primary schools; and they are bound to continue their studies uninterruptedly during the whole period. Each secondary school is to be provided with a library, maps, and charts, and the mathematical instruments requisite for teaching.

3*dly*, Of a university, in which instruction will be given in the form of lectures. 1. In literature and philosophy; 2. In theology; 3. In law; 4. Civil engineering—and in which, after a course of study of four years' duration, degrees will be conferred, after proper examination, in the different faculties.

As the primary schools are a preparation for the secondary, so are the latter required to be for the university; and, for the advantage of those young men, whose early education has not been duly attended to, and who are desirous of preparing themselves for the university, the secondary school, in the town of Corfu, is to be constituted as a college, with a boarding establishment belonging to it, formed by the government, for the accommodation of young men coming from the other islands.*

* From a communication with which I have been favoured from Corfu, of the 4th of November 1840, it would appear that the college referred to above, is founded, and was then flourishing. " The success of the college (it is stated) is most gratifying. It contains at present eighty scholars, and the applications for admittance from parents and guardians are more numerous than can be favourably attended to. The expense incurred by students is exceedingly moderate, amounting only to eight, ten, and twelve dollars a-month, for the first, second, and third years."

It is added, " The expense to government, in the first instance, was, as anticipated, heavy ; but the institution now pays its own expenses, and with the increase in the number of scholars, there will be a surplus, which will permit the establishment to be extended and improved without farther expense to the country." My informant continues, " It is under the direction of Professor Orioli, a man of European reputation, whose services his excellency (Sir Howard Douglas) was fortunate enough to acquire, three years ago, for the chair of natural philosophy."

Alluding to the expected advantages of the college, he remarks, " The moral good to be derived from this establishment is great ; the political no less so. It will bring together in Corfu, the capital of the

The following was the actual state of public instruction in the various branches, in 1838, as specified in an official return, bearing date of the 13th January of that year.*

states, the youth of the several islands. Mingling together at an early age, pursuing the same studies, imbibing the same ideas, at a moment when the mind is most accessible to impressions, island and provincial jealousies and prejudices will be softened, and gradually destroyed ; there will be no rivalry but to excel." A hope is expressed " that the most proficient will be provided for in the public service;" with the farther remark, that " a national feeling will be centralized in and towards this capital (Corfu), as the place of their education ; and this feeling is already fostering by the universal popularity of the measure, and by the contentment of the parents and connexions of the youths educated at the college."

" For the further encouragement of science and learning (it is stated in the same communication), that Sir Howard Douglas had determined to found, out of his own private funds, two prize-medals for ever [since carried into effect ; they are represented in the wood-cut at the end of this chapter], one to be given to the best essays on those important branches of learning—mathematics, natural philosophy, and law ; and the Senate, following the example set by him, have decreed two other prizes to be given for essays on such subjects as the " Commission for public instruction" may choose. Of these two medals, one I am informed is gold, for the university ; the other silver, for the collegiate school. Copies of the prize-essays are required to be transmitted to the founder and his heirs after him—a judicious condition—especially considering the distant awardment of the prizes.

* The Baron Theotoki, a native of Corfu, and more than once president of the Senate, in his " *Details sur Corfou,*" published in 1826, remarks, under the head of public education—" Les trois quarts des habitans ne savent ni lire ni écrire. Une grande partie d'affaires ne se fait que par des promesses verbales, ou par l'entremise de deux temoins, qui signent l'obligation des contractans : ce qui donne souvent lieu à des procès embrouilles où il n'est nullement facile de reconnoître les preuves nécessaires pour établir les pretentions des parties intéressées."—P 58.

University, ... 1	Professors, 9	Vacancies, 4	No. of Scholars, } 150
Secondary schools, . 8	Preceptors, 47	... 12	... 542
Lancastrian schools, in all, . . . } 102	... 111	To be established, } 28	... 4342
Female schools, . . 10	... 17	...	... 615
Day and boarding schools, . . } 2	... 13	...	... 80
123	197	44	5735

The secondary, Lancastrian, and female schools belong to the different islands; the day and boarding-schools are in the town of Corfu, one of which, said to be exceedingly well conducted, and highly useful, is under the charge of an English lady, Mrs Falconer, where young ladies are instructed; the other is a boys' school.

In addition, it requires to be noticed, that a seminary for the education of priests has been established in Corfu, by an act of the Ionian Parliament, in 1827, for the special purpose, as is stated in the seventh article of the act, " of forming ministers of religion competent for their high and important duties, and possessed of that knowledge which is requisite to make them worthy and useful pastors. * This

* The author last quoted remarks, in the same work—" Assez généralement l'on se plaint de la paresse des prêtres, et du retard que les lumières out mis à se répandre parmi eux; tout cela pourtant n'est pas fondé. Pendant quelques siècles, il n'y a pas eu un seul seminaire, où les jeunes gens qui se vouoient à l'autel, pussent recevoir une idée de leur langue, ou de leur devoir. Pourroit-on les taxer d'ignorance?"—P. 41.

In another part he says—" Des institutions dogmatiques, des psaumes, et des prières sans fin, dans une langue inintelligible à l'élève, aussi bien qu'au maître, c'étoit, généralement parlant, tout ce qu'on appeloit *exercices spirituel*, ou doctrine theologique."—P. 58.

seminary, which is supported at the public expense, is considered as a branch of the university. It is intended that the number of novitiates should be limited, and not exceed fifty-two,—a number, it is supposed, adequate to supply ministers to all the churches of the Ionian Islands, as vacancies may occur.

The university and the collegiate school are provided with apartments at Port-Raymond, in the building belonging to the public, which was previously employed as a barrack, it having been necessary to vacate the old palace in the citadel. The divinity school has been put in possession of the Casino, or country villa of the Lord High Commissioner, at Castrades, a building and locality considered peculiarly commodious for the seminary—an obligation conferred on it by Sir Howard Douglas.

The general system of education, of which the preceding is a brief sketch, has been entirely organized by government. The superintendence of it is " vested in the supreme authority of the Senate, and the Lord High Commissioner;" and the immediate charge of it is placed in a commission composed of an archon, and two other gentlemen, under the authority of the Senate, with an eforo, or vice-chancellor, who is always to be a professor, in immediate charge of the university, and an inspector-general, to perform the same duty in relation to the secondary and Lancastrian schools, each of which he is to visit yearly, and report on to the commission.

This scheme of education appears to be liberal, and well adapted to most of the wants of the people; and, if steadily carried on, cannot fail to have an excellent effect. A word of doubt, on such a subject, is disagreeable to use; but, when the brief history of the attempts which have been made to introduce education into the Ionian Islands is considered, it is somewhat difficult to have that degree of confidence in its durability which could be wished. When I first visited Corfu, in 1824, the late Earl of Guildford was presiding as chancellor over the university which he had established, with the sanction and assistance of the government. Twenty-one professorships were then founded, several of the professors had commenced their duties, and were lecturing to respectable classes, at least as far as numbers were concerned. An excellent library was formed and opened; and a building, the old palace in the citadel, was appropriated for the use of the establishment. In brief, it then bore all the marks of an institution likely to be fixed and durable, instead of ephemeral, as it proved, and depending on the life of an individual. Before I left Corfu, in 1828, Lord Guildford died, and an immediate change came over the establishment. A university, founded on the magnificent scale of Oxford and Cambridge, including amongst its professors a professor of music, was thought to be inappropriate, beyond the means of the government to support, and above the wants of the people, for whom it was designed. It was then cut down on a very economical plan; four professors only were allowed to teach in those branches of knowledge which were considered most useful; but, at the same time, secondary schools were formed for elementary education, which previously had been too much neglected, and the number of Lancastrian schools was increased. This alteration was mainly effected by the then Lord High Commissioner, Sir Frederick Adam, who, whilst he took a deep interest in the important subject, regarded it soberly and practically. Perhaps the change made was too sudden and great. It must have shaken public confidence, and must have annoyed the friends of the noble founder; and further, it had the injurious effect of depriving the Ionian Islands of the valuable library, formed by that nobleman, principally for the use of the university, and which, it was understood, was bequeathed to it, provided certain conditions connected with its foundation were complied with.

It may also be a question, whether the present scheme of university education, which is different both from that of Lord Guilford and of Sir Frederick Adam, is as complete as is desirable—considering merely the wants of the people. In both the former plans medical education was included; in the present, it will be perceived, it is omitted—but why, I have never yet heard explained. Were there an hospital established in Corfu, as would seem to be desirable, where clinical medicine and surgery could be practically taught, with an anatomical theatre attached, a foundation would be laid for a school of practical medicine; and were professors judiciously chosen, it is probable that a school might be formed which might prove of the highest utility to the islands, corresponding in its effects to the seminary for the education of priests. At present, most of the villages in the Ionian Islands are without medical men; and the people at large, excepting in towns, as in Corfu, Zante, Argostoli, Lixuri, and in two or three more, are entirely destitute of medical aid. Were a sound medical education easily attainable, and at a cheap rate, it may be reasonably supposed there would be no lack of students, and that very soon the deficiency alluded to would be supplied. Moreover, were there a poor-house, or *ospizio*, as an asylum for the aged poor, the lame, and the blind, and those labouring under chronic incurable diseases,* from whence the anatomical theatre could be supplied with subjects (proper regulations being enacted to prevent abuses, and insure respectful Christian burial), it seems not improbable that such a school, well taught, might rise in importance, and be resorted to from continental Greece. Theoretical

* An excellent institution of the kind above referred to exists in Malta, in which many hundred persons of the description alluded to are supported in comfort. In 1835, the number of inmates, of both sexes, was about eight hundred; and then there were several hundreds on the list of applicants. The majority of those received, and of the candidates for admission, were married: their not being allowed to live together was not then considered a hardship; but, though occupying different parts of the building, it may be mentioned that, being under the same roof, they had an opportunity of seeing each other daily, and of holding friendly intercourse.

medicine, apart from practical medicine, is vain and illusive; and the teaching of medicine in this way was one of the many mistakes committed at the opening of the university by Lord Guilford, and which, it may be conjectured, led to the total abandonment of medical instruction.

As the Greeks of the Ionian Islands, like the Greeks in general, have active minds and a facility in acquiring knowledge, the prospect which is opening, in the increased extension of education, is not a little cheering. If the system is persevered in; if the priesthood become enlightened; if they zealously perform their duties, aided by the labours of the masters in the primary and secondary schools—it may be confidently expected that the people generally will improve and become enlightened also—at least in degree—to which the education of females, now beginning to be attended to, is likely greatly to conduce. Two hundred years ago, the people of the Lowlands of Scotland were as deeply immersed in ignorance as are the inhabitants of these islands at present; what the parochial school-system accomplished for the former, the system now coming into operation may effect for the latter: but, to insure this, there must be the same earnestness exercised— and a constant vigilance to prevent abuse and that degeneracy to which all institutions are liable which do not grow up with the people,* especially in the

* Even in Scotland, the parochial school teaching is considered less efficient than it was some years ago. In a report of the Ayrshire Edu-

south of Europe, where the tendency to evil in all things, excepting in matters of taste and manners, apart from morals, seems to be peculiarly strong.*

cational Association, recently published, it is stated that " education in the parochial, and therefore in the subordinate schools, has materially declined from the standard which was originally assigned to it.'

* Santa Maura affords an instance of the tendency to abuse, referred to above. The writer before quoted, speaking of the manner of conducting the schools in this island, says—" But the mode of conducting the schools " (it should be remembered when he wrote, viz. in 1835) " is most to be deplored. An Italian of notorious character is at the head of the secondary school, in which are educated all the young nobles and those who are to be the future leaders, rulers, and magistrates of the people. Though this Italian master is not troubled with any superfluous delicacy or sense of propriety, he expresses the greatest horror at the *depravity* of his pupils. A sad prospect for the next generation. As to any sentiment of religion, morality, or honour, I hold preceptor and pupils to be equally destitute.

" The primary or normal school has for its master a lad related to the bishop, but whose character is so bad as to occasion his being turned out of that worthy prelate's house. This unworthy subject was placed at the head of the schools by means of some protector at Corfu ; and, to make room for him, the excellent person who had first introduced the system of mutual instruction, and is a priest universally venerated for his character, was removed without any cause being assigned for it ; neither was the local government ever made acquainted with the reason. Under such guidance, if guidance it can be called, are the schools of Santa Maura; consequently, there is a total want of discipline, of encouragement, and of every principle which ought to influence the education of youth. A general committee at Corfu having taken this important branch out of the hands of the local government, and as they are too remote and too indifferent to pay any attention to either teachers or pupils, a general disorder and neglect (as regards Santa Maura) are evident.

" Thus, though I consider the schools to be neglected, and in some instances to be doing more harm than good, I am most happy to bear testimony to the very excellent spirit that animates the peasantry.

The aptitude of the people for education, and the
facility of carrying measures of education into effect,
was well exemplified in Cerigo whilst Major Macphail was Resident of that island.   When I visited
Cerigo, in the summer of 1827, there was the large
proportion of 1300 boys and girls, out of a population
of 13,000, at school.   The schools, eight in number
(besides six private schools), were all conducted on
the Lancastrian plan, and at a cost of about L.370.
One of them was exclusively for females, and was
attended by 120 scholars, who were taught by a mistress and an assistant, and by an old priest, reading,
writing, and arithmetic ; and by the former " the Bri-

When country schools were first established among them, great clamour
and opposition arose.   Yet, on making a tour of the island last year
[1834], the elders of almost every village came forward, and strenuously
entreated for schools and roads, offering to pay, according to their
respective *means*, for the *education* of *their own children*, and to *contribute* towards the expense required for their *poorer neighbours*.   Little
as has been effected hitherto, I consider this delightful fact as a splendid triumph in the cause of civilization ; for it proves that a barbarous
and most prejudiced peasantry can, in the space of a very few years,
and under a very defective system, not only be convinced of the
advantages attending even an imperfect education, but now become
advocates for the extension of its benefits to others.

" In the knowledge that this admirable spirit is almost general
among the peasantry, I feel certain that, instead of three or four hundred, at least two thousand might be placed in the schools, who ought
not only to be educated in the usual branches of learning, but also in
their religious and moral duties, the elements of horticulture and
agriculture, a knowledge of their rights as citizens, and of such local
laws as more immediately affect the agricultural proprietor.

" I know of no measure that would so readily form and elevate the
very debased character of this naturally clever people."

tish system of needle-work," which the mistress herself had learnt from a translation made from the English into modern Greek by the judge of the island. The scholars were principally the children of refugees from the Morea, then invaded by the Egyptians under Ibrahim Pasha, and from the islands of the Archipelago. Neatly dressed in the particular costume of their respective native places, they presented a very singular and interesting appearance; and the order and propriety observed, and the advances which they had made in the course of from two to three years, were highly creditable to themselves and their teachers; whilst their alacrity and energy of manner in applying themselves to their work, and in answering questions when examined, impressed one strongly, and very favourably, in regard to their intellectual character and capacity. From a return of Schools in Cerigo, bearing date of the 31st December 1826, it appears that the total expenses of this very useful school amounted for that year only to L.50, 11s. 7d., according to the following detail:—Salary of master, L.18, 4s.; of mistress, L.13; of assistant-teacher, L.7, 5s.; house-rent, L.4, 6s. 8d.; rewards to scholars, L.3, 15s. 6d.; lessons, slates, books, L.4, 5s.

I have alluded to the tendency there is in all useful institutions to degenerate, and to the necessity of vigilant guard over them to keep up their efficiency. Systems of education are peculiarly prone to decline —to lose their spirit and become empty forms. Every university offers examples of this in different degrees. If, in consequence of the exertion of influence, and the setting aside of merit, a feeble or worthless professor is appointed to a chair, the interests of the university will naturally suffer; his class will fall off; allowance will be made in the examinations for his inefficiency—and so far they will cease to be 'a test of qualification. If, moreover, from any cause, the examiners should relax in their important duties, and not exercise their functions with that impartial and firm justice which is absolutely necessary, it will soon be perceived by the students, and there will be a corresponding relaxation in their exertions. And if favour is shown on the part of the examiners, the students will become more intent to secure that than to merit distinction. In a small society, where interest is so easily exerted, and where unusual firmness is required to do justice, in opposition to the solicitations of friends, great danger may be apprehended from favouritism of this kind, and from the dereliction of duty in examination for degrees. In Malta, I have witnessed the effects; and what I have observed there have chiefly induced me to offer these remarks, which I believe to be applicable, from analogy of institution, to the Ionian Islands. In Malta there is a regularly organized university, in which degrees are granted in divinity, law, and medicine, after examinations by the professors and by individuals specially appointed. From my official situation as a member

of the council which had the superintendence of the
university, I had an opportunity of watching the
working of this system. It was instructive to observe
how careless teaching, and careless study, and careless
examination were connected; and how, as the examinations became more stringent, the teaching improved, and the students improved. It was melancholy to observe, too, that tendency, before referred
to, to favouritism, and consequent ruin. I may mention an instance in point, and also to show that,
unless there is firm principle, the ballot may be
abused, and become the means of mischief. I should
premise, that the decision of the Medical College (as
the body of medical examiners is there called), is determined by ballot. The instance was this:—A student
for a medical degree, subjected to a *viva voce* examination, showed himself deplorably ignorant; his mistakes
called forth remark; the examiners could not conceal
their disapprobation; they expressed it both by their
looks and words. However, as a matter of form,
the ballot-box was sent round, and, strange to say,
the number of white balls prevailed. I took it for
granted this was by mistake. The box was again
sent round; the result was the same; the rejected
by word and look was approved of by ballot. I
requested, in private, an explanation from one of the
professors. He candidly said that he had put in a
white ball against his conscience; that he had been
solicited by the friends of the young man; that he

was kindly disposed towards him, and could not bear to pain him, and, as he expressed it, " blight his prospects."   And such, probably, are the feelings commonly, by which the welfare of a school, or college, or university, depending on examinations for its efficacy, is most endangered in a small community.

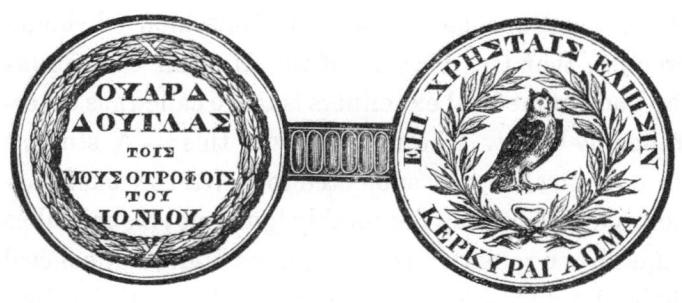

CHAPTER VI.

ON THE CHARITABLE INSTITUTIONS OF THE IONIAN ISLANDS.

Smallness of their Number. Monti di Pietà. Civil Hospitals. Lunatic Asylum. Desiderata in regard to Medical Institutions. Foundling-Hospital. Remarks relative to its former Abuses. Observations on the Condition of the Indigent Poor. Remarks on the Population.

THE charitable institutions of these islands are few in number, and, with one or two exceptions, generally of little efficacy. They are comprised in a small civil hospital, one in Corfu and one in Zante; in a foundling-hospital, one in each of these islands; in a Monte di Pietà, one also in each; and in a lunatic asylum.

The Monti di Pietà are, I believe, well conducted, and deserving of all praise. Small sums of money are lent from them to the necessitous, on pawn of articles of jewellery or wearing apparel, on the moderate interest of four per cent. for a certain time, agreeably to the system of rules by which the business of the institution is strictly conducted. As in Italy and in France, so in the Ionian Islands and in

Malta, these banks, wherever established, have entirely put a stop to the business of pawnbrokers in the hands of private individuals, with all the grinding evils and incitements to crime too often connected with the system.

The civil hospitals in Corfu and Zante are very inadequate to the wants of the people, and are nowise creditable to the government. A lunatic asylum has lately been established at St Roque-in the neighbourhood of the town of Corfu, at the expense and under the direction of government. It is the first that has been opened in these islands : it is said to be well founded and well conducted, and to give general satisfaction.* Were hospitals on a similar liberal footing established in the different islands, especially in the larger, and more especially in Corfu, the effects could hardly fail being in many respects beneficial, both directly as regards affording medical aid to the poor, and indirectly as schools of medicine and surgery. And with the same view, also, dispensaries might be instituted, of which at present there are none, and which, at a comparatively trifling expense, might be of great service to the lower classes of the inhabitants, particularly from the country, who at home are out of the reach of medical advice

---

* According to the latest information I have received of this institution, the number of patients of both sexes is sixty, who are divided into two classes—one indigent, for whom no payment is made; the other, for whom payment is made. The building, it is said, is not sufficiently ample for the wants of the islands, seeming thereby to indicate that mental disease is prevalent amongst the inhabitants.

and may be too poor to procure it, were they to come into town in quest of it.*

The foundling-hospitals in Corfu and Zante were for a long time in a very imperfect state; so conducted that they were to be considered rather as positive evils than as useful institutions. All the infants brought and deposited in the revolving-box for their reception, were taken in without inquiry. They were said to be of three classes: illegitimate offspring of clandestine amours, whose mothers were intent on hiding their disgrace; the offspring of women of the town, careless of their children, and considering them a burden; and thirdly, those of poor married women, who from their poverty had difficulty in rearing them, and who hoped, by collusion, to have them sent them to nurse. The mortality amongst these infants, forsaken by their parents, was appalling: in a paper before me, on the subject, it is stated that the deaths which took place amongst them

---

* As regards medical relief for the poor and working classes, Malta may be very advantageously compared with the Ionian Islands. The civil hospital in Valetta, supported by government, yearly receives about 3000 patients; no one requiring medical aid who applies, is refused admission,—no certificate, no recommendation is requisite. The dispensary in Valetta, instituted, at my suggestion, has not been less extensive in its operation: at the cost of two or three hundred pounds (I write from recollection), it has afforded aid to above four thousand poor people yearly. In the civil hospital, it is worthy of remark that the spiritual wants of the people are as amply provided for as their bodily; four chaplains are attached to the establishment, one of whom is always on duty, at night as well as by day, having an apartment in the building.

in five years, ending the 1st May 1835, amounted to
seventy-five per cent. of those received; and that from
the 31st May 1835 to the 31st October 1837, the
number of deaths had been fifty, namely, twenty male
infants and thirty females.* The writer of the paper
in question, pointing out the bad effects of the old
system, in relation to the cloak it afforded to licen-
tiousness and the deadening of moral principle and
natural affection, and urging reform, powerfully com-
bats the argument, that an alteration might lead to
child-murder, by the remark, of the almost impossibility of the crime ever being so destructive of human
life as the existing remedy. I have spoken of the
evils of this institution in the past tense, with the
hope that they are past: Sir Howard Douglas, in a
recent speech to the parliament, alludes to some
reform having been made, and to a complete reform
which he contemplated.

The Ionian Islands are without any legal provision
for the destitute poor; they are entirely without
almshouses, or a place of any description for the
reception of paupers. Baron Theotoki, under the
head of " Enfans Abandonnés," remarks:—" Il y en

---

* In Malta, the mortality in the foundling-hospital, for many
.years, was as great, I believe, as in the Ionian Islands, so long as
goats' milk was given to the infants. Before I left the island, a
reform was attempted, nurses were provided, but not liberally, one
nurse occasionally having had to suckle two children. Establishments
of this kind seem to be doomed to mismanagement and abuse, as if
labouring under a curse, and who shall say not merited, as in their
general tendency likely to do much more evil than good.

a une bonne quantité (de 5 jusqu' à 10 et 12 ans) qui courent la ville, et couchent sur la pavé, puisqu'il n'y a point d'etablissement où l'on puisse les recevoir." He adds,—" L'astuce, l'effronterie, l'éscroquerie, la mendicité, tirent d'ici leur origine."* The poor in distress are almost entirely dependent on casual charity, and are under the necessity of becoming beggars. In churches, it is true, collections are made for their relief; but although it is said the service is often disturbed by the importunity of beggars, —the amount contributed is so inconsiderable as not to be deserving of mention. From his addresses to the parliament, the late Lord High Commissioner, Sir Howard Douglas, appears to have been fully alive to the necessity of some active measures being taken to afford relief to the poor, and seems to have had in contemplation the establishing of almshouses, and providing constant funds for their maintenance.†

* Details sur Corfou, p. 110.

† Sir Charles Napier considers the revenue from the convent-lands as the appropriate means for supporting the poor. He says, these possessions, which are extensive, " have been acquired in legacies made by the devout and the repentant, for the use of the poor. To this use (he adds) I applied them, and had I not been interfered with, there would have been, in a few years, no destitute person in Cephalonia." And, in another place, he says :—" Had it been continued six years, no labourer in Cephalonia would have been without a competence; by which I mean, that every industrious man might have a cottage of his own, a garden of his own, be able to buy a pound of bread for 1½d., a pound of meat for 2½d., and a bottle of wine for 1d.,—in all, 5d. a-day; and receive from 10d. to 15d. a-day for his labour. When it is recollected that no firing and very little clothing are purchased in this hot climate, and that a Cephalonian

One poor-house, I am informed, he did establish at Corfu, on a small scale, by way of trial, before his departure, which, if report be correct, has since been abolished, and its inmates turned out. As the proportional population is small, and wages high, and subsistence cheap, the number of beggars is inconsiderable, and the evils of unrelieved distress of no great amount, otherwise, probably, their correction would have been sooner attended to.

The population of the Ionian Islands are an example of a people left to the natural checks, moral and physical, to its augmentation, and they appear to be perfectly adequate. As regards numbers, it is doubtful if there has been any considerable increase during the last century,* or any material improvement

has no rent to pay, I think this as good a condition as any labouring man can expect, in addition to certain refuge in a convent, when disabled by bodily affliction. And, there may be added, that every dollar he saves, he can, at once, turn to profit in small mercantile speculations. I maintain what a long residence in the island has convinced me to be practicable; but till the peasant is liberated from the grasp of oppression, and agriculture taught, this state of ease will not have place. Poverty and idleness will continue, and must continue."

* Baron Theotoki expresses an opinion to the same effect; he observes, in the absence of positive facts deducible from accurate registers, that all that is known leads to the belief, 1st, that the number of births does not exceed the number of deaths; 2d, that a very large number of children die under the age of fourteen; 3d, that a large number of women die in child-bed, particularly in the towns; 4th, that in the country six marriages take place in every thousand of the inhabitants, and in the city four; 5th, that in the country each marriage gives six children, and in the town four.

of condition. High wages have commonly been met by idleness; a mild temperature by malaria; fruitfulness of mothers in the labouring class, by carelessness towards their offspring, and great mortality in early life. In the upper classes, not exposed to these physical checks, others have acted and have had a similar effect, especially celibacy and late marriages. Baron Theotoki, under the head of "Celibataires," gives a striking picture of the consequences, amongst which he enumerates the degeneracy of some families, the total extinction of others, and a miserable state of society from an accumulation, in a small city, of old maids and old beaus.* He contrasts the town with the country, in which, he says, celibacy is almost entirely unknown, and where even most of the priests are married, as were also commonly, of old, the saints, martyrs, and bishops.

* "L'effet le plus pernicieux de ce système est qu' un millier de femmes bien nées, ne pouvant pas se marier avantageusement, et n'aimant pas descendre de la condition où le sort les a placées, demeurent, sans un état positif dans la société. Or l'influence, *dans une petite Ville*, de cette masse de vieilles vierges, revèches et hargneuses (ajoutée à la communauté laique des vieux garçons, dégoutés d'aller à la quête d'aventures, au milieu d'un monde qui ne leur appartient point, et qui ne veut plus d'eux) est facile à deduire."—Op. Cit. p. 125.

CHAPTER VII.

ON THE CHARACTER AND GENERAL CONDITION OF THE PEOPLE OF THE IONIAN ISLANDS.

General Resemblance of the People of the different Islands. Points of Difference. Habits and Manners of the Inhabitants divided into Classes. Notice of the Principal Towns; of the Houses of the Upper Class; their Furniture and Household Economy. Amusements and Recreations. Dress of the Peasantry. Other particulars respecting them. Numerous Holidays. Neglect of the Sabbath. Condition of the Women. Marriage Rites. Funerals. Neglected State of Grave-yards, and Want of Respect to the Dead. Remarks on the Character of the People. Extracts from Authors, relative to the same, contrasted.

A PEOPLE speaking the same language, belonging to the same race, inhabiting islands similar in climate, and generally similar in soil and productions, under the control of one government, and under the influence of the same religious as well as civil institutions, may be expected to exhibit one character, or that general similarity of manners, habits, and modes of thinking and acting, which constitutes national character. As far as my observations extended, such a similarity exists amongst the inhabitants of these islands, with some modifications, however, and differences, probably justly referable to what is peculiar in the circumstances or condition of the people of the different islands, and, in some instances, of the different parts of the same island.

It is hardly necessary to observe, that the inhabitants of the country are more ignorant and ruder, and more primitive in their manners, than those of the towns; and that, amongst the former, the difference in these particulars is most strongly marked amongst the mountaineers and the dwellers in the small islands off the coasts of the larger ones, in both which situations there is much seclusion, and all the circumstances are equally unfavourable to change and to improvement.

Of the larger islands generally considered, the inhabitants of the southern ones, in which the currant-vine is cultivated, are held to be more industrious, active, and intelligent, than those of the northern, in which the olive is the principal produce,—which, too, is no more than might be expected, taking into account how habits are formed, and how the one species of cultivation requires, and therefore promotes, industry,—and how the other, requiring but little labour and exertion, has a contrary effect.

Of the inhabitants of the olive-growing islands, those of Paxo are considered as distinguished for mild and amiable manners, and for absence of vice. Their olive-plantations are better attended to than those of Corfu and Santa Maura, probably in consequence of more attention to them being absolutely necessary, the trees being planted not in plains and in a deep soil, where neglect can be borne, but, as already observed, in little terraces, amongst rocks, cut out of the steep sides of hills. The fruit, too, is more carefully gathered and is better preserved, and the oil made is of a superior quality and higher price; and the consequence of this is (most of them being small proprietors), that they are in easy circumstances, favourable for that character which they have earned by their conduct.

It has been already mentioned, that the inhabitants of Cephalonia and of Ithaca have shown a more enterprizing spirit than any of the other islanders, leading them to engage in adventure and foreign commerce; and it may be added, that the Cephaloniots have also shown more freedom of will and love of liberty, prompting them to resist oppression and to break out into acts of insubordination; and that the natives of the mountainous parts of Zante, of Santa Maura, of Ithaca, and of Cerigo, partake more or less of the same character. The disposition to freedom and license in these people, has been fostered by circumstances; without fortresses excepting on a small scale, and of little strength; never occupied by any large military force, they have been very much their own masters; and from their vicinity to continental Greece, and constant intercourse with that country (that land of liberty of old, and of license in modern times, under the Turkish yoke), they have probably been infected by example, to hold

authority light and hold law in contempt. Till within
a few years, arms were generally carried by the
people—the gun, the sword, and dagger—in the use
of which they were dexterous. This circumstance,
too, it need hardly be remarked, promoted turbu-
lence and insubordination. The klepthes (the re-
putable robbers, as they esteemed themselves), of the
mountains of Zante, and of the adjoining islands
before enumerated, identified themselves with those
of Albania, and are said, for many years, during the
period of Venetian rule, to have taken common part
with them. Moreover, the kind of feudal system
which prevailed in the larger islands, and most
strongly in the largest of all Cephalonia, in which a
few great landed-proprietors were almost independent, and were disposed to make their will their law,
must have conduced, in no inconsiderable degree, to
impart that character to the inhabitants which has
just now been alluded to.*

* Sir Charles Napier, in his work on the Ionian Islands, strongly
depicts the feudal state in Cephalonia, especially in the following
passage:—" The reader must know that, in Cephalonia, every village chiefly consists of a family, and generally bears the family
name; the peasants all live in villages; no man ventures to live in
an isolated house; to mutual defence every member of the family is
pledged; each village has one or two feudal chiefs, whose influence
extends over one or several villages; when there are two chiefs in the
same village, there are generally two factions (for these chiefs seldom
smell to the same rose, as the kings of Brentford did), and the force
of this feudal influence may be judged of by the following anec-
dote:—When I was first appointed Resident of Cephalonia, an officer
on public duty (named Maclean) was very much insulted by some

As regards the manners and habits of the different classes of which the population of these islands consists, marked differences, of course, are observable.

The higher class, those constituting the gentry, many of them of Italian descent, and commonly speaking the Italian language, are so very Italian as to have called forth the remark on the part of the Baron Theotoki, that a stranger coming amongst them would have difficulty in believing them to be Greeks.* This observation, however, it should be mentioned, was made of the Corfiots; it is less applicable to persons of the same order in Zante, Cephalonia, and Ithaca, and least of all to the ladies of these islands. That it should apply rather to the men is what might be expected, considering that very

men of a village, who, indeed, would have knocked him on the head, had not his presence of mind and resolution saved him. I happened to be at dinner with the Countess Anino (to whom this village belongs, a lady meriting that I should speak of her with the greatest respect, as one whose character is as noble as her rank is distinguished), when a message came to her from the village, to inform her of the quarrel, and to know if she chose to allow the government to arrest the culprits or not; her answer was, ' *that they were to obey the government, even if it demanded their sucking children.*' The message and the answer exhibit the state of society. The Countess Anino is the greatest feudal proprietor in the island, and could, at any moment, have opposed the government with four thousand men."

* The Baron Theotoki calls the Italian spoken " un jargon poissard tiré du patois Venitien ;" and patriotically remarks, after commenting on the evil influence of the practice, " Point de langue nationale—Point de Patrie," adding—" Il suffira de dire, pour dire assez, que les étrangers qui arrivent dans cette ville ont de la peine à croire, que la noblesse y soit grecque."

many of the gentlemen, and the most influential, all who have been well educated, hitherto received their education in Italy; and that from Italy, almost exclusively, has been introduced all that has given them distinction, whether titles, or literature, or music, and even furniture and dress.

Comparing the individuals of this class in the different islands, perhaps it may be said that those of Corfu are most Italian, those of Zante most Levantine, and those of Cephalonia and Ithaca most Greek. In Corfu, long a garrison town, and the seat of government, there is a freedom in society, and an easy intercourse, quite unknown in the other islands. There a gentleman may pay a morning visit to a lady without impropriety. In Zante, where the society has been left very much to itself, there is great restraint, especially in relation to the sex; and to call on a Zantiot lady would be considered contrary to the rules of good-breeding, and probably might be held to be an insult. In the other islands there is a medium; the intercourse is less formal and restrained than in the one, and less free and more ceremonious than in the other; the ladies are not excluded from society, nor are they objects of gallantry; they have never been accustomed to their *cavalier servente*,* as

* The Baron Theotoki mentions this trait of his countrywomen of the higher class in Corfu—but for their credit, I am glad to say, in the past tense—with some other particulars not reflecting credit on them, and in accordance with the common opinion of their being addicted to gallantry. He states that, besides thinking it improper to

in Corfu; nor have they been under the necessity of paying visits, shut up and concealed in litters and sedan-chairs as in Zante.*   As hitherto, the best part of female education has been neglected in these islands—the cultivation of their minds—their intellectual and moral improvement—it is not surprising that they have taken no worthy part in society, and exercised no worthy influence, and that the tone of society has been very defective, either stupid and uninteresting, or frivolous and too often dissipated.

In the habits of life of this class there is nothing very peculiar or distinctive from the Italians.   Their hours of eating are early, as in the south of Europe generally; a cup of coffee or of chocolate, with a biscuit, constitutes their ordinary breakfast at rising; about one o'clock they sit down to dinner; and after dinner indulge in a siesta, reposing in bed until about five; when they rise, the men smoke two or three cigars; and take a cup of coffee and dress; after

go out with their husbands, and that each required an established *cavaliere servente;* they painted their cheeks, stained their hair and eye-lashes; and avoided suckling their children, from a fear of spoiling their forms.—P. 76.

* This is mentioned, by Conte Paolo Mercati, in the little work already referred to. He notices the retired habits of the ladies of Zante as the most remarkable circumstance in the society of that place; adding, that young ladies betrothed are not permitted to see their destined husbands till three days before the celebration of the marriage rites. They spend their time chiefly in their own apartments, in company with their children and female servants, employed in needle-work, especially embroidery; going out seldom, excepting to church, and there accommodated with a gallery apart, concealed by a close lattice-work from the male congregation below.

which they walk or ride, and spend the remainder of the evening till eleven, twelve, or one o'clock, either in conversation, play, or reading, as each may feel inclined. They are fond of cards and games of chance, as are the generality of idle people; and they are also fond of field-sports, and are keen *cacciatòri*.

Their dwellings may be briefly mentioned. They, too, accord with the Italian style; generally much alike,—they vary, however, in quality in the towns of the different islands.

Zante, in any part of Europe, would be considered as a handsome town. Subject to earthquakes, from which it has so often suffered, unusual care has been taken in the construction of the buildings; they are commonly strongly built, of a light freestone; the streets are regular and well-disposed; and the houses generally good, and convenient, and well fitted for a warm climate.

The town of Corfu does not admit of the same praise. Beautifully situated, and picturesque in appearance, it is generally ill built. The Baron Theotoki passes his censure on it—on its irregular and narrow streets,—till recently, ill lighted and extremely dirty.* " The houses ill built, of brick or rubble;

---

* Botta, in his account of Corfu, written shortly before the islands came under British protection, specially notices the filthy condition of the town, when expressing surprise at its comparative healthiness, notwithstanding certain apparent causes to the contrary, which he enumerates :—

" A ciò si deve aggiungere, che e grande l'immondizie di essa città, non usando quegli abitanti nissuna diligenza per trasportare via le

without conveniences; the apartments small; without courts, or cellars, or gardens, or stables, or chimneys; ill floored; with bad exposures, unprotected equally from the heat of summer and the rigour of winter."*

The other towns approach more or less to these two in their character. Argostoli and Lixuri are substantially built, and have a fair proportion of good and commodious houses; as has also the beautifully-situated little town of Vathi, in Ithaca, combining in its character in perfection the sea-port and the country town or village. Vessels, on one side, moored close to its houses, and thrusting their bowsprits into the street, pleasantly contrasted with vineyards and gardens skirting and indenting it on the other, both characteristic of the tastes and habits of the natives, most of whom are sailors till thirty or forty, and afterwards cultivators—cultivating some little property which their earnings have enabled them to purchase.

In all the towns the houses are without fire-places in the sitting-rooms; and the inhabitants are obliged to trust to warm clothing as a protection from the

sozzure, che dalle finestre sogliono per ogni dove gettare nelle contrade; ond'è, che non puoi dare due passi per una qualche contrada, sensa che t'incontri o in un mucchio di escrementi, o in una fogna che sbocca, e che ti mandano al naso un orribile lezzo."

* Op. Cit., p. 22. Improvements in the town of Corfu are now in progress, and very great ones, I am informed, are planned, especially the building of a new street on the sea-shore, in the direction of Castrades. This, indeed, is commenced.

cold of winter, or to unwholesome charcoal fires in braziers. The writer whom I have so often quoted places in the list of prejudices the aversion of the higher class of his countrymen to a fire.* The towns, too, have other faults in common—greatly interfering with health and comfort, and that propriety and cleanliness so conducive to both. I allude chiefly to the want of sewers—to means of receiving and carrying off filth and impurities—and to a due supply of that first necessary of life, water. In Corfu, where these evils were most felt, there the correction of them has been first begun. Thanks to Sir Frederick Adam, that town, as has been already noticed, is now abundantly supplied with water by means of an acqueduct, as is also Zante; and other improvements are in progress.

Of the furniture of their houses, and the manner of keeping them in regard to neatness and cleanliness, little can be said in compliment. The furniture is commonly old, often mean and ricketty and rarely elegant. The floors are commonly uncarpeted and unwashed. It is mentioned by Polybius that the supposed crime of Philip of Macedon, of poisoning Ara-

---

* Baron Theotoki, after enumerating some of their prejudices, proceeds—" Les autres sont, de croire que les vents du Sud, et les hivers pluvieux sont utiles ; de préférer les petites chambres aux grandes ; de se surcharger d'habits, et de lourds manteaux ; de craindre le feu, et de ne point s'approcher des cheminées." He adds—" Tout cela cependant n est que la portage de la ville, et de ses alentours. Les habitans de la campagne au contraire aiment le feu, et preferent le tems sec à l'humide, qu' ils appellent σαπρὸς, *pourri*."—P. 76.

tus, was discovered by the peculiar appearance of the spittle of the latter when he was ill, attracting the attention of an old servant as it hung from the wall. This is a trait of want of delicacy and of cleanliness in the ancient Greeks ; and the same may be remarked amongst the moderns, who spit, not only on the floors of their rooms, but when in bed, like the sick Aratus, against the walls.*   And even in some of the best houses, certain insects, which with us are considered as disreputable, are not uncommon, nor are they held in abhorrence.†   But in these circumstances the people of the Ionian Islands are not peculiar ; in

---

* The Baron Theotoki, speaking of the prejudices of his countrymen, alludes to this habit, expressing, at the same time, his opinion that the English abstain from it, not because they mind spoiling their carpets, as is commonly thought, but really from a sense of propriety and regard for health. His words are—" Un autre prejugé, très-répandu, et bien contraire à la santé, c'est de cracher sans cesse, dans la crainte que la salive n'aille affoiblir l'estomac ; tandis que cette liqueur résolutive est trop précieux pour ne pas être ménagée. Généralement on croit, que les Anglois ne crachent jamais, de peur de gâter leur tapis : ce qui n'est nullement vrai ; car c'est plutôt par ce qu'ils trouvent dans cette habitude, quelque chose de contraire, autant à la bienséance, qu'à la santé. Et je pense qu'ils ont grande raison."— P. 77. This habit of spitting on the floors, it may be remarked, is very commonly associated with the absence of carpets—which, no doubt, gave rise to the fancy of the Ionian Greeks. alluded to by the Baron Theotoki. Excepting the Turks, I know no other people of the south and east of Europe who accord with the English in their aversion to spitting—and they use carpets.

† The Baron Theotoki, describing the prognostics of the seasons in Corfu, mentions—" Les pays ans connoissent que le tems doi changer lorsque les *puces* remuent tout-à-coup, dans leur sein, ou depuis le cou jusqu' aux reins."—P. 112.

Italy they are much the same; in southern Italy hardly a shade better: and in Sicily as bad. In no one of the islands, when I was there, was there a public bath, and sea-bathing was little in use.*

Their amusements and recreations are few, and commonly little interesting—little worthy of a cultivated and enlightened society. The great season of gaiety is the masquerading time of carnival ;† and the

* In disinclination to use the bath, the Greeks commonly, and especially of the Ionian Islands, are strongly contrasted with the Turks and other oriental people. From Greece to India, a rising gradation may be marked in point of cleanliness. The people of these islands are dirty in person and dress; the lower classes seldom have recourse to ablution, sleep in their clothes, and often wear them out without changing them. The Turks are cleanly in their persons, but, excepting the affluent, not in their clothing—their religion exacting the use of the bath and daily ablution, but not change of raiment. The Hindus are scrupulously clean in both respects. In Greece and Turkey vermin abound—fleas, lice, and bugs—sadly to the annoyance of the traveller, and to a degree that can hardly be imagined by the inexperienced. In India, the exemption from these insects in the dwellings of the natives (with some exceptions) is hardly less remarkable. In Ceylon, to which my personal experience is limited, I believe it may be owing to the paste of cow-dung with which the women frequently smear the floors of their cottages.

† During Carnival-time, especially in Zante, gambling is practised to a great, and often ruinous, extent. The habit, probably, was derived from Venice, where, during this season, it was a fashion, and where, towards the latter end of the republic, Daru relates, it had become so serious an evil, that it was considered necessary to prohibit it. We are also informed by him, that the prohibition was of short duration: so low was public virtue then in Venice, that it was thought impolitic to diminish any of the attractions to strangers which the city held out   At Aix-la-Chapelle, under the moral government of Prussia, the gaming-house of that watering place is freely open to all strangers, but shut to the inhabitants and the officers of the troops stationed

other principal occasions are the vigils of saints' days and their feste. In all the Ionian Islands there is not a single place of public amusement, excepting in Corfu, where there is a theatre, chiefly supported by government, in which operas and ballets are the principal performances,* designed to amuse, without regard to propriety, and much less to moral feeling and improvement, and which, it is presumed, have exerted, if any, an injurious influence on manners.

From the superior class let us now turn to the inferior, in which national character is better marked, and is more distinct and entire. The language which they speak is modern Greek, or Romaick ; their dress, too, is like that of their countrymen in continental Greece ; and their modes of life and usages, habits and manners, are very similar.

Their dress, both that of the men and women, is eminently graceful and picturesque ; similar, and yet various ; equally fitted to cover, and display to advantage the persons of the wearers. The articles composing the dress of the women in Corfu (where, perhaps, most attention is paid to dress, and it is most elaborate) consists of a short open habit—of a buttoned corslet or waistcoat, and of a long full plaited

---

there ; and no doubt for the same reason as in Venice, not to render it less attractive to strangers.

* Des *opéras buffons*, écrit en très mauvaise Italien, qui blessoient l'honnêteté et la modestie, des farces qui ne ménageoit point la pudeur, et des ballets qui faisaient frémir les mœurs." Such is Baron Theotoki's notice of them.—Op. Cit., p. 58.

petticoat and short apron, with sandals or shoes, and a head-dress, of which there are two or three forms in different parts of the island, and which imparts a distinctive appearance to the inhabitants. In the northern division, it is a white cloth, carefully bleached, so applied as to form a kind of trencher-cap, its broad end pendent hanging over the back. In the southern, it is formed of yellow muslin, wrapped about the head in the shape of a turban, and confining the long hair. Of the dress of the men, the principal articles consist of a jacket, waistcoat, breeches (*brachi largi*) and sash, shoes, or sandals, a small cap, brown or red, frequently confined by a shawl or a shawl turban, worn muffled about the neck. Varieties of dress, as regards the forms of the articles, occur in the other islands, which it would be tedious to enumerate. The women, it may be mentioned, are fond of ornaments, which, becomingly applied and worn, heighten much the gorgeous effect of their gala attire, which is often in part richly embroidered; namely, the sleeves of the habit and the corslet. Their favourite ornaments are ear-rings of silver and gold, gold chains, necklaces, in the instance of the wealthier, of precious stones, pins, brooches, bracelets, and a silver girdle. A pin, surmounted with a silver cock, is often used to confine the folds of the headdress. On public occasions, when a large number of people are assembled together, especially at Corfu, the appearance exhibited, from the variety and beauty, and richness of colouring of the different dresses of both sexes is eminently striking, and can hardly fail to excite admiration. A native writer, who dwells with manifest pleasure on the subject, pictures such an assemblage, in summer, which is the common festal season, collected on the green turf, under the shade of an olive-grove—broken by various accidents of light—and points it out truly as a scene well fitted for the study of the artist ; and especially, it may be added, when it is animated by the peculiar circular dance of the country and the music of the tambourin and pipe.

The manner of living of the small proprietors and the more substantial individuals of this class, differs but little from that of the higher order ; and the hours for their repasts are much the same, as, indeed, are those of the poorest. The food of the common people consists chiefly of bread, onions, garlic, cheese, Sardinias, and other salted fish ; of oil, wine, and wild herbs. In Corfu and Santa Maura, bread or cake of Indian corn is more used than wheaten bread. Butcher's-meat and poultry are very little used—seldom, excepting on festal occasions.

They generally reside in the villages, probably for the sake of greater security from pirates and brigands, at least formerly they had this reason—rarely in detached houses. Each village has its church and belfry; and from the trees, especially the cypress, intermixed with the houses, is commonly of very picturesque appearance. In Corfu some of the villages are, from their fine situation and the accessories, beautiful objects in the landscape; their site is most frequently the summit of a hill, or its ridge or steep declivity, and difficult of access, from the rugged nature of the ground—such as the village of Calafationes, in Corfu, the subject of the frontispiece to this volume.

Their houses are commonly substantially built, but they seldom contain much furniture. The labourer is considered well off, if, when married, he has a bed, formed of boards and trestles, and a large chest; in the better houses there may be a few tables and chairs. Their bedding, to their credit, is almost invariably clean. The napkin is placed on the plate at meals; and, even in the country, occasionally silver forks and spoons are in use. Fire-places, even in the country, and in the dwellings of the opulent farmers, are rarely seen; and often the windows are unglazed.

During the fine season, whether glazed or not, they are almost constantly kept open by day—allowing the swallows to fly in and out. In Greece, I may observe, these birds are almost domestic; cherished and protected, their nests are commonly to be seen in the farm-houses, not only outside, under the eaves, but also within, in rows along the beams of the principal room. Their presence is held to be of good omen; and their arrival in spring, which is regular almost to a day, is welcomed as such, as well as a proof of the pleasant time it ushers in.

The condition of the people, as regards means of subsistence, varies considerably in the different islands. It is best in the southern islands, where there is the largest number of small proprietors, or coloni, and where the price of labour is highest; and perhaps worst in Corfu; but even there the industrious can easily earn comfortable support, the field-labourers' pay being, as already remarked, about fifteen-pence a-day. Their habits are so frugal, and their food so cheap, that it is calculated that three or four days' work are sufficient to yield subsistence to a man and his family. Such facility of living engenders idleness, which is encouraged by the monstrous proportion of saints' days in the calendar. Amusement is indulged in by them to excess; I never was amongst a people so prone to it, and who had such apparent enjoyment in their sports. The dance is their favourite diversion in Corfu, in which both sexes join, to the wild music of a rustic pipe, and sometimes of the violin.* In Zante and in Cephalonia the wine-shop is more frequented, and boisterous conviviality practised; in the streets the riotous drunken chorus is common, interrupting the better-conducted serenaders, who, on a fine evening, are frequently to be heard, making very agreeable music,—little parties of young men, singing to the sound of the guitar, which, in the towns, where

* A rude drum, resembling an Indian tom-tom, is sometimes used by the villagers. On one occasion, when examining the coast of Corfu, on our boat approaching Point Avilla, the head-man (the primate) of the adjoining village came down with a party to oppose our landing, marching in military array to the sound of the pipe and tom-tom. The display of a Sanità flag averted their hostility, and, on landing, we found them very civil. Their military equipment was sufficiently picturesque—old long fowling-pieces, powder-flasks of gourds, suspended by cords, and cane bullet-cases.

Italian music is cultivated, is, with the violin, a favourite instrument.

So many holidays are made during the week, that it is not perhaps surprising that Sunday is hardly kept holy and made a day of rest. Baron Theotoki complains of one and of the other, and points out the evils resulting, injurious to industry and morals ; and he holds up to his countrymen the example of England—recommending that Sunday should be observed as a Sabbath, according to the law of Constantine,* and that the only other holidays kept should be the canonical ones, which, according to him, are not numerous. The just medium of relaxation and amusement for the labouring class is necessarily a difficult problem. In this country we have passed into the opposite extreme ; the people are over-tasked, and, it is to be feared, are too often rendered thereby moody and discontented, and, it may be, dissipated and seditious.

Wherever a people is little advanced in civilization, the lot of the female sex is commonly hard; and, I fear, this remark holds true of the women, at least of the inferior class, in these islands.† They are

---

* " Que tous les juges, tous les habitans, tous les artisans, se reposent le jour du soleil, à l'exception seulement des gens de la càmpagne, qui pourront travailler *en cas* de nécessité pendant le tems de la moisson et des vendanges, n'étant pas juste de laisser périr les biens que la Providence nous donne." This quotation is from the author referred to above.

† I have heard a lady, long resident in these islands, and well acquainted with female manners, speaking of the women generally in

subjected to much domestic drudgery; in some parts of the country, they have not only to convey water for the use of their families, but also to collect and gather wood. Where a fountain is situated at a convenient distance in a town or village, or its vicinity, and is of easy access, the task of water-carrying is an easy and agreeable one; it is commonly performed after sunset or in the early morning, and is made the occasion of gossip and often of merriment. It is a pleasant sight to see a party of women, assembled about the well or fountain, waiting their turn, well content with delay; or walking home in company, gracefully carrying their earthen-ware pitchers, of classical forms, nicely poised on their heads, their hands and arms free, if not employed in knitting or spinning. But if the distance is considerable, as is often the case, particularly in the mountainous parts of the islands, and the paths steep and rugged, and instead of the earthen vase, supported on the head, with the myrtle branch to prevent splashing, it is necessary to use a barrel and carry it on the back, then the labour is often severe, and the sight of the bent form toiling under its burthen is anything but

Zante and Santa Maura, divide them into three classes: those of the higher order in independent circumstances; those of the lower, having no objection to go out and be employed in service; and an intermediate class, supporting themselves in part or entirely by needlework and embroidery, and who, like the upper class in these islands, lead a very secluded life. She made the distinction in reference to a medical officer, who unreasonably expected that women of the second class, for whom he had to prescribe, should come to his hospital.

pleasing, as is also the effect on the carriage and shape of the women.*

On the ceremonies of marriage, baptism, and burial, a few remarks may suffice. They are performed according to the forms of the Greek Church, occasionally intermixed with superstitious usages, some of which probably have descended from ancient times. The priest, in Zante, commences the marriage-rite with a declaration of excommunication against any enemy of the betrothed, who may practise magic to prevent a happy union. On returning to his house with the bride, the bridegroom carefully avoids the way by which he came. On entering the door of the house, the mother is in waiting to present a spoonful of honey and pomegranate, of which they partake,— expressing the hope that they may be as sweet as the one and as united as the other. At the marriage-dinner, a pair of roasted pigeons is placed before them, of which they eat together, emblematic of that love which becomes the marriage-state. Even amongst the lower classes, marriages are made by contract, managed by the friends,† and are commonly inde-

---

* In manners this class is commonly civil, respectful, and courteous, and consequently they appear to much advantage to strangers. They are generally a handsome people, peculiarly graceful in their carriage, and easy in all their movements: the mildness of the climate, the form of dress, the light shoe or sandal, all conduce to ease and gracefulness of motion, excepting in the instances just before mentioned, of the females compelled to the toil of carrying water and wood on the back.

† Baron Theotoki, under the head of marriages, remarks—"Dans

pendent of courtship; the first advance is made by the family of the bridegroom, and when preliminaries are settled, he presents some trinket to the bride, through the hands of his mother or sister. In fixing her dower, the articles included are either in threes or fives, even numbers being considered unlucky. The coronals or garlands of myrtle or olive, which are used in the marriage-ceremony, are commonly carefully preserved, attached to the wall of the sleeping-apartment, above the head of the bed, sometimes one on each side of a print of a patron saint.

The respect shown to the dead in the Ionian Islands is not great: the interment commonly takes place within twenty-four hours from the fatal event. The body, after having been washed and dressed for the occasion, is carried on a bier, the face exposed to the gaze of the multitude. After the religious rite is over, the most affecting part is left to hired care, the mourners retire before the body is committed to the earth. The practice prevails of burying in churches;* the body, without a coffin, is deposited in

la ville, assez généralment, ce sont les courtiers qui font les mariages, et à la campagne les prêtres, les vieilles femmes, et les pères de famille d'une probité reconnue. C'est qu'effectivement les gens de la ville, le plus souvent *épousent la dot*, et necessairement s'adressent à ceux, qui ne s'y entendent pas mal: les autres *épousent la fille*, et désirent avoir un garant, responsible en quelque sorte, de sa valeur personnelle. Aussi, sur cent mariages de la ville, il y en a toujours un, romper, cassé, ou dissous: et sur mille de la campagne, il y en aura, tout au plus un qui réclamera les soins paternels de l'autorité ecclésiastique.' —P. 120.

* Recently a cemetery has been formed for the town of Corfu, in

a common grave; the individual, however worthy, however respected, however much loved, in his grave receives no marks either of public or of private regard; no inscription commemorates his virtues, not a stone even marks the spot. Where grave-yards are used, as they are in some parts of the country, they are totally neglected, and were we not informed, in passing, of their object, it would be impossible, from their appearance, to conjecture it. One of the greatest men of ancient Greece declared to the Athenian people, " that where the greatest rewards are proposed for virtue, there the best patriots are ever to be found." This was said in a funeral oration in honour of men who had died in the service of their country; how worthy is this excellent truth and noble sentiment of the attention of the moderns, especially in these islands, where it appears to be entirely unknown, or, what is equivalent, disjoined from practice and conduct.

Many superstitions are connected with the dead, commonly of a kind to excite fear and abhorrence, and very unworthy of reflecting minds: some of them have been already alluded to. Probably were minute inquiry made, vestiges of ancient usages would be

the neighbourhood of Castrades, for which the people are indebted, amongst other important works, to Sir Howard Douglas. I am informed that the prejudice against it, and in favour of the old bad practice of burying in churches, is wearing away, and that it is rapidly coming into general use. It was opened in September 1840; the number of interments in it, up to January 1842, I am informed, have been 501.

found to exist in the manner of treating the dead, notwithstanding all that is honourable and distinctive has passed away. I may mention one little incident which has come to my knowledge : in the island of Fanò, the friends of the deceased who attend the funeral, before they part, drink a portion of a cup of wine in the church, and pour the remainder into the grave.

In any of the preceding remarks seeming to imply censure, I would not wish to be understood as expressing an opinion, that these people are deficient in natural affection, or in tender regard to departed friends : my remarks are directed to the absence of public demonstrations of these feelings. According to the forms of their religion, they perform masses for the dead ; and some, it is said, commemorate the event ever after, annually.

As further illustrative of the manners of this class, in the next chapter I shall give an account of a little tour which I made through the mountainous district of Zante, in the summer of 1824, a portion of the island seldom visited,—and where, in consequence of seclusion, the native manners are to be seen least adulterated.

Of the moral character of the people, of their virtues and vices, it may be better at present to avoid discussion. For a number of years ill-governed,— subject to a code of laws (the old Venetian laws) which have been described by competent judges as disgraceful to common sense and justice,—uneducated and ignorant,—under the influence of an illiterate, bigoted, and superstitious priesthood,—it would be nowise reasonable to expect to find them distinguished for a fine moral sense, integrity of purpose, and correctness of conduct; one might as well expect to find cleanliness of habits in a town where water is sold, as was the case in Corfu before the construction of its aqueduct, or literary and scientific tastes and habits, where there are no institutions to form them. That they have excellent natural abilities, is unquestionable; fine senses, lively feelings; a great aptitude to learn. It may be hoped, therefore, that, under good institutions, they will become an enlightened, honest, and respectable people. The new codes of civil and criminal law, lately brought into use,—the extension of education, now in progress,—and the diffusion of useful knowledge,—must be powerfully instrumental in effecting improvement; and if religious and moral instruction keep pace,—if the priesthood become qualified for their high office, and gain the respect of their flock, and perform their duties conscientiously,—the regeneration alluded to can hardly fail to take place; but of this latter part, not much reasonable hope can be entertained, unless the Greek Church in the Ionian Islands is rendered independent of the patriarch of Constantinople, and of that injurious influence and control which has been commonly exercised by him and his agents,—too often, it is believed, in connexion with political intrigue, exciting dissension, and occasionally promoting conspiracy and rebellion.

The same motive that induces me to avoid the discussion of the subjects just alluded to,—the moral features, the vices and virtues of this people,—prompts me to make some extracts from the writings of others, to show how very differently their character has been estimated, and what very little reliance is to be placed in sweeping conclusions on points of such extreme difficulty, in relation to the ascertaining of truth. Moreover, I do hope, should this work reach the Ionian Islands and be read by any of their inhabitants, that both the accounts of the vices and virtues attributed to them, may have a beneficial effect,—in the one instance, in exciting an honest indignation with a determination to prove, by their conduct, that they have been aspersed; and in the other, in producing an opposite feeling,—an ambition, to prove themselves worthy of the praises bestowed on them, and to show that it has not been unearned or dealt out as flattery.

The author whose opinion I shall first notice, is the late Dr Hennen,—an individual of some talent, but whose own knowledge of the people he described was very limited: in his " Sketches of the Medical Topography of the Mediterranean," when treating of Corfu, under the head of "Morals," he thus expresses himself of the Ionian Greeks in general :—

" It would be unphilosophical and unjust to deny that many individuals of strict integrity and unblemished honour may be found among the Ionian islanders ; but the concurrent testimony of all who have governed, resided among, or trafficked with them, justify us in asserting that the national character is the very lowest in Europe.

Vanity is the predominant characteristic of almost every individual, however low in rank he may be. But of what are they vain? Among them, before they came under British protection, justice was openly sold to the highest bidders; public faith was unknown; and as to individual veracity, Greek falsehood (*Græcia mendax*) is proverbial. The instances are rare in which these islanders do not exhibit an uncontrolled propensity to revenge, litigation, and political intrigue, cloaked under the thin veil of patriotic enthusiasm for the national glory. These objects they pursue with all the pertinacity of vice, and with scarcely one redeeming qualification. Tyrannical to their inferiors, they are to their equals and superiors what Juvenal long since described them:—

" Adulandi gens prudentissima."

Their clergy are taken from the very scum of the population, and are, with few exceptions, illiterate, superstitious, and immoral. Their nobles are without honour, their merchants without integrity, and their peasantry ignorant and degraded to the most abject degree."

" Whence (he proceeds) this lamentable decadence may have proceeded, this is not the place to investigate. It pervades all ranks, from the palace (and every house of more than ordinary size is called a palace) to the cottage. That the Greek character, in general, has been greatly debased by their long endurance of Turkish tyranny and Venetian prostitution, as exerted on the continent and in the islands, is agreed on all sides, and is consonant with what the history of man has, in every age, presented to our view; but one of the principal causes is to be found in the depravity and ignorance of their clergy. Many of these persons can barely read their breviary. Few, if any, acts of private atrocity or rebellion have occurred in the islands, which have not been planned, and in fact executed by the priests; and there are few gangs of robbers or pirates which have not their chaplain. I know many who publicly keep concubines, although a wife is allowed them by their religion;* and yet some of these reverend sinners pretend to a sanctity and chastity quite superhuman."

Contrasted with this account, is that of another medical writer, Dr Lazaro de Mordo, for many years

* " Marriage does not hinder any person, if he be not otherwise unqualified, from being put into holy orders; nor is such a one obliged to live from his wife. But the general practice of the church is

proto-medico of Corfu, and who, in 1808, published
a short account of the island, for a perusal of which

against marriage after orders; so that, if any priest, once married,
should marry a second time, much more if a priest, not before married, should enter into this state, they are liable to censures; and, as
if the character imprinted upon them, when they were made priests,
were by this act razed out, they are esteemed as mere Laicks, and accounted Παρά νομοι or flagitious persons, and transgressors of the laws
and canons of the church."—An Account of the Greek Church, by
T. Smith, B. D. London, 1680. Speaking of the clergy generally,
this writer observes:—" Considering the poverty of the Greek
church, and the scanty provisions (on the voluntary system, be it kept
in recollection), made for such as enter into holy orders, there being
no rich livings to invite them to do so, it must only be a principle of
conscience, at first, that makes them willing to take up that holy
calling, which deprives them of all other ways and means of getting
a subsistence. For the clergy must be content with their allowance,
and not think to better their condition by busying themselves in any
secular employment, as being altogether inconsistent with their holy
profession. But custom and long use make things most troublesome
and difficult to be borne, easy at last. It is accounted a good prefer-
ment, if, in a country village, the poor priest can make, in the whole
year, forty crowns, out of which he pays a proportion to his bishop.
For there being no lands belonging to the church besides the small
allowance agreed upon at first by him and the people, they pay him
so many aspers for christening their children, giving them the sacrament upon extraordinary occasions, burying their dead, and performing other funeral rites, an the like. And, on the great festivals, they
present him with money, or what is money-worth, that he may expressly mention their names, or their relations, whether alive or
dead, when he comes to that part of the liturgick-service in the celebration of the sacrament, where such commemorations are used, as believing such a recommendation, made by the priest at that solemn
time, to be of great force and efficacy." The author wrote of the
Greek church amongst the Mohammedans, of which, in his travels, he
appears to have had good opportunities of judging; but most of the
above remarks are at present applicable to the clergy of this church
in the Ionian Islands.

I am indebted to a gentleman well acquainted with him, who informs me that he was generally respected for his worth and integrity. According to this author, the characteristic of the Corfiots is good sense. He says they are fond of letters, easily reconciled, readily forget an offence; are grateful and prudent. The lower classes, especially the peasantry (villani), are extremely punctilious, fond of praise, and are unwearied in exertion to obtain it. The Corfiots, he remarks, are accused of two faults principally—inhospitality and vain-glory. The first charge he considers as altogether unjust; and in proof, he asserts that there is no country, in proportion to its population, in which there are so many resident foreigners as in Corfu, and he declares that at least two-thirds of all the possessions in the island have passed into the hands of strangers. The other charge, that of vain-glory, he partially admits, prefacing the admission with the saying of Gerbellio, "*E chi non ha difetti?*" He considers and extenuates it as a relict of their ancient glory, supported, in its decline, by the preference given to them, amongst the islanders, by their Venetian rulers, with whom it was not an uncommon thing to be connected by marriage; and in relation to this, he observes, how great is the pleasure to a man of any feeling, to see one nearly allied to him filling the office of Bailo, of Provveditore, and of other high functionaries;—to look on the portraits of their ancestors dressed *alla grande*, and adorned magnificently! He adds, in confirmation, that in his

time, there were preserved in Corfiot families the
colours of the galleys which, on many occasions, had
been armed at the expense of private individuals;
and he goes on to say, that in the last revolution (I
suppose he alludes to that which was fatal to the
republic) the strongest proof was given of the gener-
ous feeling excited: all were faithful to the sovereign
power.*

Dr Lazaro de Mordo was a Jew. The next author
whose opinion I shall give, was also a native, and of
Corfu, the Baron Theotoki, whom I have already so
often quoted.

"*Hommes.* L'on voit rarement sur les visages des habitans des
traits indécis, grossiers, ou irréguliers : au contraire tout ce qui les
caractérise est noble et spirituel. La forme de leur visage est advan-
tageuse, précise et décidée; toutes les parties s'accordent et sont en
harmonie avec le tout. Ils ont assez généralement les cheveux châtains, ou noirs, et rarement blonds: la peau brune claire, le teint
coloré, les yeux noirs, le regard pénétrant, la physionomie intéréss-
sante. Le genre de beauté est achevé, dans tous les classes. La tête
d'un pâtre et d'un forgeron, figureroient dans un tableau aussi bien
que celle de Thésée et de Platon. Les têtes des viellards sur tout,
sont distinguées : la grande taille n'y est point rare, et tout son
developpment est remarquable.

" Le partage moral est un esprit fin, subtil, vif, imperieux : beaucoup de bile d'ou parte une irritabilitée subite, et véhémente : une
penetration immediate : un desir très-animé pour le merveilleux :
et ce doux penchant à la melancholie, qui renferme les germes du
génie.

" Le manque d'émulation, la pauvreté, la servitude de quelques
siécles, et les calamités qui l'accompagnent y ont pu laisser les esprits
et les âmes sans ressort. L'ignorance a dû prevaloir : et des vices

---

* Nozioni Miscellanee intorno a Corcira, esposte dal Medico fisico
Collegiato Lazaro de Mordo.

necessaires chez un peuple, rempli de forces morales nullement appli-
quees, et entouré d'exemples contagieux, devoient plus ou moins
glisser et s'y enraciner. Mais tout cela n'a été, et n'est, qu' accessoire
et momentane. Le fond du caractère observé en physicien impartial,
est effectivement celui que je viens d'exposer." *

The last opinion I shall extract is that of Sir

* The Baron Theotoki's description of his countrywomen may amuse
the reader ; and in reading it, let him keep in recollection that the
author was twice President of the Senate, the highest office that a
native of the islands can fill, and second only to that of the Lord
High Commissioner.

" *Femmes.*—Les femmes sont Grecques ; savoir belles femmes et
jolies. Généralement, sous des sourcils bruns, des yeux radians,
roulent une prunelle noire enflammée. L'éclat des charmes d'un
visage ovale, inquiet, mysterieux, et negatif, les environne comme
des rayons de lumière. Leur taille est avantageuse et svelte. Elles
ont assez ordinairement le teint brun clair, le front ouvert, le nez
affilé et delicat, les joues animées, les cheveux châtains dorés, ou
noirs touffus, le corps adroit, agile, bien fait. Tout y annonce l'air
ingénu d'une virilité florissante, et d'une santé inalterable.

" Le plus léger duvet trahit l'âge et le sexe, et ombrage quelquefois le dessus de la lèvre supérieure, et les bras: ce qui fait ressortir
de toute la personne une teinte de ferocité intrepide, d'un effet ener-
gique et piquant.

" Leur voix est passionée, flexible, et en même tems étendue, de-
licé, agréable. Les poëtes diroient que c'est la plainte de Zéphyr sur
des collines de neige.

" Elles portent la tête levée, comme pour admirer la beauté de leur
ciel ; si elles s'inclinent quelquefois, c'est, pour laisser échapper des
soupirs, essor naturel d'une âme fervente et active.

" Quant au caractère, elles réunissent des qualités qui paroissent
opposées ; mais qui decoulent, dans leur source, d'un seul element.
Franches, simples, sobres, dociles, reservées, elles ont une intelligence
délicate et habile, une phantaisie romanesque, et une vivacité que l'on
irrite par la moindre violence ; mais aussi faciles à emouvoir qu' à ap-
paiser, elles sont très-aisées à conduire, et à engager dans les entre-
prises les plus dangereuse ; surtout s'il agit de religion, de patrie, ou
de famille."

Baron Theotoki enters further into their character; but as his pic-

Charles Napier, expressed in the opening of the pre-
face to his singular work on the Ionian Islands.   His
words are :—

"Having for many years governed the largest of the Ionian Islands,
and gained some experience with regard to the character of the people,
and their resources, I naturally feel much interested in their fate.
However full of faults the Ionians may be, I maintain that they have
not more than might be expected from the corruptness of the Venetian
domination, from those human frailties which are so conspicuous in
small societies, and from a natural vehemence of character that dis-
tinguishes the Greek people : but, on the other hand, they are endowed
with virtues that are no less prominent ; if they have received much
evil from education, they have received much good from nature ; and
I found more of the latter than the state of society led me to expect.
The richer classes are lively and agreeable in their manners ; and,
among the men, many are well informed.   The women possess both
beauty and wit in abundance, but their education has been, generally
speaking, much neglected.   The poor are not less industrious than
other southern nations ; and an extraordinary degree of intelligence
characterises all ranks.   A spirit of commercial enterprise distin-
guishes the hardy mountaineers of Cephalonia ; they are full of pleasant humour and vivacity, and their resemblance to the Irish people
is striking, in every thing but their sobriety ; for, though the Cephalonian labourer drinks freely of the potent wines which his mountains
so abundantly produce, yet a drunken man is seldom to be seen, and
among the rich inebriety is unknown.   Such is the character of the
people with whom I have passed the most pleasant years of my life."

---

ture may be considered somewhat poetical, I shall transcribe only one
other paragraph, and that a concluding one.   Referring to his eulogies of his countrywomen, he says :—

"Il ne faut pas, cependant, en chercher beaucoup (de l'espèce de-
crite par cet article) dans la ville, où assez generalement une éduca-
tion sotte, pedantesque, et stérile, fâne et detruit les germes d'une
beauté jeune et delicate, aussi bien que les éléments des dispositions
morales les plus heureuse.   Il faut plutôt aller les admirer à la campagne, où l'on permet à la nature d'étaler ses forces en tous sens, et de
montrer tout ce qu' elle peut, en faveur de cette portion précieuse de
l'humanité."

CHAPTER VIII.

NOTICE OF A JOURNEY THROUGH THE MOUNTAINOUS
DISTRICT OF ZANTE IN 1824.

This District hitherto imperfectly known. Particulars of Catastari.
Monastery of Speliotissa. Character of the adjoining Hilly
Country. Volimes. Pitiable Condition of the Sick. Total Des-
titution of Medical Aid. Free, independent Life of the Inhabi-
tants. Monastery of St Georgio. Bay of Vromi. Prospects
from the Heights of Vrachiona. Village of Maries. Houses and
Habits of the Villagers. Cisterns of Oxicora and its basin-like
Valley. St Leo. Instances of remarkable Longevity. Large
Apiary. Basin-like Valley of Luca. Coldness of its Climate.
Monastery of Madonna Paragato. Woodcock Shooting. Gilli-
amano. Village School. Neglected Grave-Yard. House of the
Priest. Farther Particulars respecting the Occupations of the
People. Comparative Severity of the Winter Season. Villages
of Ambelo and Chieri. Malaria of the former. Manner of
Snaring Doves. Diglidani's Leap. Cultivation and Peculiarities
of the Currant-Vine in the Valley of the Pitch-Springs. Appear-
ance and Dress of the People in the Mountain Villages.

IN the former chapter I have alluded to the great
seclusion of the mountainous or hilly district of
Zante; and in proof, I may mention that the gentleman with whom I had the pleasure to visit it, although
he had been many years in the island, and filled
a situation connected with its revenue—and, more-

over, was fond of inquiry, yet, in common with the majority of the inhabitants of the city, he had never penetrated into its recesses—to him, as to them, it was a terra incognita, vaguely known only by report.

We set out together on this little exploring excursion on horseback. It was the height of summer when we started, the 26th of August—the time of the currant-gathering—when a continuance of dry weather, then so important, is looked for with confidence, and when the country, from the activity prevailing in consequence, is seen to advantage.

Crossing the beautiful plain, we stopped for the night at the village of Catastari, close to the bay of the same name, and almost skirting the mountain barrier. It has been before mentioned, that scattered solitary houses, with a few exceptions, are very uncommon in these islands, and that the natives residing in this country live chiefly in villages. The most remarkable exception to this is the plain of Zante; and it owes very much of its peculiar beauty to the villas and farm-houses dotting its surface, each commonly white-washed—in the midst of trees—the cypress and orange the most conspicuous, and frequently enclosed by a fence of aloes. At that time a macadamized road was only just commenced; the island was without a carriage-road; we met mules, in rapid succession, coming towards the town, laden with bags of new currants, each led by an attendant. On our way we called at the villas of several of the proprietors, most of whom we found at home, super intending the gathering of their valuable crop; at one we were received by the lady of the house, in the absence of her husband; she was young and handsome—indeed, the reputed belle of Zante, and withal a countess. She was at the door when we arrived with some female servants, her infant in her arms, and so plainly attired, as to be hardly distinguishable by her dress.

It was twilight when we reached Catastari. We were shown into a good house, belonging to the capo; it was newly built, clean, and well furnished; and the middle, " the upper room " (the reception, eating, and sitting-room combined), " the guest-chamber," was well lighted by the common lamp of the country, fed with olive-oil.* My friend had sent his servants on before; and we found the table laid with clean linen, napkins, &c., belonging to the family. After washing off the dust, an operation which was performed very much in the eastern manner, by the pouring of water by a domestic from a vase on the hands held over a ewer, without much delay we sat down to table, in company with three others, one the son of our host; who was the notary of the village : another a native belonging to the office of my friend, a stout, jolly fellow, well acquainted with the country, having had to travel through it twice a-year for the purpose of collecting certain government dues, and whom we intended to take with

* A figure of this kind of lamp is given in Plate VI.

us as interpreter and purveyor; and the third, a Sicilian, in the employment of government, in charge
of the adjoining salines. The repast was a substantial
one, according to usage, consisting of roast turkey,*
ham, and fowls, with abundance of wine of the place,
of an agreeable flavour, but too new to be wholesome.
During the meal, the conversation was chiefly concerning the village, which is the largest in the island,
possessing about three hundred families,† many of
them in easy, and some of them in opulent, circumstances. In common with other villages, besides a
capo, or primate, it has three inspectors, who are
selected by the head of the island police, with the
approval of the local government. The duty of the
capo is to receive and execute the orders of government, and to arbitrate upon and settle the disputes of
the inhabitants, with the aid of the inspectors. I
have mentioned there was a notary, as there is in
most of the large villages; there were two medical
men, several priests, many blacksmiths and carpenters,
but no shopkeepers—the villagers supplying themselves with all the necessaries of life, and procuring

* The turkey is a favourite article of the table in Zante, and is
consumed in large numbers by the wealthy class. Few are bred in
the island. In prosperous times, before the invasion of the Morea by
the Egyptians, the usual number imported from that quarter annually
was 15,000; a flock of them is frequently to be seen in charge of a
boy—who, with a long white rod in his hand, keeping them before
him, drives them about.

† According to the census of 1839, the number of inhabitants of this
village was 1136; or, including that of the contiguous little village of
Centato, considered as belonging to it, 1321.

from *the city*, as the town is called, all their super-
fluities and luxuries, which, indeed, are very few.   I
saw one of the medical men, a native, and conversed
with him in Latin, which he spoke pretty fluently.
He appeared to be an intelligent man, considering the
few opportunities he had for improving himself.   He
had studied, he said, only the theoretical part of medicine; had never seen a dissection; and had never
been in Italy.   He spoke in praise of the salubrity
of the place; the ordinary diseases, he said, in summer, were intermittent and remittent fever, which he
attributed to the effect of the wind from the plain;
and in winter and spring pneumonia and rheumatism.
At ten o'clock we retired to rest, and had good clean
beds.   The bed-rooms, four in number, of small dimensions, opened into the hall or middle room; they
were tolerably neat and clean, and free from vermin;
had the floors been washed, they would have been
almost unexceptionable; but it appears to be contrary
to the custom of the natives either to paint or to
wash, and, in consequence, their floors and wainscot
are neat only when new.

On the following morning, after breakfast, we
continued our journey, and in about three hours,
after a rather laborious ascent through a rugged pass,
at the foot of which the marl formation of the plain
is succeeded by mountain limestone, we arrived at
the monastery of Speliotissa, situated in a hollow of
the mountains, and distant, it is reckoned, from
Catastari about nine and a-half miles   The contrast

between the luxuriant plain we had just before left, and the surrounding hills, was striking: the vegetation was scanty and stunted, and confined chiefly to the fissures of the rocks of grey limestone; the arbutus was the common shrub; the myrtle did not reach so high; heath and wild thyme were abundant. Excepting a small space of arable ground in which the monastery stood, then in stubble and in possession of a large flock of goats, not a single spot bearing marks of cultivation was visible   The monastery is a pretty extensive building, in the form of a hollow square, within which is a neat chapel, containing a picture of the Virgin Mary, said to have been found in an adjoining cave, and in honour of which the edifice was erected.   The establishment supports a priest and thirteen calloyers or lay-brothers, the main occupation of the latter of whom is to till the ground and look after the flocks.   Here we rested and took some refreshment during the heat of the day, and experienced much civility from the inmates, one of whose duties is to receive strangers, for which an allowance is made by government,—a humane and very necessary measure, in a wild and thinly peopled country, without inns or rest-houses.   Before taking leave, the Papa brought me a patient—a little boy, a relative of his own—labouring under chronic disease of the abdominal viscera, the consequence of fever contracted in the plain, who, on coming to me, prettily kissed my hand, according to the graceful usage of the country.

About one o'clock we renewed our journey, directing our course towards the village of Volimes, on the
way to another monastery, that of St Georgio, where
it was our intention to pass the night. Proceeding
by a winding bridle-path along the sides of the hills,
we passed by some patches of vineyard, and observed
that the bottom of the glen was similarly cultivated
by means of terraces, in which the soil was confined
by stone-walls. These vineyards are the property of
the monastery. We saw no houses,—only a few
stone-huts, of the rudest construction, to shelter
cattle; each, in fact, was a pile of stones, in the form
of a hollow dome.

There are three villages of the name of Volimes,
Upper, Middle, and Lower. Upper Volimes is about
three miles from Speliotissa; it is small and neatly
built, but without trees. Passing through and crossing
some corn-fields, we came to Middle Volimes, a larger
village than the former, and containing some good
houses. By the way, we were led to a spot where, it
is said, gold was once found, in scales mixed with
the soil. The proprietor of the field had covered the
spot with a heap of earth, to prevent others from
collecting the imaginary treasure, and not without
apprehension that the government would seize on it.
From the appearance of the soil, I had little doubt
that the presence of a little mica, in minute plates,
had given rise to the opinion. During the few
minutes we stopped in the village, I was asked to
visit a poor man supposed to be dying; I found him

in a small, close, dark room, with a light burning, and three women in attendance; one, his wife, who was on the bed with him sitting, supporting his head: he was in the last stage of debility, from a neglected diarrhœa: during his illness he had used little else than bread and water; he died the following day. Neither in this nor in any other village amongst the mountains, as I afterwards found, is there a medical man; nor can the inhabitants procure any medicine or advice nearer than Catastari; consequently, almost all their complaints, of any duration, are left to take their natural course,—for, with the exception of a dose of rhubarb or an enema, there is seldom any interference, unless, perhaps, at the commencement of illness, when, as our Greek interpreter informed me, it was usual to take a large draught of wine, about a pint, in which a bulky crust of toasted or burnt bread had been extinguished, eating at the same time the bread. I was also consulted by a man labouring under serious organic disease of some of the abdominal viscera, the effect of a severe blow received a year and half ago. I here began to make inquiry relative to the occurrence of earthquakes above the Plain, and was assured that, in this village, as well as in the other highland villages, a shock was rarely felt, and that the great earthquake of 1821, which did so much damage in the town, was only just perceived. This part of the country is without springs; and each house has its own cistern or cisterns for receiving and retaining rain-water. No rain had fallen since April. The view around was peculiar, and not uncharacteristic: both Upper and Lower Volimes may be seen at once,—collections of stone-buildings, without a single tree, with two or three wind-mills on the heights in their neighbourhood. The adjoining country equally destitute of wood, is divided by stone-walls into large fields, in which cattle and sheep were feeding, apparently on the stones which are scattered over the surface in abundance, —I say apparently, for the surface was completely parched ; and on minute observation, very little was to be seen excepting a few dried blades of grass and a little stubble, all the cultivated ground here being arable. The general appearance of the country reminded my companion of some parts of Portugal.

We did not visit Lower Volimes (a very inconsiderable village situated near the sea), but proceeded direct to the monastery of St Georgio, distant about three miles from Middle Volimes. In descending, we passed several vineyards on the sides of the hills and in the lower parts of the valleys, and observed also a good deal of ground lying waste, probably admitting of easy cultivation. We met a party of villagers, who, with their dogs and guns, had been out shooting; they had killed a hare, which the Capo, who was of the party, very civilly sent us as a present. The liberty which these mountaineers enjoy, must give a great charm to the kind of life which they follow, and attach them strongly to their native place. Almost all

are on an equality; they must live quite independent
and free; and their general air and manner betokened
it.   They have no game-laws,—no great landed proprietors,—no gentlemen; they are all cultivators and
labourers, ploughing their own fields, tending their
own flocks; and he must become richest who is most
industrious, and who has most children to assist him.
Descending gradually, the turn of a hill brought us
suddenly in sight of a pretty extensive grove of firs,
which, being of a lively green, made a very agreeable
appearance: they seemed to be growing wild, and re-
sembled the Scotch fir. The air was strongly perfumed
by the resin which exuded from them, and the smell
was more like that of myrrh than of turpentine.
Crossing this grove, we arrived at the monastery of
St Georgio, where we found excellent quarters.

We were tempted by the freshness of the air, the
proximity of the sea, and the noble appearance which
the Black Mountain, just opposite, in Cephalonia,
made, to descend almost immediately to the shore,
about a mile or less distant.   The sea scenery we
found very magnificent; the cliffs almost white, from
two to three or four hundred feet high, in many
places perpendicular, very irregular from their projecting headlands and bendings, fringed above by
wild shrubs, and occasionally with fir-trees, and
washed by a bright blue sea, which was beautifully
clear, excepting where rendered slightly of a milky
hue by the disintegration of the soft calcareous rock,
from the action of the waves.   The most conspicuous

of the near objects was a bold headland, of singular and grand appearance, almost detached from the adjoining cliff, which, we were informed, was formerly the site of the monastery of St George. The ancient monastery, of which there are now no traces remaining, excepting eighteen cisterns, is said to have been founded seven hundred years ago,—four hundred before the present building, which was erected by the Spaniards, and by them fortified with a tower.

Observing a little arched-way in a small valley running down towards the sea, we descended to examine it; it proved to be a small cavern in the limestone rock, luxuriantly shaded with wild myrtle, rosemary, and arbutus; above which was another cave of larger dimensions, partly lighted by a perforation in its roof. Here we were assured that Saint Jerasimo took refuge when he was ill-treated and pelted with stones by the inhabitants of Plemcnario, a neighbouring village, and that from hence he crossed over to Cephalonia, of which island he became the tutelary saint.

The monastery of St Georgio has the reputation of being the oldest as well as the best in the island. It supports two monks and twelve lay-brothers. The latter are allowed a ration of bread and oil daily, a small sum monthly to purchase shoes, ten dollars a year, and an apartment each in the convent. As the situation is an easy one, it is in request amongst the lower orders: celibacy is required of them, and daily attendance, during divine service, in the church of

the monastery, when at home and not employed. I
was requested to visit one of them, whom I found
labouring under a slight attack of pneumonia; he
occupied a small cell, without a window and without
a fire-place, and furnished only with a bed and a
chest. As the style of architecture of the monastery
indicates, it has been built at different times; the
oldest part of it is a round tower, evidently designed
for defence, now in a state of decay. The chapel,
neat and in good repair, a newer structure, contains
a relic of St George, contributed, at some distant
period, by the Patriarch of Constantinople, and also
a picture of the warrior saint on horseback, armed
cap-a-piè, trampling on the dragon. Behind the
chapel is a small cemetery, where the monks are
buried; after three or four years the skulls are taken
up and placed under a shed; they may amount to
about forty. On the wall close to the entrance, is
the following inscription, rudely cut in stone:—

> Viator chi guardi in su
> Io son stato come sei tu
> Sarai come son io
> Pensa a te, e va con Dio.

The part of the building which we occupied was
quite new and good, consisting of two storeys. The
upper one, set apart for strangers, is entered by a
flight of steps and a small balcony, the roof of which
is supported by neat stone pillars. It consists of a
large hall, tolerably well furnished, and of two small
bed-rooms, provided with good beds and clean linen,

and has adjoining requisite offices, as kitchen and stable.   After the close heat of the town, we found the cool fresh air of this place particularly agreeable and refreshing, especially in the morning early, and after sunset; at half-past nine, the first evening we were here, the thermometer was at 70°; and the following morning at six it was as low as 68°.

From hence, on the 28th, we went to the little bay of Vromi, returning to sleep at the monastery. Passing over some naked hills, where we saw a good deal of ground cultivated, chiefly arable, with a few vineyards here and there, we came to the village of Plemonario, about two miles from the monastery, situated rather low, and in its lowest part skirted by some fields, having a deep red soil, in which are many olive-trees of considerable size, and apparently very old.   The tradition is, that the Saint of Cephalonia, in consequence of the treatment which he experienced here, pronounced a malediction on the place, owing to which a great part of the population was soon swept off by disease, and the village never after flourished.   Now it is thought to be reviving; but still it has a cursed appearance, and looks sufficiently miserable.   About a mile nearer the sea, we came to the monastery of Santa Madonna Annafonitra, a hollow square building like that of St Georgio, and provided with a similar round tower: it is finely situated in a small plain surrounded by bold hills, which to the eastward are covered with wood, chiefly low pines.   Beyond the monastery, the road proved, excessively bad; we were mounted on mules, having left our horses to rest at the convent; it was so steep and rocky, as to be hardly passable by them; and when we came to the brow of the hill above Vromi, it was necessary to dismount and scramble down to the shore on foot. This part of the country is generally covered with brushwood, with clumps of firs interspersed; the ground is almost mountainous; the valleys deep, their sides precipitous, without traces of cultivation. The shore has the same bold character as that in the neighbourhood of St Georgio, and the cliffs are similarly composed, and as lofty; in more than one place, they present an escarpment towards the land, and a precipice towards the sea. The bay of Vromi is a narrow inlet, not a quarter of a mile deep, open to the south-west, and without a landing-place, excepting two spots of sandy beach practicable for a boat. Its shore is rocky and precipitous, and its water apparently deep. It is said to be the resort of smugglers; but of this we saw no indications. As it may probably afford shelter to small craft, and perhaps to large vessels with particular winds, it may be deserving of being carefully surveyed. The approach to it, it may be remarked, is rendered more difficult by the islet of the same name contiguous.

After breakfast on the 29th, we left St Georgio, and proceeded to Maries, about four or five miles distant, a very pretty and considerable village, situated towards the head of a fine valley,—a great part of it cultivated, either covered with vineyards or

spotted with olive-trees, the cypress and fir intermixed. Even in the village, the cypress was common; and in graceful clumps amongst neat white-
washed houses, in company with the vine and fig-
tree, imparted peculiar beauty to the spot, the sense
of which, perhaps, was heightened by the wild and
rocky barrier of hill on each side. We took up
our quarters in the best house in the place, belonging to a wealthy farmer, said to be worth thirty
thousand Spanish dollars, though, from the meanness
of his appearance, it might be supposed he was not
worth one. When we inquired why he was so
meanly dressed, we were told it was the custom of
the country, and that he took pride in seeing his
children well dressed, rather than in being so himself. As soon as mules could be procured, and after
I had prescribed for some sick people, we set out to
ascend Vrachiona, reputed to be the highest mountain in the island. The ascent was not difficult, and
was pretty gradual, excepting where we crossed two
small plains, or rather concavities, which in winter are
under water, having no outlet, and in spring become dry
from evaporation. Vrachiona has two summits, separated by a moderately deep valley, and about a mile
and half asunder. It is commonly said that that to the
northward is the highest; but this is doubtful, judging
from the indications of the barometer.*

* At eleven A.M., at Maries, the barometer was 28.78; thermometer attached, 76°; not attached, 75°.

At two and a-half P.M., on the northern summit of Vrachiona, the

The views from these two heights were very different; that from the northern summit included a great part of the plain of Zante, and most of the northern coast of the island, and was not uninteresting or uninstructive, though too much of a bird's eye view, map-like, to be very pleasing; but, from the other summit, extended over the eastern and southern part of the island, all of it high ground, and being much nearer, its features were distinct. We could see several villages, the mountain village of Giri, about two or three miles off, very prettily situated, the most elevated in the island, and Upper Volimes, and the cultivated grounds of several others, which were themselves hid by the hills which sheltered them. We were surprised at the considerable extent of vineyards, reaching in some places very high up the mountain side, and made with great labour. They are generally in patches, and enclosed by strong stone walls. The rock on each summit was similar, a white limestone, compact, and of very fine grain, which dissolved almost entirely in nitric acid. The upper surface of the mountain, which was very stony and rocky, was covered with heath and low plants, amongst which thyme abounded. Whilst stopping to take some refreshment, an old goatherd, whose goats were browsing close by, came to us, and

barometer was 27.61; thermometer attached, 72°; not attached, 69°.

At four P.M., on the other summit, the barometer was 27.50; the thermometer attached, 71°; not attached, 71°.

being invited, willingly partook of our fare. The flock he was looking after was his own, amounting to about three hundred; but our interpreter, who knew him well, assured us it was only a small part of his wealth; that he was worth at least 25,000 dollars: he was seventy-five, and in the full enjoyment of all his faculties.

We returned to Maries about five o'clock, and spent the night there. Before supper I was requested to see three persons at their houses; one the Capo of the village, who was labouring under a slight feverish attack of a few hours' duration; another, the nephew of our host, who had in the morning an attack of ague (a relapse), and the third a woman, I believe the wife of the Capo, dangerously ill with symptoms of remittent fever, complicated with distressing cough. She had been about fifteen days labouring under the complaint, which had been almost entirely neglected. During the whole time she had used little else than bread and water. I ordered her to take a small dose of a medicine, which I happened to have with me, in a basin of chicken-broth, and to encourage perspiration. It acted very beneficially, occasioned profuse sweating, and greatly relieved her cough. I left directions for her further treatment. The other cases were comparatively slight, yet I had some difficulty to prescribe for them, and for several more that came to me labouring under chronic complaints, there being no medicine in the place, and none to be procured in any of the adjoining villages. I was obliged to have recourse to wood ashes, salt-water, sulphuretted water, and some simples within their reach. Such demands for medical aid might at first give rise to the idea that the place is unhealthy, which I believe is not the case. I probably saw all the sick of the village; curiosity, as well as the hope of obtaining relief, might induce them to apply, and the impulse was not checked by any economical motive, as they were sure of having advice gratis. I mention this, because our interpreter, well acquainted with their habits, described them as a frugal people, indeed parsimonious, so as to grudge very much giving a fee, or even laying out any money on drugs. My professional visits afforded me an opportunity of seeing them nearer than I should have otherwise done, and what I saw generally was in their favour. Their houses were good, and tolerably furnished, and would have been very comfortable, if a little neater and cleaner. Their beds were invariably good, and the linen clean; some of them were ornamented with a kind of lace-work, the manufacture of Venice. Our host's house was the largest in the village, and the best. He had three daughters alive, and as many sons. Two of his daughters were married, one to a farmer at Catastari, with a portion of seven hundred Spanish dollars; another to a farmer in the same village, with five hundred dollars—a smaller sum, because being so near home, she received other assistance. One son only was married; he, according to custom, lives with his wife and children, under the father's roof; and, if all the sons had been married, they would have had only one establishment; and, on the death of the parents, the property would be divided amongst them.   They appeared to live together in sufficient harmony.   All of them were very industrious, never idle.   In the morning it rained heavily, and the old people came into the room where we were, accompanied by their two daughters, and daughter-in-law; the married daughter, for the purpose of consulting me on account of some ailment. They brought their work with them.   The old man was knitting a coarse kind of sack to hold currants to send to the market in town, and a large pile of the dried fruit in the room, lying uncovered, might have stimulated his industry.   The old woman was spinning coarse woollen thread, with the primitive spindle and distaff.*   The unmarried daughter was knitting stockings, and the two other women were

---

* *Vide* Plate IV., figs. 8, 9. The spindle and distaff used by the old woman were each about a foot long; the former was terminated by a slender wire-hook, by which the cotton that is spun and wound about the middle of the instrument is made fast.   The distaff is formed of wood, or is merely a straight slender branch, stripped of its bark, and cut obliquely at the end, to which the raw cotton is loosely attached. The forms of both instruments somewhat vary; the distaff is occasionally seen terminating in a fork, and the spindle provided with a circular weight.   This, I believe, is most used in spinning flax.   The Ionian women acquire great dexterity in using these simple instruments.   They are almost constantly so employed, at least when not more seriously engaged; so that it must be to them, as it were, a relaxation.   In walking the streets, and sitting or standing by their doors, gossiping with their neighbours, the spindle bears them company, and is ever active.

spinning fine cotton thread. I was rather amused with the manner of the woman who consulted me relative to her health. When I asked her age, she said she did not know, and referred to her father; he observed she was forty-five, at which she expressed some surprise, and said, " Surely, I am not so old; if I am, I shall have no more children;" and this she uttered in a tone of regret, although she had already given birth to twelve. Such regret is easily accounted for, amongst a people so primitive, whose children form part of their wealth, and where women are almost exempt from the curse bestowed on the mother of mankind, bearing with little suffering, and often up, it is said, the next day, following their usual occupations.

The weather clearing after breakfast,* we proceeded on our journey. Descending a little from Maries, the road led through a cultivated valley, a great part of it arable land, till it brought us to Oxicora, a considerable and well-built village. In approaching, and close to it, we passed a large collection of cisterns, sixty in number, made in a clay deposit that had collected in a shallow hollow, from which there is no outlet, and which, in the rainy season, is consequently under water. These cisterns, which supply the village with water, are merely pits roofed over with stones, but not lined with puzzolana. Oxicora, not being more

---

* On the 30th August, at Maries, at 6 A. M. after a thunder storm, attended with a heavy shower, the thermometer, exposed to the wind, which was northerly, fell to 66° ; the barometer was 28.66.

than a mile and half from Maries, we did not stop,
but went on to Cambi, an inconsiderable village near
the sea, about two or three miles distant from the
preceding. We descended the greater part of the
way, for it stands on a much lower level. We passed
through some arable land, but saw no vineyards,
which seem to be confined chiefly to the higher
grounds. As we rode along, we had partial views of
the coast. It exhibited the same character as at
St Georgio and Vromi, and was little less bold, and
here as there a great deal of land lying waste, appeared to admit of easy cultivation. On quitting
Cambi, we saw a village boundary-stone: it was a
column about eight feet high, neatly surmounted by
a niche, in which stood a small cross. From Cambi,
returning again inland, we went to St Leo, by a
very rugged steep mountain road. These villages are
about two miles apart; and the intermediate country,
excepting a few spots of vineyards, is barren, and
covered with loose stones.

St Leo is rather a pretty village; it stands nearly
as high as Maries, and is almost as large. There is
a good deal of arable land and some vineyard round
it, but few trees, and these the cypress and the olive.
We rested here a short time, in a good house, in
every room of which there was a pile of currants, the
produce of the neighbourhood.* Here we saw an old
man, aged 110, whose name was Stelleanò, a native

* At St Leo, at noon, the barometer was 28.72°; the barometer,
free and attached, 75°.

of the place, and a goatherd, who had spent the
greater part of his life in the adjoining mountains
attending his flock, excepting a short time that he
was in the Morea, where he served during the first
struggle made by the Greeks to recover their liberty.
He retained all his vigour till he was 80; and when
we saw him, he did not bear marks of such great age.
The hair of his head was light brown, and scarcely a
gray hair was to be distinguished; his beard was a
mixture of gray and sandy; he had four front teeth
remaining in his upper jaw; his hearing was unim-
paired; and he had the use of all his limbs. He
walked into the room, using a stick, and seated himself on a low stool, from which, when questioned
relative to his strength, he rose, without his stick or
any assistance, stood erect, walked across the room,
placed himself in a firm attitude, and said, if he could
see well he could walk to the city, and again seated
himself, without aid, on a stool not more than a foot
high. He had lost the sight of one eye in consequence of cataract, and the vision of the other was
considerably impaired from the same disease. He
was about five feet five inches high, of spare habit,
light blue eyes, and of a very cheerful disposition,
much given to joke and laughter, and taking every
thing said to him in good part. His chest was rather
narrow, but deep; and when I examined it, he put
his hand on his heart, and exclaimed, " all is right
there." His ancles did not swell; in fact, he laboured
under no perceptible disease affecting his general

health ; had a good appetite, and seemed still to enjoy life ; indeed, so satisfied was he with the life which he had led, that he said he wished he could live it over again. He was once married, and had seven children, respecting whom we did not make any particular inquiries. He had always been needy in his circumstances, and had lived in a very frugal manner, his diet consisting chiefly of bread and garlic. In the same village there were many more old people, several between seventy and ninety.

After stopping about half-an-hour at St Leo, we went on towards Luca, still ascending the mountain. We saw very little cultivation, excepting at a distance, and passed by only two or three small vineyards. In one of these, by the road-side, was a large apiary, consisting of perhaps seventy or eighty hives ; and the proprietor, who was living with his family in a stone-hut in the vineyard, was at that time employed in collecting the honey, which we tasted and found very rich. The hives generally consisted of a piece of the trunk of an olive-tree, about a foot and half high, hollow, with two cross sticks within, placed horizontally, to give support to the combs ; they stood on flat stones, an inch or two from the ground, and were covered with a thin piece of stone, brought from Langadachia, which, from its slaty and porous texture, must be a bad conductor of heat, and very well adapted to the purpose to which it was thus applied. There was a cistern in the vineyard, and small troughs to water the bees ; the supplying them with water is the most important part of the whole economy, and demands constant attention ; it kept employed two or three people.

The village of Luca, about a mile and half from St Leo, is small, but pretty well built, judging from its appearance at a little distance, for we did not enter it.   It is situated on the side of a hill, at the upper end of a valley that has no outlet, the largest of the kind I had yet seen.   It may be a mile long, and nearly a quarter of a mile wide where widest ; and the greater part of it is cultivated and arable land.   In winter it is overflowed and converted into a lake ; in the dry season the water evaporates, excepting what is collected in the cisterns, fifty-five in number, situated nearly in the middle of the plain. The soil is a red clay, and of considerable depth ; the cisterns, which are mere pits in it, are from fifteen to twenty feet deep.   I found the temperature of the water just drawn so low as 58°.   We afterwards learnt, at Gilliamano, that Luca is considered the coldest spot in the island ; and it was remarked that the inhabitants are obliged to wear their warm capotes even in June ; and that every winter the lake is frozen, and continues frozen three or four days.   Such severity of cold, probably, is not owing to altitude alone ;—probably evaporation and radiation aid, for both which the local circumstances are peculiarly favourable ; for the former, an extensive surface of shallow water and saturated clay ; for the latter, the form of the valley, not unlike a concave mirror.

Ascending from this valley, we proceeded to the monastery of Madonna Paragato, about two miles and half from the village of Luca, finely situated at the declivity of a hill covered with oaks (the ilex) of considerable size, and opposite another hill covered with firs, with a cultivated plain of some extent intermediate, partly corn land, partly vineyard. The monastery, though very inferior to that of St Georgio, afforded tolerable accommodation, and we spent the night in it. It belongs to an establishment of the same name in Egypt, the head of which appoints a monk to it as a benefice, on the condition of transmitting certain dues to the parent monastery. In the adjoining woods there is excellent woodcock shooting in November, the month in which the great flights of this bird take place in the Mediterranean, on their passage to winter in Africa. Our interpreter said he had killed here six brace in an hour. The sportsmen go out early, and return soon after sunrise, when the birds become very wild. My travelling companion went out before breakfast, and sent in a small squirrel which he shot, of a light mouse colour. It is a rare animal in Zante, and the servants showed a dread of touching it. The evening and morning were both very cool; just after sunset, in the plain, the thermometer fell to 64°; and it was the same the following morning, just before sunrise.*

After breakfast, on the 31st, we took our departure

---

* August 31, 6¼ A.M., the barometer was 28.32°; thermometer attached, 69°: not attached, 64°; cistern-water, 60°.

from the monastery for the village of Gilliamano,
standing nearly on the same level, a hill intervening,
and about two miles and half distant.   The intermediate country is wild and picturesque, well adapted
for field sports.   As we rode along, we noticed a
small dark brown owl, close to the road, and within
shot, but the natives would not fire at it, saying it
was unlucky to kill either an owl or a crow.   We
saw several of the latter flying at some distance, and
two large birds that appeared to be kites.   On our
way we passed through the small valley of Trapies,
about two miles from the monastery, similar in its
formation to that of Luca, and containing several
cisterns.   Water from one was of the temperature
56°, of another 58°.   When we arrived at the wells,
two women were drawing water, and became very
angry at our taking a draught and giving a little to
our animals; apprehensive, no doubt, that the stock
might be exhausted before the dry season was concluded ; our interpreter, however, soon silenced them
by becoming angry himself, and threatening to throw
them into the water they were so unwilling to spare.
From these cisterns the adjoining village of Gilliamano is partly supplied ; a low neck of land, connecting two hills only, intervenes.

We arrived at Gilliamano early ; took up our quarters in a large good house belonging to the priest of
the village, and remained there during the heat of
the day, busily occupied in looking about and in prescribing for patients, so that there was scarcely time

to dine. Our interpreter had stood godfather to the grandchild of our host ; in consequence, he was considered as a relation, and we were all welcome on his account. On entering, we found some six or seven boys in an open porch, learning their lessons ; one boy, who had misbehaved, was on his knees as a punishment. The books they used were pamphlets, of a few sheets, neatly stitched together; and to preserve them from being soiled and torn, they were attached to pieces of reed as handles—thus :—

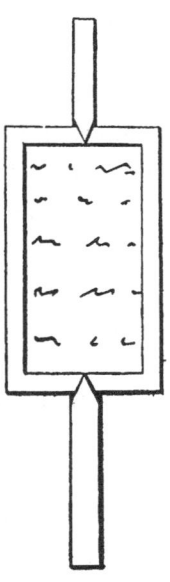

The children were all neatly dressed, with shoes and stockings, and they appeared to be very orderly ; the senior boy acted as a monitor and heard them read. The village, generally, is neatly built ; it contains some good houses and a large church, rather richly ornamented, at the time undergoing a thorough repair, under the direction of an Italian artist, who was restoring the gilding, &c., with a good deal of skill, paid out of a fund raised by voluntary contribution. Here they do not bury the dead in the church, but in the small yard in which it stands, which is without tomb-stones, exhibiting no marks of pious care and regard—a dirty, neglected surface, defiled with impurities not to be mentioned.

Amongst the visits we paid, one was to an old woman said to be 110. She was very infirm and deaf, and quite of a different disposition from the old man of St Leo, apparently very melancholy and miserable, and life a burden to her. She burst into tears on our asking some question respecting her strength, and wrung her hands, saying the time was when she was as strong and as gay as any present. There were with her her daughter, grand-daughter, and great-grand-daughter, so that we saw at once assembled under the same roof four generations. The daughter said she was sixty-five, but she looked much older, the grand-daughter was twenty-eight, and her child was four.

The house in which we stopped was a good example of the houses of the villages amongst the mountains of the better kind. It had been built thirty years, as an inscription in front indicated. It consisted of two storeys, and, with the outhouses, formed a hollow square. The entrance was by an arched way, in which were small ornamented niches for holding water-vessels. On the ground-floor were the sleeping apartments, in each of which was a good bed, without curtains; and in one of them, besides the bed, there was a loom. They had separate entrances, so as to be well adapted for different families. On the upper floor, approached by a flight of stone steps, was a large hall, containing one or two presses, several large chests, and a sufficient number of chairs and tables—all in pretty good order, and of tolerable quality; and ranged round the walls were pictures of the Virgin, of saints, and monasteries; and opposite the principal picture a lamp was suspended, and kept constantly burning.   Off this hall, and communicating with it, there were four small bed-rooms, well provided with beds.   In none of the rooms was there any fire-place.   The kitchen was a large room, a separate building in the rear, well provided, as it appeared, with culinary utensils, as spits, pots, &c. It had two ovens, one large, the other small, of the common construction, provided with holes below for holding ashes, with small recesses above, with a shelf on each.   In another part of the room was the hearth, with low seats on each side of it, forming a square. The fire was kindled in the middle of the enclosed space, and the smoke had no vent, excepting through the door, as there was no opening in the roof above, and, if I recollect rightly, no windows.   The firewood was piled on the other side of the room.   The only utensil that attracted my attention particularly was a small hand-mill (Plate VI., fig. 4), composed of two circular pieces of rough sandstone from Cephalonia, used to grind grain for soup, similar in construction to the hand-mill of Ceylon and of the continent of India, and to the quern of old of England and Scotland, and which is still in use in some parts of the Highlands.   In another building adjoining was an olive-press, exactly of the same kind as that used in the town; and in a third building there was a cornmill, of the common construction, which the proprietor let out, receiving in payment a certain portion of the grain ground   It was at work at the time; two

women, in a kind of harness, assisted a horse in turning it.   The sight was sufficiently degrading; it was,
however, a labour they were accustomed to, and
they did not seem to mind it;—their hands were
busily employed at the same time in spinning.   This
was not the only time and place where we saw women
so occupied; at Oxicora we first noticed it; there
we witnessed six in harness, labouring at the mill,
and spinning as they ran round.

I availed myself of this opportunity, considering it
a favourable one, to make inquiries respecting the
occupations of the people, their agriculture and farm-
ing utensils.   In preparing the ground, the only
implements they use are the plough and hoe.   They
sow corn, as wheat, barley, or oats, every second
year, in the same ground, and have a crop of hay, or
allow it to remain fallow the intermediate year: they
manure for hay, but not for corn.   The year round,
their occupations are nearly as follow:—In October,
after the rains, they plough; in November, sow; in
December and January, they gather the olives and
make oil; in February, they turn over the soil in the
vineyards; and in March, they do the same round
the olive-trees; in April, they cut hay; in May and
June, their different kinds of corn; in July, they
level the ground about the vines; in August, they
gather and dry their currants; and in September,
they gather their grapes and make wine.   When
there are no olives (of which they expect a crop
only every alternate year) in January and February,

they make lime, an article with which the mountains supply the town and plain.   Besides these their principal occupations, there are many minor ones.   The women are even more busily employed than the men, and as variously; spinning, weaving, and knitting may be considered almost as their amusements and recreations, after the more important and laborious labours of the day.   They spin both cotton and worsted thread, and also goat-hair; knit very good stockings; and weave hair-cloth for bags, cotton cloth for dress and household purposes, and some carpeting, of which I saw two or three very pretty samples in the form of rugs.

At dinner we were attended by the daughter-in-law of our host, a fine active young woman, perfectly modest, without being in the least bashful. Her easy manner indicated that it was the custom of the country,—that she considered it a duty,—and that she was used to it as well as not displeased with it.

Here, at ten o'clock in the forenoon, the barometer was 28.39; the thermometer attached and free, 72°; water of a cistern, 62°; so that this village is nearly on the same level as Paragato. It is as high, if not higher, than the adjoining little valley of Trapies, where the temperature of the cistern water was so low, 6° lower than in this place,—a circumstance favourable to the idea, that evaporation is in part concerned with radiation in producing the comparatively great degree of cold experienced in these valleys. I may here add a few other particulars relative to the severity of the winter-season in this mountainous region, collected in conversation with the most intelligent of the villagers. We were told at Paragato that there is frost every winter there,— that it lasts two or three days at a time,—and that the ice is often two fingers thick. Here, at Gilliamano, we were informed that, in the very cold winter of 1813-14, they had a frost which continued a month, and that even the wine in the barrels froze;—that every year they have ice an inch or two thick, and that the water in the neighbouring valley is covered with ice.*

In the afternoon we set out for Kieri, with the intention of sleeping there. At the distance of about three miles and a-half, we passed through the neat small village of Agala, situated at the upper end of a cultivated valley. From hence, descending by a very rugged path, we next came to the small village of Ambelo, at about an equal distance, and the country, like that between Agala and Gilliamano. in great part lying waste. Near the village, on the rocky side of a hill where there were some cisterns, we saw a large apiary; probably there were not less than

---

* If this information be correct, and there is no reason to doubt it, it occurred to us at the time, that it might be easy to supply the town of Zante with the luxury of ice from hence, laying it up in store, in winter, in an ice-house in the village ; and in summer, when required, transporting it to an ice-house, in town, on mules, which might be done with great ease by way of Lagapada, and in the short space of three hours.

seventy hives; we inquired the exact number; the reply was, they did not know; it was unlucky to count them.

Ambelo is in bad repute; it is considered the most unhealthy spot in the island, and is particularly liable, towards the end of summer and the beginning of autumn, to intermittent and remittent fevers.   At this time, we were told that in every family there was one or more sick.   It is situated pretty high, close to a valley without an outlet, where the soil is deep and water stagnates in winter, and which is planted with olive-trees that have attained a great size, and produce a dense shade.   The water used by the inhabitants is partly from cisterns in the village, and partly from those in the valley just mentioned; it appeared to be good.   They blame the air, and are of opinion that the malaria is wafted up from the valley of the pitch springs, which is also notoriously unhealthy; the distance is about two or three miles.

The village of Kieri is about two miles from Ambelo; the road is difficult, the worst we passed over, very rocky, and in one place it winds along a precipice.   The intermediate country is quite uncultivated.   It was moonlight when we arrived, and the bold scenery around appeared to great advantage. In neatness this village is very inferior to the other mountain villages, and we experienced here much less civility; our interpreter gave the inhabitants a bad character.   It is ill supplied with water, the number of cisterns being comparatively few, owing to want of industry; and, in consequence, when little rain falls in the winter, there is a great scarcity in the dry season. The fir-tree abounds in the neighbourhood. Although situated high up, on the steep side of a hill, its absolute height above the level of the sea is not considerable;* and we experienced very distinctly at night the change of climate from diminished elevation, and once more began to perspire sensibly when not taking exercise. In the morning early we descended to the shore, which is not more than a mile distant. The cliffs are very bold, and having a descent from their summit inland (a common feature of the shores of the Ionian Islands), they have the appearance of sections of hills. By the way, we passed through a small grove of fir-trees in an adjoining valley tolerably cultivated, in quest of doves which resort here, in great numbers, in September and October, and are now beginning to make their appearance. They are shot by the natives, and caught in snares of a very simple construction. The snare is a running loop of twisted horse-hair, which is attached to the bare branch of a tree, alighting on which the birds are entangled or are caught by the feet. About the same time, quails in large flocks migrating southward, alight on the neighbouring

---

* Here, on the 1st September, five and a-half A.M., the barometer was 29.23; thermometer attached, 73°; not attached, 69°; water of a cistern, 69°.

shore, and spreading over the adjoining hills, afford
the fowler, it is said, excellent sport.   We were
led to a spot on the cliff called Diglidani's Leap.
About five or six feet from the margin of the cliff,
and about twelve feet below, a mass of crumbling
rock projects upwards, terminating almost in a point.
The exploit which has given this spot celebrity
amongst the country-people, was performed about
120 years ago by a native whose name it bears,—
a man of extraordinary activity, strength, and dar-
ing.   By way of display, the story goes, he jumped
on the pinnacle just mentioned, alighting like a bird,
and there not being sufficient space to turn, he leapt
back backwards.   The height of the cliff here is
between two and three hundred feet: the detached
mass, however, when the extraordinary feat was performed, it is said, was on a level with the boundary
margin.   His descendants still reside in his native
village, and possess the tar-springs in the adjoining
valley, which were originally granted to him for
some service of difficulty which he performed for
the Venetian government, and which at that time,
when the value of the produce was much greater
than at present (now bringing only about thirty
or forty dollars a-year), must have been a high
reward.

After breakfast we proceeded on our way to town:
crossing a pretty lofty hill which divides the valley
of Kieri from that in which the pitch-springs are
situated, and defends the village from its malaria, or

the wind blowing from it, we descended to the latter
by a very bad and steep path, and visited the two
springs which, for so long a period, have attracted
the attention of the curious.   Having already described them, I shall here add only such particulars
as now came under observation, not previously introduced.   Notwithstanding the extreme insalubrity of
the air of this valley, according to popular belief, it
is not entirely uncultivated.   The dry parts are
planted with olive-trees, which appear to flourish.
Along the sides of the morass, pretty extensive plantations of the currant-vine have been formed by
ditching and draining,—and as any one who pleases
may cultivate the marsh, they are extending.   We
saw two men employed in reclaiming a piece of the
swamp, to plant vines in ; they were labouring hard,
their heads uncovered, exposed to the mid-day sun,
up to their knees in black fetid water, throwing up
mud and decomposing vegetable matter, and forming
at the same time a bed and a ditch.   This cultivation is said to be very productive ; but, as might be
expected under such circumstances, with so little
regard to precaution, very unwholesome and hazard-
ous, fever being almost an inevitable consequence of
engaging in it.   The enterprising and careless labourers
do not live on the spot, but belong to the village of
Kieri.   The currant-vine here, in this rich soil of
moist vegetable matter, is very precocious, rapidly
coming to perfection, and as rapidly decaying ; it
bears fruit, it is said, on the third year from its

planting, and perishes in about twelve or fifteen years; in the intermediate time, whilst in vigour, yielding a great profusion of fine fruit.

It has been mentioned before, that the hills forming the valley of the tar-springs consist of limestone, and form a part of the great limestone range, constituting the mountainous district. Advancing towards the town, on descending into the next valley in which there is a small rivulet, conglomerate rock presented itself, resting on limestone on one side and marl on the other, from whence the latter continues into the plain. At and near its junction with the limestone or conglomerate, the marl in this place was more or less indurated, approaching in appearance to shale; and such is its general character, as far as my observations extended, all along the boundary-line of the two districts.*

I shall conclude the journal of this little excursion, which was one of uninterrupted gratification and amusement, with a few observations on the inhabitants of the villages we visited. Generally they are better looking than the inhabitants of the town and plain, and decidedly fairer: very many of them indeed have light-blue and hazel eyes, and light hair. We saw several women possessed of considerable

* The morning after our return to town, on the 2d September, at eight A.M., in my house, only a few feet above the level of the sea, the barometer used on the journey was 30.148; thermometer 80° attached, and the same unattached: on the 8th of the same month, at eleven A.M., the former was 29.851; the latter 82°.

beauty, and not a few with good clear complexions, and some colour. The dress of the men was very similar to that used by the same class in town. The covering of the head is a small skull-cap, the prevailing colour of which is brown. The hair is allowed to flow over the shoulders (at least of the young men), and shaved about the temples. The growth of hair over the upper lip is encouraged, but not beneath, nor is the whisker tolerated : they pride themselves on their mustaches, and would consider it a very great indignity to be deprived of them. When our Greek interpreter asked the old Stelleano, if he should cut them off, he replied with some briskness, drawing his hand across his throat, that he should cut that first· They wear a double-breasted waistcoat, and a jacket made to fit neatly. The former is commonly very smart; the latter, in warm weather, is thrown over the shoulder. The neck is left bare; the shirt-collar is turned down, displaying it. Their breeches are made like our dress small-clothes, to button at the knee, and stockings are worn by them, and either shoes, with large buckles, or sandals of goats-skin, laced about the foot. The most peculiar part of the womens' dress is a white scarf, worn so as to envelope the head and cover the shoulders, for which sometimes a handkerchief is substituted, simply wrapped round the head. Their gown is long, with long sleeves, tight about the waist, and high, concealing the bosom. When formally dressed, they wear stockings and shoes, and very large shoe-buckles. On ordinary occasions, they commonly go barefooted, at least about the house.   They are under little restraint, appear to be quite at liberty to show themselves, and in their manners very much resemble women of the same class in England.

CHAPTER IX.

MISCELLANEOUS REMARKS; WITH EXTRACTS FROM
JOURNALS, IN FARTHER ILLUSTRATION OF THE
STATE OF THE PEOPLE IN THE IONIAN ISLANDS.

Notice of a Visit to the Monastery of Taffeo, in Cephalonia, and how
entertained there. A Medical Consultation in the same Island.
Excursions from Cephalonia and Santa Maura to Ithaca. Primitive Reception and Hospitality. Particulars respecting the Island
of Meganisi. Notice of the desert Islet of Tiglia. Particulars of Leftimo, a district of Corfu. Excursion to Sidari, on
the north coast of Corfu. Particulars of Fanò, and other Islets,
off the north-west coast of Corfu. Notice of the Island of Paxo.
Its cisterns. Bishop of Paxo. Manners of the Inhabitants.

WITH the same intent as that with which the preceding journal has been given, I shall, in this chapter,
insert some extracts from other journals, with the
hope that they may not be unacceptable to the reader,
and that, however imperfectly written, they may aid
in giving more correct ideas than can be derived from
general descriptions.

In the chapter on the geology of the Ionian
Islands, mention is made of the cavern of Dracon-
dispilo, in Cephalonia, near the monastery of Taffeo.
The visit was made with Captain, now Lieutenant-
Colonel R., and a Greek gentleman, a native of Ar-

gostoli, who was well acquainted with the Economo
of the monastery, where we passed the night, and
where we experienced a most hospitable reception.
Our supper was not uncharacteristic. It consisted of
that excellent pastoral dish, a roast lamb (it was in
the month of January), roasted whole,* and of stewed
fowls, with a white sauce made of lemon-juice and
egg beat up together. Bread was the only vegetable
substance at table, except a sallad made of turnip-tops.
Cheese of the convent, of a high and peculiar flavour,
followed, and a dessert of walnuts, which one of the
attendants, without any idea of the least impropriety,
cracked with his teeth in the room; and, after all, we
were served with a cup of coffee each, and a glass of
liquor, intensely strong, and highly flavoured by the
essential oil of aniseed. The coffee-spoons were perforated with little holes, to answer, as was explained,

* In Greece and Asia Minor, the lamb or sheep roasted whole, is
well known to the traveller, and is an almost indispensable article of
liberal hospitality. In the wildest country, where most acceptable,
the preparing and cooking process is most amusing and picturesque.
The last time I saw it practised was in a deep wooded valley, opening
on the Black Sea, on its southern shore. After a visit from the chief
of the district, a Mohammedan, a sheep was brought from him as a present, led by a cord, which was attached to a belt girding its loins.
In a surprisingly short time (it was the hungry time of evening,
and our people were short of provisions), the animal was killed,
skinned, and spitted on the branch of a tree cut for the purpose, and
roasting (the spit resting on two forked sticks, driven into the ground),
over a powerful fire of glowing embers, the produce of a bonfire that
lighted up the valley, made in the most reckless way. It was basted
with the tail fastened to a long stick, knowingly applied by the man
who took the lead in the business.

the better for taking up and removing any intrusive
flies, or offending matters.   Wine was drunk (wine of
the country), both during the repast and after; and
many a toast was given, and many a hearty *viva* pronounced, and several songs sung, the best by our mu-
leteers, one of whom had an excellent voice.   The
people who came with us, and those of the monastery, for none were excluded, enjoyed the merry-
making.   Their manner was uncommonly free; yet,
from a certain dash of respect in it, and great natural
good humour, it was nowise offensive.   One man, a
villager, belonging to an estate of our Greek friend,
took unusual liberties in the capacity of waiting-man,
and very often patted us on the shoulder.   The
Economo, or head of the convent, was not the least
cheerful of the party; he joined in the songs and
merriment *con amore*.   The evening was cold, and it
froze during the night; there was no fire-place in the
room ; we were indebted for warmth to a pan (and
that a frying-pan) of charcoal placed underneath the
table; and, for warmth in bed, there being no blankets,
only sheets and a quilted coverlit, we slept with our
clothes on.

It has been mentioned under how much less restraint the women of Cephalonia and Ithaca live than
those of the same class in Zante.   I allude to the
upper order.   An instance may be given in illustration, and to show, at the same time, the manner of
holding a medical consultation.   Whilst I was stationed in Cephalonia, one of the wealthiest merchants

of Argostoli, a native, was seized with fever, and became so dangerously ill that his life was despaired of. I was requested to see him in consultation. In the ante-room of the patient's bed-chamber, the family were assembled, the ladies regularly seated as on an occasion of ceremony. Three physicians of the town were present. After examining the sick man, who, strange to say, considered himself then actually dead, and spoke of the folly of prescribing for a dead man, and who, in consequence, after his recovery, was facetiously called by his friends, *il morto*,—after inquiring into his present symptoms, we adjourned to the ante room, and in the presence of the assembled company, discussed the case; and this was done by the Greek physicians in the most formal manner, each in turn giving a kind of clinical lecture, in which the history of the disease was traced, the rationale of the symptoms given, the supposed exact nature of the malady, and its nosological place assigned, and a mode of treatment proposed, founded on the views taken. It was an ingenious theoretical display of ability, each striving to appear to most advantage; but it need hardly be observed, that it was better adapted to impress the audience with the cleverness of the speakers, than to be of practical use to the patient. In the discussion there was no reserve in the use of terms, on account of female ears; no indelicacies seem to have been imagined by either party.

Till within a few years, there were no roads in

Ithaca. When I visited that island in the winter of
1825, I was assured by the then respectable Resident, the late Captain Knox, that, before the roads
which he was engaged in were opened, it was usual
for women to be employed in carrying bags of currants—a labour since performed by donkeys.

The state of Cephalonia and of Ithaca, in relation to
communication, is very similar to that of the remote
Highlands of Scotland and the islets adjoining, where
steam navigation has not been introduced, and the
same remark applies to most of the other Ionian
Islands.   In the winter above referred to, I crossed in
a small open boat from the little port of St Euphemia, in Cephalonia, to Opiso Aitos, in Ithaca, a distance of about three miles. The guardiano at this latter
place, was a boy, who acted in the double capacity of
Sanità guard and of guide.   He had no hesitation in
leaving his post, and accompanying us with his ass,
carrying our little baggage across the mountain to the
town of Vathi.   By the way we met with a shepherd
who made the rocks resound to the wild and stirring
music of his clossoscambuno, the bagpipe of the Ionian
Islands, already noticed.   My travelling companion
was a Greek of Cephalonia, who, like myself, was a
complete stranger in Ithaca.   We went, on our arrival in town, to the house of a friend of his father's,
and were received with the most hearty and primitive
hospitality, not only with shaking of hands, but also
with kissing of cheeks; and presently we were regaled
with a repast consisting of eggs, bread, wine, cheese,

salt-fish, and coffee, served in the sleeping-room ; and our kind hostess, in picturesque, though coarse attire, the hair loose, falling on her shoulders, presented us with roses.

In the month of March of the same year, I paid another visit to Ithaca; this time from Santa Maura, and in a manner not less primitive. Through the kindness of the late Major Temple, then Resident of the latter island, I was allowed the use of a government boat, called a scampa-via, somewhat of the construction of an ancient galley, adapted equally to rowing or sailing, broad of beam, and of little draft of water, fitted for encountering the gale by day, and for seeking shelter by night, wherever a landing-place could be found, according to the manner of ancient navigation. We started from Santa Maura, on the 18th of March, and entered the port of Vathi, on the 20th, after a rough, but far from unpleasant passage,— the beauty of the wild scenery, in this inland sea, and the novelty of the kind of life, and its enterprise, more than compensating for its inconveniences. The first night we stopped at Meganisi, and had an opportunity of seeing a considerable portion of that poor and barren island, with a population of about five hundred souls, collected in three villages, in a ruder condition than the inhabitants of the wildest parts of the mountainous district of Zante, generally poor, squalid, and dirty, the men said to be very idle, the women laborious and over-worked ; without cisterns, and depending for water on two wells close to the sea-

shore, at some distance from the villages.* The next
night we stopped at the desert little islet of Tiglia,
situated in the narrow channel between the eastern
extremity of Meganisi and the northern one of Santa
Maura.   It was a good example of the many islets
which contribute so much to the beauty of this lake-
like sea.   About a mile and half in circumference, of
irregular hilly surface, it was a wilderness of shrub-
berry,—an arborescent heath, of white and sweet
flower, then in bloom, the myrtle and arbutus growing luxuriantly intermixed, were the most conspicuous plants.   Our boat was drawn up on the shore
of a little cove ; a bed was spread on deck, under
cover of a temporary awning, and we supped and
breakfasted on a stone-table, a slab-like mass of white
lime-stone (the latter meal consisting of cold meat,
bread, and wine), in a hut literally of myrtle, made by
the crew of the scampa-via, who often put in here.
The scenery, at all times beautiful, at this season was
heightened in its charms by the striking contrast of
colours, between the many mountain ridges and summits, still covered with the snows of winter, and the

* A subaltern officer from the garrison of Santa Maura, was generally stationed in this island, with a detachment of twenty or thirty
men.   There was also there a Sanitá officer, with a capo, in each of the
three villages, two or three constables, and a person to look after the⁻
vineyards, and prevent the trespassing of cattle. This office was taken
in turn by the villagers, armed with a stick with an enormous head ;
and it was incumbent on him, according to his instructions, rigorously
to kill any trespasser, even though his own cattle, and on his own
property.

adjoining shores and lower hills bright in the verdure of early spring.

The district of Leftimo, in Corfu, comprising its southern extremity, which terminates in the bold headland Cape Bianco, the ancient Leucimna, where the Athenians erected a trophy for their first naval victory on the breaking out of the Peloponnesian war, is in many respects peculiar. The soil is almost entirely marl; the principal produce oil; its villages, once flourishing, as the size and description of houses indicate, are now in decay; many of the buildings in ruins; most of them out of repair;* the streets filthy; the people of miserable appearance, generally ill dressed and dirty; many of them in rags; most of them diseased. Agues are very common among them; so is scurvy, particularly amongst the men, and dropsy and visceral disease. It is remarkable that they are also very subject to gout, a complaint generally extremely rare in these islands. I was told that, in the whole population of the five principal villages, which are contiguous, amounting to about 2000, there were, when I visited it, in the spring of 1825, forty cases of the complaint, many of them severe and chronic. I saw one man a complete martyr to the disease, who had been confined to bed three or four years, a cripple from concretions of lithate of soda in the joints of his hands and feet.† The very sickly state of these vil-

* Such is the deficiency of stone in this marl-district, that it is said the stone of which the villages are built is imported from the opposite continental coast.

† A remarkable contrast, in relation to gout, is exhibited between

lages is referred principally to situation, which is low, with stagnant water in their neighbourhood; and, in confirmation, it is said that Potamo, which lies lowest, and along the bank of a canal, is much more unwholesome than the next and adjoining village of Teodoro. It is referred also to the bad quality of the water used, which is generally hard ; and the prevalency of scurvy is supposed to be, in part, owing to the use which the natives make of the wild plants, which are said to be saline. These circumstances may have some effect, but perhaps still more is owing to the common habits of the people, and their mode of living. Besides being dirty, they are reported to be generally very idle and licentious, especially those of Potamo ; they drink much wine and ardent spirit; they use very little animal food, and subsist chiefly on bread made of Indian corn, on beans, wild vegetables, and oil. The quantity of oil they consume is great. During the time that they are making oil, I was assured they use from one to two pounds a-day, and that, when there is no scarcity of the article, they may use about six ounces a-day ; during the year in which no oil is made, and it is scarce, about

---

the wretched inhabitants of the above mentioned district, and of the flourishing and opulent capital of Austria. In Vienna, I was assured by a high medical authority, and excellent pathologist, that true gout is unknown. In the valuable collection of morbid anatomy attached to the great civil Hospital, there is not a single specimen of gouty concretion ; and the physician referred to, who has the charge of it, told me he had never, in all his *post mortem* researches, met with an example of such concretion.

two ounces.   They have the character of being ferocious in their manners, and resentful.   Before the population was disarmed, they seldom had recourse to the laws, generally avenged their own injuries, and sometimes resisted the orders of the government ; so that, when any government measure of an unpopular nature was proposed, it was common to say that cannot be carried into effect in Leftimo.   Compared with the inhabitants of Zante, whether health or reputed morals are considered, and whether of the hilly district or of the plain, they present a remarkable contrast.   The Zantiots may, in every respect, be held up as a favourable example of the Ionian people, the Corfiots of Leftimo as the very reverse. The decay of their villages is said to have commenced, after suffering from the plague in 1813 ; but probably there were special causes which then came into operation, to which the effect rather was owing ; and a stop or check to smuggling, about that time, was probably one of them.

Other parts of Corfu might be as favourably contrasted with Leftimo as Zante, especially some of the hilly and mountainous districts.   In the month of October of the same year I had an opportunity of witnessing an example of the kind, in a little excursion to Sidari, situated on the northern coast of the island.   Our party consisted of three English officers and a Greek gentleman, well acquainted with the country and its inhabitants, and whose presence insured us, wherever we went, a kind reception.   Although absent only two days, we saw, travelling on horseback at our leisure, a considerable portion of the island, and some of its most beautiful parts. The village where we slept and supped was Carusades, situated near the sea-shore, on a steep hill, composed chiefly of sand, with a little clay intermixed, and occasional layers of sandstone. The site is healthy, and the soil fertile. Many of the inhabitants, we were assured, were between seventy and eighty years of age, and were still hale and fresh looking. The luxuriancy of vegetation was striking; looking round, from the house where we stopt, we saw the almond, the palm, vine, fig, and orange, and also the common reed growing in the same garden, and almost in a group. The house, like the majority of the best farm-houses in the country, was of two stories : the upper story, containing the dwelling-rooms, was approached by a flight of steps, and entered by a porch ; it was tolerably clean and pretty well furnished ; the lower was used as a storehouse. Having made our visit quite unexpectedly, we had an opportunity of witnessing the ordinary mode of entertaining strangers by a native, such as our host, in easy circumstances, and it impressed us very favourably. The supper to which we sat down consisted of the following dishes:— First, boiled rice, with a sauce of lemon-juice and egg beat up together ; second, stewed fowl, with a savoury sauce, and thin slices of bread soaked in it ; third, roasted chickens ; fourth, whiting and some other fish delicately fried in oil ; and lastly, a dessert of

almonds, melons, grapes, and apples, with wine of
last year, considered by the natives of the first quality, red, brisk, and slightly pricked. The master of
the house kindly gave me up his bed, which was a
very comfortable one, without curtains; at its head,
against the wall, were pictures of saints, two marriage
crowns, or circles, made of cotton, bound round and
confined by red tape, and a palm leaf, fancifully cut
and arranged, a present from the village papa on
Palm Sunday.*

Off the south-west coast of Corfu, towards the
entrance of the Adriatic, are the three islets of Fanò,
Merlera, and Samitraki: of the two former of which
Baron Theotoki has made very favourable mention,
with an account of their natural advantages, and of
the good qualities of their inhabitants—where

" Il puro a respirar aere odorato ;"

and where, in the manners of the people, he is of
opinion proof is afforded " que les bonnes mœurs
valent plus que les bonnes lois."

Having had an opportunity of visiting these spots,†
considered so favoured, I shall state here some particulars respecting them, which were collected and
noted down at the time, and shall be well pleased
should they excite curiosity and lead to more mi-

---

* According to the means of the individual, a douceur is expected
by the priest in return.

† In the summer of 1825, in company with the late Lieutenant-
Colonel Harper, Royal Engineers.

nute inquiry than a passing traveller could attempt to institute. Little societies, shut out from the world, are always curious, if not interesting objects for study; and examination into them, whilst easy, can hardly fail to be instructive; they may be viewed as experiments in political economy, and may aid in solving some of its difficult problems.

The three islets mentioned constitute a barony, and are the property of a Venetian, who claims one-tenth of their produce, and draws from them an annual rent of about 800 dollars. Their joint population may amount to about 1300, of both sexes, and of all ages. In Fanò there are fifteen small villages or hamlets; in Merlera seventy-five scattered houses; and in Samitraki thirty-five. The houses bear the names of their proprietors, as is also the usage in the island of Paxo. This circumstance, and that just mentioned relative to the distribution of the population, would seem to indicate that they have been comparatively recently peopled, and during a period when little was to be dreaded from piratical depredation. The story, indeed, is, that the first settlers, the original stock from whence the present settlers have descended, were a party of twelve pirates obliged to fly from Paxo, having been outlawed; and who, on settling in Fanò, following the example of the early Romans in procuring wives, went to the nearest part of the Albanian coast, and, on the pretence of buying linen, seized and carried off the women who brought it to their boats; and the tale proceeds further to say that they took the same measure to procure a priest, whom, after the performance of the marriage-rites for which he was brought, they impatiently threw into the sea in returning, and drowned.

Fanò, of the three islets, is considerably the largest, about twelve and a half miles in circumference, of an irregular form, which has been compared to that óf a shoulder of mutton; its greatest length is about four and a half miles; and its breadth about two and a quarter. Merlera, in form not unlike a horse-shoe, is about three miles long, and nearly as many broad. Samitraki, about six miles in circumference, is about two and a half miles in length, and about half-a-mile only broad.

Fanò, in geological structure and disposition of ground, somewhat resembles Zante. It consists of two parts; one mountainous, rising to the height of about a thousand feet above the sea, the summit of which, Maraviglia, may be five or six hundred feet higher, and including a mountain valley, of basin-like form, without an outlet, already described; the other, an irregular low hilly surface, entirely destitute of plain. The former, as already remarked, is composed of limestone; the latter chiefly of marl and sandstone; the one without springs; the other, the marl district, abounding in them.

Merlera and Samitraki are without any mountain limestone; they rise to no considerable height, not perhaps above two hundred feet; are hilly, like the lower part of Fanò; and, like it, consist principally of marl and of sandstone—the former greatly preponderating. Baron Theotoki mentions, amongst the excellent qualities of Merlera, that it has abundance of good water, and very many springs, and little streams. The information I obtained on the spot was not in accordance with this. I was told that the inhabitants are dependent on one spring—that, fortunately, a copious spring—and that there was no other. His remark is more justly applicable to Samitraki, where there are five perennial springs of good water; and where, I was assured, in winter and spring, springs are innumerable—a curious circumstance, considering the very limited extent of the islet and its distance from Corfu.

Although the population of these islands is so limited, it is considered rather in excess, in relation to produce and the means of subsistence.* Most of the inhabitants have portions of land in *colonia*—paying, as already mentioned, a portion of the produce to the lord. None of them are rich; few of them are very poor; the majority of them, although above want, are in rather straitened circumstances, and have more or less difficulty in living. They live in a very

* The men, it is said, seldom marry under thirty; the women earlier. The marriage ceremonies, especially the feastings, practised on the occasion, are expensive, which, with providing bedding, &c., must act as a check on improvident marriages, and tend to preserve a certain proportion between the numbers of the inhabitants and the means of subsistence; and the same causes I apprehend are in operation throughout the Ionian Islands, where the population, scanty in proportion to the space occupied, appears to be very stationary.

primitive manner. In Fano there are two priests; in Merlera, one; they have no medical men; no lawyers; no artificers; no shopkeepers; they make their own ploughs, and even their own boats. In each island the cultivation is of a mixed kind. In Fano, the olive is extensively grown. In the two other islands there are few olive-trees; the vine is principally cultivated, and Indian corn, both of which form also a part of the cultivation of Fano.

Belonging to the three islands there are about a hundred and fifty head of cattle, of a diminutive size, and light active form, not unlike deer, few of them exceeding four feet in height. They are bred there, and are kept chiefly for the use of the plough; no use is made of cows' milk. In Fano and Merlera there are about 1000 sheep and goats; and in Samitraki, about 150. Their milk is chiefly employed in making cheese.

Having been in quarantine with Corfu, for a long period, from which they were not released until 1819, or about that time, they have been little in habits of intercourse with that island; more with the Albanian shore. Oil and honey are the principal articles which they export; the honey of Fano is excellent, and in high repute. Their imports are very trifling indeed, and very miscellaneous—little comforts, and articles of luxury, if the term be applicable, rather than necessaries, excepting grain, which, not growing sufficient themselves, they are under the necessity of purchasing, in part, abroad.

In Fano, there is a small detachment of British troops, under the command of a subaltern officer, who performs the functions of commandant and governor, and, in his very limited sphere, is a person of consequence. To him quarrels are referred ; and, if they exceed his power to settle, the cases are brought before the tribunals in Corfu. There is a nominal militia; each party of fifty men has a leader; the people have not been disarmed; the leaders are privileged to carry large knives. I must not pass over their dwellings. Their houses are neatly and strongly built, especially in Fano, and are kept clean and in good order. In each there is commonly one bed for the married pair, and one only; others of the family sleep on the ground, as is commonly the custom amongst the Greek peasantry, sleeping in their clothes. By the bed often may be seen a little cradle of reeds, just large enough to hold an infant, suspended by cords. Amongst their household utensils may be mentioned a hand-mill, a kind of quern, for grinding corn, a pot for cooking, and a hook for suspending it over the fire; a shelf or two against the wall, on which are arranged a few plates and dishes of earthenware, and a stick, in which holes are bored, suspended from the roof, for holding wooden spoons. Their corn they store in large pots or vases, made of clay, mixed with hair or straw, fashioned with the hands, and slowly dried in the open air, from which they are cautiously removed within doors, by means of ropes ; it is said that grain will keep in them, in good condition, three or four years. Oil they preserve in vessels of baked clay; cheese in barrels, in brine; honey in glazed jars,* and also wine; and wine and oil also in skins. The spindle and distaff are in use, and the loom; a coarse cloth is made, and a coarse strong cordage, from the fibre of the broom, obtained by maceration. The women are said to lead hard laborious lives, as may be well expected, where so much is to be done at home; and it is also said that they are harshly treated. Notwithstanding the eulogies of the author just now quoted, relative to the manners of this people, they have the character, I was informed, of being envious, jealous, and rather quarrelsome. The eulogy referred to, I fear, is no better founded, in reality, than is the description of the isle of Calypso (whether it be supposed to be identical with Fano or Gozo), by Homer or Fenelon :—

> " A scene to fill
> A God from heaven with wonder and delight."

I am tempted by the recollections called up by looking over my notes of our excursion, on this occasion, to give a few more particulars, and especially of Paxo, the end of our little coasting-voyage.

* The bees are not destroyed when the honey is collected; they are driven from the hives by smoke, and return to them. This is the practice in the Mediterranean generally; a little honey is left for their subsistence. Even in winter, in fine days, the bees are abroad and busy. Should the winter season be very unfavourable for flowers, in some places, as in Malta, sugar is given them. The price of the fine honey of Fano, when we were there, was ten oboli, or about fivepence a-pound.

The south-west coast of Corfu—along which we passed, lying off and on, landing wherever we felt inclined—is well adapted to excite interest and afford pleasure; indeed, I am not acquainted with any shore more beautiful on the whole, or more varied, assuming, as it does, different characters of scenery according to the description of prevailing rock. But on these peculiarities it would be tedious to dwell here; I shall pass on to Paxo.

The island of Paxo has not yet been accurately surveyed; its circumference is considered as about twenty-seven miles, its length about seven, and its width about three. In form it approaches the oval; the outline of its north and north-east side is most irregular, where the coast is indented with little bays. It is hilly, or rather one hill, the most elevated part of which probably does not exceed 600 feet.

Its population, according to the last census, was 5300 souls, distributed in the little town of Gaja, the capital of the island, and several small villages scattered here and there, and in isolated houses, which are chiefly confined to the higher grounds. Most of the names of the villages and of the detached country-houses terminate in *atica*, as Casatica, Colmatica, Boikatica,—*atica* signifying *of*, being the termination of the genitive, and the prefix, the names of the proprietors. The houses commonly, both in the town and country, are rather neatly built, of stone of very good quality, in which the island abounds. The walls frequently are without cement, being composed of flat flags of limestone that hardly require it, at least externally. Their roofs are covered with tiles brought from Corfu: nothing of which clay is the material is made in Paxo.

The town of Gaja is very agreeably situated on a rocky declivity, at the bottom of a pretty and deep little bay, with the two islets in front of it, hiding it from the open sea,—the outermost one, the Scoglio della Madonna, where there is a little chapel erected in honour of the Virgin,—and the inner one, nearly in the middle of the bay, the isle of St Nicolo, where there is a small fort. With its neat white-washed houses, fruit-trees, and olive-trees occasionally inter-mixed, Gaja, viewed on entering, offers a very agree-able object; but it contains nothing worthy of note, excepting a large cistern, on which the inhabitants are chiefly dependent for a supply of water. The capacity of this cistern is equal to about 50,000 gal-lons; it was commenced by the Russians before the Ionian Islands were under British protection, and had not, at the time of our visit, been very long completed. The rain-water which it receives, falls on an inclined plane of stone pavement, from whence it passes into a circular gallery surrounding the reser-voir, and filters through sand, laid on a pavement of bricks without cement, into the latter. The cistern itself, cut out of the rock, is lined with bricks coated with Roman cement,* and the latter is covered with

* The cement so called, I was informed, was made of the powder

a varnish of boiled linseed oil.   After it was finished,
it was not used for twelve months.*   Before its construction, in the dry season, the inhabitants were
under the necessity of importing water from Parga
and Leftimo; indeed, I was informed that this necessity was constant throughout the year,—that the
island is without a single spring of fresh-water, and
that the cattle drink sea-water,—a very exaggerated
account.   It is true that Paxo is very deficient in
springs, but is not entirely without them.   On the
shore of Gaja there are several springs brackish in
summer, but fresh in winter and spring, the water of
which, and not sea-water, is used by the cattle; and
in the country there is a small number of springs of
fresh water.   At Papandi I saw two little wells, and
at Laka two others; and at a spot called Remitti, a
spring of running water.   This was in August, at
the height of the dry season, and, with the exception
of the last mentioned, the water was very scanty:
that spring, however, was pretty copious, and it tasted
well; but from its situation, of difficult access, it is
hardly available.†

of well-burnt bricks and virgin-lime, the powder added to the lime,
in the form of paste; it is said to set very well under water, and
makes an excellent cement.

 * Recently, during the administration of Sir Howard Douglas,
another cistern has been formed in Gaja, capable of containing 240,000
gallons of water, which to the inhabitants must be a great benefit, as
before the supply was far from equal to their wants; and in the
summer season, they were almost constantly on an allowance, like
the crew of a ship on a long voyage.

 † It is about three miles from Gaja, in a ravine about thirty feet

As regards the surface and appearance of Paxo, its characteristics are a dry, stony soil, a succession of walled terraces, and an almost continuous foliage —that of its olive-plantations, with the cypress intermixed. The cypress, rising above the olive grove, often has a very pleasing effect, particularly by the side of a belfry, of which a large number are scattered over the island.*

The traveller who may be pressed for time, on visiting Paxo, will do well to go to Papandi, nearly in the centre of the island, standing high, and commanding an extensive view. This pretty village is the bishop's residence, and contains a church, of a singular form, with two domes. The old bishop, whose history is not unlike a romance, was not at home when we called to pay our respects; but we were invited in, stopped, and took some refreshment, and had thus an opportunity, not only of seeing his house, extremely plain and homely, the principal room of which in neat order was a bed-room, as well as a sitting-room, but also of hearing something of his adventurous life. His income is about L.200 † a-year, paid by the government; and it is considered

above the sea, at present inaccessible on the land side, and, excepting in calm weather, inaccessible by sea. Were a path or road cut by which it could be approached at all times, it might be of great service to the inhabitants.

* It is said there are sixty little churches in Paxo; scattered here and there, their belfrys are picturesque objects.

† It is L.156 a-year; the above amount was the sum stated in the bishop's own house; it would be well were oral information generally so near the truth.

an ample allowance. For many years he had been
Bishop of Parga, where, in common with his countrymen, he suffered much from the cruel persecutions
of Ali Pasha, who in vain, both by favour and terror,
attempted to induce him to promote his plans, and
persuade the Pargiots to submit themselves to his
will. The bishop's relations, one after another, it is
said, were put to death; and, lastly, his house was
blown up with gunpowder. His escape, in common
language, might be called miraculous; so it was considered by the people; with the roof he was propelled
into the air, and yet sustained no injury.

The condition of the inhabitants has been already
alluded to; poverty, amounting to beggary, is uncommon amongst them; almost every one has some property of his own in the country, either in land or
olive-trees; indeed, they commonly estimate their
property by the number of their trees. There are
many instances of persons possessing olive-trees without land. This is a paradox, no doubt; the pos-
sessors have taken the liberty to plant the trees on
another man's ground; and possession for a few years
unquestioned gives a permanent right of property, so
long as the trees last.

The air of Paxo is esteemed very healthy, and
there are many instances in the island of advanced
old age; I saw one woman said to be ninety-seven.
They are a good-looking race, especially the women,
when young; but their beauty is ephemeral, seldom
surviving their teens. Their dress is somewhat dif-

ferent from that of the women either of Corfu or
Zante. The head is covered with a kerchief or two,
commonly yellow; a jacket is worn, adapted to
the form, with long sleeves, variously ornamented,
and a full petticoat, frequently of black, flounced
below. Like the men, they have the character of
being very idle and inoffensive; ignorant and superstitious, as must be the case where education is
neglected. Few of them can use the needle and
make their own clothes; they spin a little thread of
cotton, flax, or broom, and knit stockings. In proof
of the ease of circumstances which prevails in this
island, it may be mentioned that very many of the
families residing in the town have cottages in the
country, to which they often resort, especially on Sun-
days and their numerous holidays.

CHAPTER X.

ON MALARIA AND THE FEVERS OF THE IONIAN ISLANDS.

General Healthiness of the Ionian Islands, independent of Fevers of Malaria-Origin.   Tables in illustration.   Different Types of Fever described.   Summer Fever of the Mediterranean.   Remittent Fever.   Illustrative Tables.   Remarks on the Nature and Treatment of Remittent Fever.   Intermittent Fevers.   Malaria. Conjectures respecting its Nature.   Negative Evidence.   Facts in illustration of its Mysterious Origin.   Circumstances favouring its Agency.   Precautions against it.

In relation to salubrity, the principal drawback on the climate of the Ionian Islands is malaria, or that quality of atmosphere or of emanation, whatever it may be, by which the most fatal fevers of warm climates are generated.   Were it not for malaria, these islands would be superior even to our own country, and to most parts of Europe, in general healthiness, and I believe on a par, or nearly so, in regard to lowness of mortality.

In illustration and proof, the following Table is given, showing, for a series of years, the deaths from fevers and from all other diseases amongst our troops serving on this station, drawn up from authentic documents.

RETURN OF DEATHS FROM FEVERS AND ALL OTHER DISEASES AMONG
THE TROOPS SERVING IN THE IONIAN ISLANDS, DURING THE UNDER-
MENTIONED YEARS.

Year.	Average Strength.	Deaths from Fevers.	Deaths from other Diseases.	Total Deaths.
1822	3836	47	39	86
1823	3451	68	41	109
1824	3313	67	34	101
1825	3358	28	41	69
1826	3375	36	31	67
1827	3429	56	38	94
1828	4056	87	60	147
1829	4832	62	76	138
1830	4394	62	56	118
1831	3340	26	24	50
1832	3244	6	40	46
1833	3239	18	40	58
1834	3300	20	34	54
1835	3255	10	34	44
Mean,	3608	4238	42	8435

From which it appears that the average mortality of fourteen years, exclusive of fevers, has been 1.16 per cent.; and, including fevers, 2.34 per cent., or about double.

This fact of the destructiveness of the fevers of the Ionian Islands, clearly shows the importance of the subject; and the next Table that will be given, in which the degree of prevalency of different types of fevers is exhibited, as clearly proves that it is chiefly concentrated in those fevers which are most distinctly of malaria-origin.

RETURN OF CASES OF FEVER ADMITTED INTO THE MILITARY HOSPITALS
IN THE IONIAN ISLANDS, DURING THE UNDERMENTIONED YEARS, PAR-
TICULARIZING THE TYPE OF EACH AND ITS FATALITY.

Year.	Average Number of Troops.	Febris Interm. Quotidiana.		Febris Tertiana.		Feb. Quartana.	
		Admitted.	Died.	Admitted.	Died.	Admitted.	Died.
1822	3836	346	3	282	1	3	...
1823	3451	343	6	158	...	...	...
1824	3313	428	3	207	1	2	...
1825	3358	345	...	100	1	...	...
1826	3375	200	3	65	...	1	...
1827	3429	372	5	142	...	...	...
1828	4056	568	2	217	1	2	...
1829	4832	530	1	398	...	...	...
1830	4394	297	1	405	...	...	...
1831	3340	178	...	278	1	...	...
1832	3244	44	...	249	...	...	...
1833	3239	47	...	181	...	...	...
1834	3300	68	...	195	...	...	...
1835	3255	178	...	51	...	...	...
	Total,	3944	24	2928	5	8	...

TABLE—(*continued.*)

Years.	Average Number of Troops.	Febris remittens.		Febris continens.	
		Admitted.	Died.	Admitted.	Died.
1822	3836	214	30	1347	17
1823	3451	201	56	826	9
1824	3313	374	58	672	5
1825	3358	163	22	803	5
1826	3375	220	19	663	14
1827	3429	507	50	934	1
1828	4056	720	59	1118	25
1829	4832	731	46	1068	15
1830	4394	679	48	930	13
1831	3340	341	20	550	5
1832	3244	290	5	386	1
1833	3239	214	16	468	2
1834	3300	176	15	607	5
1835	3255	292	9	329	1
	Total,	4898	453	10233	118

From which it appears, that the proportional mortality from these different fevers, judging merely from the return, is in every thousand cases as follows :—

Intermittent fevers, ...	4
Remittent, ...	92
Continued, ...	11

Before entering on the obscure subject of malaria, I shall treat briefly of the different types of fever, commencing with that of the continued kind, and confining myself, as much as possible, to facts.

The common continued fever of the Ionian Islands is most prevalent in the hottest months. From this circumstance, it has been called the summer fever. And from its character, being very similar in the different stations and countries of the Mediterranean, it has been further designated as the summer fever of the Mediterranean. Its degree of frequency, during the different months of the year, is tolerably well shown in the following Table, drawn up from the monthly returns of sick of the 51st regiment.

RETURN OF CASES OF CONTINUED FEVER ADMITTED INTO THE HOSPITAL OF THE 51ST REGIMENT, MONTHLY,* DURING THE UNDERMENTIONED YEARS.

Strength,	413†	404	405	411	527	532	533	508	475	Total for nine Years.
Year,	1825.	1826.	1827.	1828.	1829.	1830.	1831.	1832.	1833.	
Station,	Cephal.	Zante.	Zante.	Corfu.	Corfu.	Corfu.	Corfu.	Corfu.	Corfu.	
January,	5	1	3	1	1	9	..	..	..	20
February,	6	2	1	3	4	9	2	3	..	30
March,	7	5	6	6	1	5	..	2	..	32
April,	9	7	8	6	7	5	4	..	5	51
May,	14	2	6	5	17	4	..	2	19	69
June,	16	3	6	20	12	41	8	7	..	113
July,	31	9	28	18	11	25	1	4	20	145
August,	36	3	20	17	21	34 1‡	1	2	10	144
September,	28	5	5	5	12	4	1	..	4	64
October,	23	15	5	2	10	2	..	1	3	61
November,	20	4	1	1	2	..	..	1	3	32
December,	2	5	..	1	3	..	..	..	3	14
Total,	197	61	89	85	101	138	17	22	67	775

This fever, in its character, approaches the ephemeral, and in many instances is purely ephemeral. It commonly terminates in health in three or four days. If protracted beyond these limits, local internal inflammation is to be apprehended. The very little danger attending it—the very trifling mortality produced by it—is clearly shown by the preceding Tables, and especially by the last; from which it appears that, of the total 775 cases which, in the course of nine years, occurred in the 51st regiment, one only had a fatal termination.

A very brief notice will suffice of the symptoms. Its invasion is sudden. It generally commences with

* The monthly period is from the 21st to the 20th—g. e., the 21st December, to the 20th January.

† Number of men at headquarters, from whom the admissions into hospital.

‡ The second number denotes a death.

some severity of symptoms, especially headach, not a little alarming to those ignorant of its nature. Beside the headach, there is usually pain in the back and limbs. The pulse is commonly much accelerated, small, and hard; the skin hot; the tongue foul, with urgent thirst and anorexia. The attack is sometimes ushered in by a slight rigor.

Considering the real mildness of its nature, the treatment of it is of little importance. The probability is, that the majority of cases would do well without any medical treatment. Owing to the same quality of mildness, I may remark, it will bear much and varied treatment with impunity; and recoveries will take place in most instances, even though the treatment should be improper.

Gentle purgative medicine, rest, and abstinence, in most instances, are the best remedial means. Bloodletting is well borne, but it is hardly required.

When the disease terminates fatally, I believe it is invariably in consequence of the existence of local inflammation, or of complication with some organic lesion; or it may be maintained, and perhaps most correctly, that the diagnosis in such cases has been incorrect, and the term continued fever, improperly applied. In illustration, I shall adduce the few fatal instances which I witnessed whilst I was on the station, altogether nine in number. The bodies were all submitted to a post-mortem examination, of which I made notes at the time.

I. Aged 21; admitted on the 26th July; died on the 12th August, of peritoneal inflammation, probably owing to a minute perforation in some part of the small intestines. The perforation was not detected ; the inference is drawn from pain of abdomen coming on suddenly, when the patient was apparently convalescent, on the 6th August, and from there being in the cavity of the abdomen, besides coagulable lymph, a considerable quantity of fluid, of an offensive odour.

II. Aged 28 ; admitted on the 8th October ; died on the 18th October, also of peritoneal inflammation, and probably depending on a minute perforation of intestine, which escaped detection. Three pints of sero-purulent fluid were found in the cavity of the abdomen, and parts of the intestines and omentum were nearly gangrenous.

III. Aged 33 ; admitted on the 12th July ; died on the 16th July, also of peritoneal inflammation, depending on perforation of the lower part of the ileum. The perforation was very small, barely admitting a fine surgeon's probe. The peritoneal coat round the perforation was dark red—the villous coat very little redder than natural ; the site of the perforation was a small ulcer, very little exceeding the cavity in its dimensions. The adjoining glandulæ aggregatæ were unusually elevated, and the solitary glands in the large intestines were larger than natural. This patient was considered convalescent on the 14th of July, when his skin was cool, and pulse slow. On the 15th he had pain and heat of forehead and fulness of epigastrium, without pain on pressure. On the 16th, at two o'clock P.M., he had severe pain in the umbilical region, rapidly followed by other symptoms of peritonitis, and at nine o'clock P.M. he expired.*

---

* Perforation of the small intestines, the effect of circumscribed ulceration is far from an uncommon occurrence in the Mediterranean, and I believe is the principal, if not the only, cause of fatal peritoneal inflammation, excluding, of course, that of traumatic origin ; whilst perforation of the stomach is exceedingly rare. In Germany, on the contrary, the latter is not uncommon, whilst the former is uncommon in a very high degree. In the extensive pathological museum attached to the great Civil Hospital in Vienna, there are several examples of perforated stomach, but not one of perforated small intestine ; and the distinguished professor who has charge of the collection, assured me he had never witnessed the latter. The locality of organic diseases, strictly investigated anatomically, is a subject which has not hitherto

IV. Aged 27 ; admitted on the 3d of May ; died on the 5th of May, of inflammation within the cavity of the cranium. Pus (tried by the optical test), was found in small quantity in the posterior cornua of the lateral ventricles, and at the base of the brain, mixed with lymph. The disease commenced with a rigor, on the 2d of May, after exposure to the sun, and an excess committed in drinking, followed by severe headach and nausea, and on the 4th, by violent delirium, which was not relieved by copious blood-letting.

V. Aged 23 ; admitted on the 5th December ; died on the 10th of December, also it is probable, of inflammation within the cavity of the cranium. Fluid was found under the arachnoid membrane ; about an ounce and half at the base of the brain, and a small quantity of lymph and puriloid fluid in one of the convolutions. The ordinary febrile symptoms were accompanied with severe delirium.

VI. Aged 25 ; admitted 16th July ; died on the 23d July ; the cause of death doubtful. The epithelium of the œsophagus was partially abraded. The stomach and intestines were distended with air, and contained a dark grumous matter, which became red on dilution with water, as if it were coloured by blood. There were no traces of inflammation either in the stomach or intestines. Jaundice preceded death, and nausea and vomiting, and a matter was thrown up not unlike coffee-grounds.

VII. Aged 22 ; admitted on the 10th of December ; died on the 17th of December, of partial inflammation of the substance of the lungs and of the bronchia generally. Portions of the lungs were found hepatized, and the bronchia very red, and smeared with muco-purulent fluid. The febrile symptoms were accompanied with cough and pain of chest.

VIII. Aged 28 ; admitted on the 2d of May ; died on the 9th of May, of inflammation of the lungs, complicated with inflammation within the cavity of the cranium. The lungs were found gorged with blood and serum, and the bronchia unusually red. The choroid plexus, in the inferior portion of each lateral ventricle, was covered with lymph, and there was a pretty thick pellicle of lymph on the pons varolii and medulla oblongata. At the commencement of the

---

received the attention which it seems to deserve. Were it fully inquired into, it might make us better acquainted with the causes of many diseases which at present are only vaguely conjectured.

attack, the febrile symptoms were attended with some pain of chest, and towards its conclusion, with deafness and delirium.

IX. Aged 35; admitted on the 28th August; died on the 15th of October, of chronic dysentery, following inflammation of lung. The inferior part of superior lobe of right lung was found densely hepatized, of a light colour, and the colon closely studded with chronic ulcers. No symptoms of pneumonia were observed during the progress of the disease. In its early stage the febrile symptoms were accompanied with jaundice, and this was succeeded by dysentery.

The remittent fever of the Ionian Islands is most prevalent, and most severe, during the summer and autumnal months. The following Table, formed from the monthly returns of sick of the 51st regiment, during a period of nine years, shows pretty well the connexion of the disease with the seasons.

RETURN OF CASES OF REMITTENT FEVERS, ADMITTED INTO THE HOSPITAL OF THE 51ST REGIMENT, MONTHLY, DURING THE UNDER MENTIONED YEARS.

Year.	1825.		1826.		1827.		1828.	1829.		1830.		1831.	1832.	1833.		Total.	
Station,	Cephal.		Zante.		Zante.		Corfu.	Corfu.		Corfu.		Corf.	Corf.	Corfu.		Admitted.	Died.
Strength,	413		404		405		411	527		532		533	508	475			
		Died.		Dieu.		Died.			Died.		D.				Died.		
Jan.	2	..	9	..	1	..	..	5	..	8	..	..	..	2	1	28	1
Feb.	..	..	2	..	1	..	..	..	1	9	..	2	..	3	..	17	..
March,	..	..	..	..	..	..	..	2	..	5	..	..	..	2	..	11	1
April,	..	..	2	..	..	..	2	5	..	5	..	4	..	..	..	18	..
May,	..	..	..	..	..	..	..	8	..	4	..	..	2	..	..	14	..
June,	..	..	4	..	..	..	..	20	2	41	..	8	7	..	..	80	..
July,	1	..	13	..	4	2	6	15	2	25	..	1	4	..	..	69	4
August,	8	1	14	1	32	2	8	28	1	34	1	1	2	..	..	128	7
Sept.,	13	..	14	1	27	4	11	25	2	4	..	1	..	5	1	100	7
Oct.,	5	..	3	1	15	..	10	24	2	2	..	..	1	3	..	63	3
Nov.	4	..	4	..	12	1	13	11	..	..	..	..	1	..	..	45	3
Dec.,	4	1	2	..	1	..	7	15	..	..	..	..	..	1	..	30	1
Total,	37	2	63	3	93	9	57	158	10	137	1	17	22	12	12	603	27

The character of this fever is very different from that of the preceding, both as regards symptoms and progress, as well as degree of danger.

Its proportional danger is indicated, in some measure, by the preceding Tables relating to it; according to the first of which, p. 220, it has proved fatal to about nine of every hundred attacked amongst the troops generally, in the different islands, during a period of fourteen years; and, according to the second, that last given, to about four of every hundred attacked in the 51st Regiment, during a period of nine years, which were, with the exception of two, unusually healthy years.

The disease commonly commences with sudden prostration of strength, and apparent diminution of all the vital energies. The pulse is almost invariably quick and feeble; the respiration quick and short; the temperature either below the natural standard, or only a little above it, accompanied with a sensation of chilliness, sometimes amounting to rigor. There is generally headach, though not severe; or a sensation of weight of head, with pains of back and of limbs. There is often nausea, occasionally vomiting; occasionally yellowness of the skin; often flatulent distension of abdomen; occasionally relaxation of the bowels.

The remittent type of the disease is commonly well marked in its progress. The exacerbation is, in most cases, of irregular occurrence, and uncertain duration—often many times in the course of the twenty-four hours, with stages of apyrexia intervening. Some cases approach the confines of fever of the intermittent type, and others of the continued.

Most commonly the exacerbation is not preceded by chilliness, nor followed by sweating. It is often accompanied with delirium.

The danger is almost invariably greater than the symptoms would indicate to the inexperienced. With the exception of flatulent distension of abdomen, all the symptoms the least distressing are easily removed, especially pain, but without diminution of danger, which is chiefly indicated by rapidity and feebleness of pulse, and by prostration of strength. When I reflect on the severe cases, no other disease occurs to me, excepting spasmodic cholera, which gives such an idea of the energies of the constitution being overpowered, as if a subtle active poison had been administered, paralyzing the nervous system, and fatal to life. The course of the fever, accordingly, is commonly rapid; when fatal, it is generally before the ninth day; often on the third or fourth.

In the fatal cases, the appearances on dissection are very various. They may be conveniently divided into three classes;—1st, Those belonging to the disease, when pure, or not distinctly complicated; 2dly, When complicated; and, 3dly, When misnamed. I shall give the results of the examinations of thirty-eight bodies, returned as having died of this disease. The cases were all under treatment in our regimental hospitals, under the care of their respective medical officers. I saw most of them in progress, and was present at each post mortem examination, and immediately made notes of the principal appearances.

TABLE, SHOWING THE PRINCIPAL APPEARANCES NOTICED IN THE UNMIXED INSTANCES OF REMITTENT FEVER, OR THOSE NOT DISTINCTLY COMPLICATED.

No.	Station.	Age of Patient.	Duration of Disease in Days.	Time of Death.	Autopsia Hours after Death.	Morbid Appearances.
1	Corfu,	25	5	Aug. 10,	6	A good deal of fluid in lateral ventricles, and at base of brain; spleen large; not unlike the crassamentum of blood, but less dark; lower portion of colon dark-red, as if from ecchymosis; partial, undue redness of stomach, and of intestines.
2	...	22	3	8,	13	Lower part of ileum redder than natural; glandulæ aggregatæ enlarged; cœcum red and rough, as if from the deposition of a little lymph: the spleen about twice its natural size; soft, like the clot of blood.
3	...	24	7	July 31,	8	Pretty much fluid in the ventricles and at base of the brain; red spots on lower portion of ileum; a few minute ulcers where the colon passes into the rectum; the spleen about thrice its natural size; like the preceding.
4	...	36	7	26,	18	The spleen about thrice its natural size, and very soft.
5	...		11	Nov. 4,	7	Skin yellow; four scruples of fluid at base of brain; gall-bladder distended with thick viscid bile; common gall-duct pervious; omentum reflected over, and adhering to, gall-bladder and stomach; stomach and intestines partially red; the spleen large, dark-red, and pretty firm.
6	...	29	4	Aug. 1,	10	Stomach and duodenum redder than natural; the spleen large, dark, and soft.
7	...	28	8	June 23,	18	Portions of the dura and pia mater more vascular than usual; pretty much fluid in the ventricles, and at the base of the brain; red patches on stomach and ileum; the spleen large and soft.
8	Zante,	34	7	Sep 6,	14	The surface of the lungs studded with vesicles distended with air, from the size of a pin's head to that of a pea; diaphragm unusually vascular: a little lymph on contiguous surface of liver; red patches near cardiac portion of stomach, from which a slight oozing of blood; a blackish fluid in stomach, like coffee-grounds (had hiccough and vomited similar fluid); duodenum redder than natural; the spleen unusually large and soft.
9	...	30	9	20,	16	Dura mater unusually vascular; much fluid at base of the brain; two ounces of yellow serum in the pericardium; the spleen large; weight about two pounds, resembling crassamentum.

TABLE—(*continued.*)

No.	Station.	Age of Patient.	Duration of Disease in Days.	Time of Death.	Autopsia. Hours after Death.	Morbid Appearances.
10	Zante,	30	11	Sept. 23,	19	(The wife of a soldier) ; inner surface of uterus very red ; a clot of blood, the size of a large pea, in left ovarium ; in right three cavities of a smaller size, containing a limpid fluid ; (she had aborted several times) ; spleen large, and extremely soft ; liver, pancreas, and kidneys soft.
11	...	30	11	Oct. 2,	14	Dura and pia mater redder than natural ; a good deal of fluid in the tissue of the pia mater, and in the ventricles, and at the base of brain. Aspera arteria throughout dark red : rough transverse stripes of a warty appearance, in many instances covering ulcers in cœcum, ascending colon, and upper part of rectum.
12	...	29	6	5,	21	The spleen large and soft. The membranes of the brain, the air passages and alimentary canal unusually red, but probably the effect of staining.
13	...	32	9	13,	6	Pretty much fluid in the ventricles and at the base of the brain ; the trachea redder than natural ; partial abrasion of epithelium of lower portion of œsophagus, with redness of its mucous coat ; slight œdema of posterior mediastinum ; the spleen large and soft.
14	...	25	5	27,	10	Pretty much fluid in the cellular tissue of the pia mater ; about an ounce and a half in the ventricles and at the base of the brain. Bubbles of air in the thoracic duct ; lower part of ileum very red, and also the lower part of rectum and its glands enlarged ; the descending colon dark red, and smeared with a thin bloody mucus, and in one spot slightly ulcerated. Spleen large and very soft, about three lbs. weight ; gall-bladder distended with bile ; spots of ecchymosis on its inner coat.
15	...	24	4	28,	9	A good deal of fluid in tissue of pia mater ; the spleen large ; not unusually soft, but friable.
16	Corfu,	36	6	July 31,	18	Pretty much serum in the ventricles and at the base of the brain ; inner coat of stomach in part dark red, and in part brown ; much bile in the gall-bladder ; liver voluminous and rather soft ; spleen large and soft. The patient died suddenly and unexpectedly, the symptoms having been mild,—an event, it may be remarked not uncommon in cases of this disease.
17	...	28	4	20,	24	Two ounces of fluid in the ventricles and at the base of the brain ; spleen large and very soft—its weight about two lbs. ; a little coagulable lymph on the surface of the liver. The blood-vessels, air and alimentary passages more or less red, probably from staining : putrefaction had commenced.
18	...	25	5	24,	12	A good deal of 'fluid in the pia mater, the ventricles, and at the base of the brain ; the spleen large and exceedingly soft, of the colour of burnt umber.

TABLE—(*continued.*)

No.	Station.	Age of Patient.	Duration of Disease in Days.	Time of Death.	Autopsia. Hours after Death.	Morbid Appearances.
19	Corfu,	30	8	Aug. 30,	24	About three ounces of serum in the pericardium ; the heart large ; the aorta diseased throughout ; its inner coat irregularly thickened ; its middle atrophied irregularly ; the spleen large, but very little softer than natural.
20	...	20	5	Oct. 5,	12	The trachea unduly red. The solitary glands of the colon unusually large ; many of the follicles of the rectum the seat of small ulcers. The spleen large, of poultaceous consistence, and extremely foetid ; putrefaction was far advanced in it ; the *foetor* from it excited nausea and a peculiar slightly acrid sensation in the pharynx.
21	Paxo,	47	5	23,	8	A good deal of fluid in the pia mater, in the ventricles, and at the base of the brain ; large fibrinous concretions in right ventricle, with a little clot ; three and a half ounces of serum in pericardium ; the spleen large and soft.
22	Zante,	31	2	Sept. 18,	14	A good deal of fluid in the ventricles and at the base of the brain ; spleen between two and three lbs. in weight ; very soft.
23	...	18	4	21,	18	Lower part of œsophagus and cardiac orifice of stomach unusually red ; spleen large and soft.
24	...	28	4	21,	18	A good deal of serum in the ventricles and at the base of the brain ; about one ounce and a half in the pericardium ; about two pints in the cavity of the abdomen ; inner coat of stomach unusually red ; the liver of unusual firmness ; its surface rough ; the spleen large and soft.

Relative to the day of death, given in the fourth column of the table, reckoning from the commencement of the fever, the numbers assigned must be considered only as approximations ; they strictly denote the time the patients were in hospital : in military practice, it is always difficult to ascertain when the early stage of any complaint commences, as soldiers are averse to come into hospital, and will generally continue in performance of their duties as long as possible.

Besides the morbid appearances noticed, other appearances were very common. The vessels of the dura and pia mater were frequently much injected with blood; but whether from what is commonly considered inflammatory action, or a post mortem effect from pressure on the great vessels from flatulent distension of the stomach and intestines, which was of common occurrence, it may be difficult to decide. The right cavities of the heart, the venæ cavæ, the vena azygos, and the depending part of the lungs, were, in most instances, more or less gorged with blood, and the blood was generally either liquid or only softly coagulated; it seldom showed a buffy coat, or, what is equivalent, fibrinous concretions.

TABLE SHOWING THE PRINCIPAL APPEARANCES NOTICED IN THE COMPLICATED INSTANCES OF REMITTENT FEVER.

No.	Station.	Age of Patient.	Duration of Disease.	Time of Death.	Autopsia. Hours after Death.	Morbid Appearances.
1	Corfu,	39	2	Oct. 31,	18	A good deal of fluid in the tissue of the pia mater, and in the ventricles and at the base of the brain; the superior portion of the corpora striata softer than natural; the inferior portion of the trachea and the bronchial tubes dark red, and spotted with coagulable lymph, producing an appearance like that of minute tubercles; the lungs loaded with dark blood, particularly inferiorly; red patches here tand there in jejunum; the spleen about twice its natural size, and unusually soft, especially its dependent portion.
2	...	28	3	Aug. 1,	22	About two ounces of fluid at the base of the brain; left lung extensively hepatized, and in part œdematous; the right similar, in a less degree; the spleen large, dark, and soft; liver soft, and easily broken; gall-bladder distended with viscid bile, and containing some curd-like substance.
3	...	23	5	Dec. 7,	6	The intestines generally and other abdominal viscera redder than natural, as if from vas-

TABLE—(*continued.*)

No.	Station.	Age of Patient.	Duration of Disease in Days.	Time of Death.	Autopsia, Hours after Death.	Morbid Appearances.
						cular fulness; lower part of ileum dark red, and studded with deep ulcers, the largest oval, about one inch and three-fourths long in diameter, with elevated edges, the valve of the colon partially destroyed by ulceration; the colon, and especially the cœcum, redder than natural; the spleen large, dark, and soft.
4	Zante,	23	12	Sept. 25,	15	Pia mater enfiltered with serum; a good deal of fluid in the ventricles and at the base of the brain, about two ounces; great sympathetic nerve rather red; portions of stomach and of small intestines redder than usual; upper portion of colon thickened from œdema of its cellular coats; its lining membrane rough, red, here and there green, with ulcerated streaks and spots; ulcerated spots in the descending colon; the rectum redder than natural.
5	...	31	11	Oct. 11,	18	More fluid than usual in tissue of pia mater, in the ventricles, and at the base of the brain; slight œdema of cellular texture of right side of neck; second ganglion of pneumo-gastric nerve unusually vascular; aspera arteria unduly red; the inferior portions of both lungs hepatized; inferior lobe of left lung very soft; weight of spleen about half a pound, very soft.

In neither of these five cases were there any symptoms noticed indicative of the unusual lesions discovered after death, excepting in the second, in which the pulmonary affection might be considered as connected with cough,—slight at first, and before death troublesome. In this last mentioned instance, the general character of remittent fever was sustained, in the well marked exacerbations and remissions of the disease. Such a masking of lesions in relation to symptoms is not uncommon, nor more than might be expected from experience in fevers generally, and especially when accompanied with delirium, or having a tendency to it. Under excitation of the brain, or the reverse, whether in mania or amentia, in furious or in low and muttering delirium, diseased states of other important organs are commonly latent, and advance often to a fatal result without materially affecting their functional actions,—at least, according to ordinary observation, unassisted by the best methods of medical examination.

TABLE, SHEWING THE PRINCIPAL APPEARANCES NOTICED IN INSTANCES RETURNED AS REMITTENT-FEVER, AND, IT IS SUPPOSED, ERRONEOUSLY SO.

No.	Station.	Age of Patient.	Duration of Disease in Days.	Time of Death.	Autopsia, Hours after Death.	Morbid Appearances.
1	Corfu,	39	69	Nov 13,	7	Much fluid in tissue of pia mater, and in the ventricles and at the base of the brain; two ounces of serum in the pericardium; the lungs exceedingly diseased, abounding in minute tubercles, in different stages of softening, and in the superior lobe of each containing an excavation; small ulcerated spots in the bronchia; dark, as it were gangrenous, patches in the lower portion of œsophagus; most of its epithelium abraded; the lower part of ileum slightly ulcerated; the larger intestines severely ulcerated, as in chronic dysentery.
2	Zante,	30	20	Sept. 20,	18	A few hydatids, the largest about the size of a hazel-nut, adhering to the posterior part of the left pleura. Several melanotic tubercles in both lungs; small vomicæ in left lung, and one large one in its inferior lobe; a few small cavities in the middle and inferior lobe of right lung; a deep ulcerated cavity, penetrating to the cartilage under the border of the left sacculus laryngis; the aspera arteria of a livid hue, with purplish spots, as if becoming gangrenous; the spleen and pancreas harder than natural.
3	Corfu,	25	5	Nov. 23,	24	Both lungs unusually red—even their upper surface—and exhibiting spots, some of a dark red, others of a florid hue; the larynx, trachea, and bronchia, also very red, even the epiglottis; gelatinous mucus in the large bronchial tubes; patches in stripes of ecchymosis, interspersed with elevated lines, as if of coagulable lymph, throughout the whole of the large intestines; the spleen of natural size, appearance, and consistence.
4	...	26	7	Sept. 27,	19	A good deal of fluid in the tissue of the pia mater and at the base of the brain; the lower part of the trachea and bronchia very red; the gall-bladder distended with black fluid, of slightly putrid odour, and without viscidity; the inner coat of gall-bladder stained

TABLE—(*continued.*)

No.	Station.	Age of Patient.	Duration of Disease in Days.	Time of Death.	Autopsia. Hours after Death.	Morbid Appearances.
						by it, as also the cystic and common duct, and a portion of the duodenum; the hepatic duct contained some orange bile; the liver appeared to be healthy; the spleen small and firm; the epithelium of œsophagus very thick, like a false membrane, and easily detached; and the subjacent surface unusually red.
5	Cephal.,	47	14	19,	10	Much fluid in the tissue of the pia mater, in the ventricles, and at the base of the brain; a hemispherical tumour, about the size of a walnut, attached to the dura mater, under the left parietal bone; that part of the cerebrum on which it pressed, not apparently diseased: the stomach very red, with bright streaks of a vermilion hue; it had a raw appearance, being without adhering mucus; the spleen was firm, of its ordinary size.
6	Corfu,	27	13	11,	8	A good deal of fluid in the ventricles and at the base of the brain; a considerable quantity of fetid serum, with some pus and coagulable lymph in the cavity of the abdomen and in the pelvis; a live round worm in the right iliac fossa, close to a perforation in the lower part of the ileum; numerous and large ulcers in the inferior part of ileum, laying bare, in some instances, the muscular coat, and in others the peritoneal; similar ulcers, but smaller, in the upper portion, and a few also in the jejunum; the contiguous folds of intestines were glued together by lymph; spleen of natural appearance.
7	...	27	10	Dec. 21,	31	Much fetid sero-purulent fluid, mixed with which was a little fæcal matter and oil, in the cavity of the abdomen; adhesion of the convolutions of the intestines; a small perforation in the upper portion of the ileum, communicating with an ulcerated spot in the mucus coat; there was no other ulcer near it; in the lower portion of the ileum there were several deep ulcers, two or three of which had nearly penetrated into the cavity of the abdomen; the glandulæ aggregatæ were enlarged; the spleen large and rather soft.
8	...	22	25	Aug. 28,	6	A good deal of fluid in the ventricles and at the base of the brain; about two ounces of purulent fluid in the cavity of the pelvis; the lower part of the ileum studded with ulcers, two of which had penetrated through all the coats of the intestine into the cavity of the abdomen; the spleen of natural firmness, and very little larger than usual.
9	...	34	2	Sept. 10,	16	Vessels of dura and pia mater very turgid; a considerable quantity of blood effused between the pia and dura mater over the cerebrum, especially of right hemisphere; a good deal of serum in the ventricles and at the base of the brain; the substance of the brain apparently natural; a slight abrasion of epithelium of œsophagus here and there; the mucous coat of a dusky red; the spleen firm, and of moderate size.

In these cases, the symptoms at the commencement were those of remittent-fever; the name of the
disease was then given; the after symptoms were of
a different description, and according, more or less,
with the principal organic lesions discovered by the
post-mortem inspection.

The remittent-fever of the Ionian Islands appears
to be of the same kind as the endemic remittent-
fever of the East and West Indies, of the tropics
generally, and of the south of Europe, including the
yellow fever of warm climates, which seems to be
merely a variety of it.

Relative to the exact nature of the disease, and
the best modes of treating it, I must confess myself
equally at a loss to give a satisfactory answer.

The symptoms of remittent-fever throw little light
on its nature, perhaps it should rather be said none,
no more than do the symptoms in cholera morbus on
that disease.   From the autopsia, it appears that the
spleen is the organ most commonly found in a diseased
state; and next to the spleen, the intestines, especially the follicular structure, the glandulæ aggregatæ
of the ileum, and the solitary glands of the large
intestines.   But, comparatively, what little relation
is there between the lesions discovered after death,
the symptoms during life, and the fatal event.

Whether the blood is the main seat of the disease
is deserving of careful inquiry.   It is not indicated
by the appearance of that fluid drawn in the early
stage, which then often has the character of healthy

blood.   In the Ionian Islands I did not examine the
blood after death ; but on the occasion of an endemic
fever which occurred at Malta in the autumn of
1829, of the remittent kind, and in many instances
accompanied with yellowness of the skin, I made a
partial examination of it, and in several cases found
it to contain urea; in these cases death was preceded
by suppression of urine, or by a greatly diminished
secretion of it.

If the nature of the disease be obscure and unde-
termined, it is not surprising that the treatment of
it should be matter of hesitation and doubt.   I have
witnessed the trial of various modes of treatment,
anxiously and carefully made, but I cannot say that
I have seen any happy general results—any tolerably
uniform success from any special method.   At present it is more easy to say what is injurious than what
is beneficial.   It is proved, I believe, by very extensive experience, that blood-letting, excepting in small
quantities, and under peculiar circumstances, is decidedly injurious.   Experience, too, as far as I could
learn, is against the use of calomel in large doses, or
of mercury, with the intent of producing ptyalism,
though this is more doubtful.   Experience also seems
to be against the administration of bark and of sul-
phate of quinine, excepting with great caution, and
in very moderate doses.   From all I witnessed I
was disposed at last to prefer the mildest treatment ;
watching symptoms, and attempting the relief of
them ; paying particular attention to the bowels and

their evacuations, and administering the gentlest aperients, especially the oleaginous.   Nursing, in the
remittent-fever, is of very great importance; the patients require peculiar attention.   When the disease
is at all severe, they should be kept strictly in the
horizontal posture ; a bed-pan should be used ; there
are many instances which have come to my knowledge of sudden and unexpected death, apparently
from syncope, produced by assuming the erect posture, and especially after an alvine evacuation.

Independent of the reasons already assigned for
expressing myself with hesitation relative to the treatment of remittent-fever, there is another deserving of
consideration, namely, that in different situations, and
in different years, it may, more or less, vary, if not
in type and character, at least in intensity and complications, so that the remedial means which may
have been found on one occasion to be useful, may
fail on another.

The proportional prevalency of intermittent-fever
is shown by the table in page 220 ; as is also the
degree of prevalency of its three varieties, the quotidian, tertian, and quartan.

The following Table is inserted, for the purpose of
showing the connexion of these forms of fever with the
seasons of the year.   It is drawn up from the monthly
returns of the sick of the 51st regiment, and embraces
a period of eight years.   Quartan fever is, in no instance, mentioned ; but whether because it never
occurred, or because, on account of its great rareness'

it was not thought deserving of special notice, I cannot undertake to say.

RETURN OF CASES OF QUOTIDIAN AND TERTIAN INTERMITTENT-FEVER, ADMITTED INTO THE HOSPITAL OF THE 51ST REGIMENT MONTHLY, DURING THE UNDER-MENTIONED YEARS.

Year, . .	1825.		1826.		1827.		1828.		1829.		1830.		1831.		1832.		Totals.	
Station, . .	Cephal.		Zante.		Zante.		Corfu.		Corfu.		Corfu.		Corfu.		Corfu.			
Strength, .	413		404		405		411		527		532		533		508			
Months.	Q.	T.	Q.	T.	Q.	T.	Q.	T.	Q.	T.	Q.	T.	Q.	T.	Q.	T.	Q.	T.
January, . .	16	..	1	..	3	..	8	..	..	..	..	2	4	..	2	..	34	2
February, .	2	2	2	..	1	..	2	4	2	3	..	..	..	1	..	..	10	10
March, .	6	..	1	..	5	..	3	6	3	2	..	1	..	3	..	4	18	16
April, . .	14	..	1	..	1	5	6	5	5	2	1	2	2	..	..	..	30	14
May, . .	15	..	2	..	1	5	2	3	3	2	2	..	..	..	..	..	25	12
June, . .	22	..	1	..	2	..	1	1	..	1	5	..	..	..	..	..	31	2
July, . .	20	..	4	..	2	1	1	4	..	..	1	..	..	1	..	..	28	6
August, .	6	..	8	..	7	2	1	..	..	..	..	..	..	2	..	1	22	5
September, .	7	..	4	..	3	3	..	1	3	..	1	..	..	2	..	..	18	6
October, .	6	.2	4	..	2	..	1	..	2	..	..	5	1	..	..	1	16	6
November, .	..	2	5	..	4	2	1	1	..	2	..	2	..	1	..	..	10	10
December, .	4	..	4	..	9	3	..	..	..	2	..	3	2	..	..	1	19	9
Totals,	120	4	39	..	40	21	26	25	18	14	10	15	9	10	2	7	261	98

Of all the cases of intermittent-fever which occurred in the 51st regiment, amounting to 359 in eight years, not one appears to have proved fatal, offering a remarkable contrast, in relation to result, when compared with remittent-fever in the same corps. The Table, too, in page 220 shows how small the mortality is from this form of fever : and were it possible to analyze all the fatal cases referred to intermittent-fever, whether quotidian or tertian, I have little doubt that the number of genuine instances would be found very much smaller. This conclusion is the result of necroscopic evidence. I shall briefly notice the principal morbid appearances which were observed in five cases, returned as intermittent, at the inspection of which I was present, in confirmation of the remark just made.

I. Aged thirty-eight; admitted on the 8th February; supposed to be labouring under tertian ague, which shortly assumed the character of remittent-fever, and proved fatal on the 14th of the same month. No distinct morbid appearance was discovered, excepting in the spleen, which was enlarged and soft, like a mass of stale crassamentum.

II. Aged thirty-two; a chronic case of intermittent-fever; died August 1. About a pint and half of serum was found in each pleura; about four ounces of serum in the pericardium; the spleen large, weighing about two lbs.; of firm consistence, and containing masses of a light hue, either yellowish or pinkish, slightly fibrous, not unlike, in appearance, the substance of the udder of the cow; the pancreas of unusual firmness; about six ounces of serum in the cavity of the abdomen; the large intestines throughout spotted with minute ulcers and small cicatrices of ulcers of a bluish hue, and unusually vascular. The left testis, it may be added, was extremely atrophied; hardly a vestige of it remained; a small bony concretion was found in the tunica vaginalis adhering to it, composed of phosphate and carbonate of lime and animal matter; it was of a crystalline structure and slightly diaphonous.

III. Aged twenty-one; admitted on the 27th May, supposed to be labouring under intermittent-fever; dysentery preceded death, which took place on the 24th June. The bronchial and œsophagial glands were found very much enlarged, without consolidation of, or tubercles in the lungs; the spleen was larger and firmer than usual; the lower part of the ileum was red, and its villous coat was slightly ulcerated; the cœcum was nearly of natural appearance; the rest of the colon was red and ulcerated,—not unlike the skin in small-pox, when the eruption is declining, being studded with small ulcers little larger than the flat surface of a split pea; the lumber glands were enlarged, but in a less degree than the thoracic.

IV. Aged twenty-six; admitted on the 19th May, supposed to be labouring under quotidian ague; died on the 13th of June. A small quantity of serum was found in the left pleura; the left lung was partially hepatized; the liver was adhering to the diaphragm and colon; the spleen was enlarged, and contained three soft, cheese-like tubercles, the largest about the size of an almond.

V. Aged twenty; admitted on the 6th June, supposed to be labouring under quotidian ague; died on the 22d of June. A large vomica or cavity of an abscess was found in the upper parts of the superior lobe of right lung,—its walls irregular, sloughing, fetid, almost gangrenous; the substance of the lung adjoining was hepatized to some extent; no well-marked tubercle in either lung; but in the right, independent of the hepatization, there was a deposit not unlike curd in appearance, but firmer and diffused.

In accordance with these results, I believe it may be laid down as a general fact, that when intermittent-fever terminates fatally, it is either in consequence of its passing into the remittent form, or owing to organic disease either arising out of it from some peculiarity of constitution, or accidentally associated with it; or, it may be, the organic disease having been ushered in by rigors, the existence of ague has been erroneously assumed.

I shall now proceed to offer a few remarks on malaria, the presumed cause of intermittent and remittent-fever, and, according to some medical men, of the continued and ephemeral fevers also of warm climates.

What is malaria?—I apprehend were it not for the fevers above mentioned, the word would not be in use; and that the only idea we can at present with propriety connect with it, is that of a certain something, an agent in the atmosphere, the cause of these fevers.

The great obscurity of the subject is manifest from

this, that there is little agreement amongst authors respecting it.

Some have supposed that the substantial cause is principally light carburetted hydrogen,—the gas of marshes, generated by the fermentation and decay of vegetable matter under water, or at least in a moist state, at a certain temperature. Others have supposed that it is sulphuretted hydrogen produced by the decomposition of salts containing sulphuric acid, by the agency of decomposing vegetable matter: others, that it is aqueous vapour and a high temperature combined; and a fourth class of inquirers have attributed the effects to vicissitudes of temperature successively heating and chilling the animal body.

But these views appear to be partial, and not sufficiently supported by facts, or, in brief, are not an induction from established facts.

That the light carburetted hydrogen of marshes is not the gas constituting malaria, seems to be well proved by the experience gained in laboratories and in collieries; and I am of opinion that a similar remark is applicable to sulphuretted hydrogen and all other known gases which have been made the subject of research, and have been breathed more or less in conducting experiments.*

* Mr Daniell, in an ingenious paper " On the Spontaneous Evolution of Sulphuretted Hydrogen in the Waters of the Western Coast of Africa," (*Phil. Mag.* July 1841), has endeavoured to prove that this gas, which he considers as derived from the action of decomposing vegetable matter on the sulphates contained in sea-water, is the principal cause of the remittent fevers which so often prevail there, and

The other views of the nature of the cause of these fevers are also opposed by strong negative evidence:

are so dreadfully destructive. That sulphuretted hydrogen, in a certain quantity, is injurious to health, and even fatal to life, is well known; but I am not aware of any fact in proof of its being capable of producing either remittent or intermittent fever. How many watering-places may be mentioned, in which the atmosphere is partially tainted with sulphuretted hydrogen, and yet exempt from these fevers. How many other places might be named, subject occasionally to severe malaria fevers, the atmosphere of which is not perceptibly contaminated with this gas. The expedition to the Congo, under Captain Tuckey, was as disastrous as the recent one up the Niger, directed by Captain Trotter. In the account of the fever, no mention, I believe, is made of offensive mephitic effluvia, or indeed of any circumstance to which the dreadful malady could be plausibly referred. I could enumerate many instances of the production of sulphuretted hydrogen, in the manner supposed by Mr Daniell, unattended by any sensible bad effect, especially to the extent requisite on his hypothesis. With perfect confidence in the accuracy of his experimental results, a suspicion has arisen in my mind, that the sulphuretted hydrogen he detected, in so many instances, may have been produced by the action of the cork undergoing decay in the water. I have examined at different times, samples of water from the ocean, hundreds of miles from land, from tracts of it where the effects of malaria have never been witnessed, and yet, in most instances, I have found the specimens fetid, from sulphuretted hydrogen, the production of which I have hitherto been in the habit of attributing to the cause just assigned. Mr Daniell does not state how the specimens of water which he examined were preserved. If confined, as is probable, by corks, then the fallacy I have alluded to was present, and further inquiry may be necessary, using water preserved in bottles, with glass stoppers, to determine the question of the presence or evolution of sulphuretted hydrogen in the waters of the western coast of Africa. A large river, from the wooded hills and jungles of the interior of Ceylon, flows into the sea, between Colombo and Negombo; the former town is hardly three miles from its mouth; both towns, in common with the whole south-west coast of the island, are ex-

no constant association of the presumed cause and
effects can be traced. At a certain elevation in a
mountainous region, even within the tropics, and in
situations where the plains are extremely unwholesome, and intermittent and remittent fevers of common occurrence, these diseases cease to appear, though
the changes of temperature by day and night are
great and sudden, very much more so than in the
valleys beneath or in the lower levels.   And, at a
certain distance from land, in the tropical ocean,
there is a like exemption, though moisture often
abounds and the heat is great, as in the region of
squalls, towards and under the equator, where the
gusts of wind, followed by calms, are usually accompanied by drenching rain.

It is far more easy to say what malaria is not, than
what it is. All that relates to its production appears
to be enveloped in profound mystery. I am not
aware of a single circumstance, excepting one, which

empt, in a remarkable manner, from intermittent and remittent
fevers.   Moreover, the worst parts of the western coast of Africa, are
not constantly equally unhealthy.   Occasionally, for months together, there is an exemption from the destructive fever ; but we
cannot suppose that, at the same time, there is any cessation of the
decomposition of vegetable matter, or of its action on the salts of the
brackish or salt-water, or of the production of sulphuretted hydrogen, as a consequence of that action.   On such an obscure subject
as malaria, it is advisable that speculation should be conducted with
extreme caution, especially with a view to practical results, and the
offering of suggestions with a hope of protection.   If the hypothesis
be false, the suggestions founded on it may not only be of no avail,
but, by imparting undue confidence, tempting exposure, and leading
to neglect of other precautionary measures, may do harm.

with propriety can be called a common one, always existing where there is malaria, or where there are fevers attributable to it, and this is warmth, or a certain temperature many degrees above the freezing point; its exact limit is not easily defined.

I shall mention some facts tending to show the mysterious nature of malaria,—facts which have led me to the above conclusion.

1. The most striking fact, perhaps, in relation to the mysterious origin of malaria, and which is unquestionable, is the irregularity of its occurrence, and this even in situations where it occasionally operates with extraordinary intensity and violence, and in regions remarkable for equability of climate, as in Sierra Leone, the West Indies, the interior of Ceylon, and the islands of the Mediterranean, and especially the Ionian Islands. I have known a tract of country in the interior of Ceylon, free from fever for three or four years, and peculiarly healthy, and suddenly, without any apparent cause, become the reverse,— the weather as before, and all the circumstances of life of the inhabitants as before, so far as they were appreciable. For a few months, destructive remittent-fever has scourged the population, converting a flourishing district almost into a desert; and then, still without apparent change of climate or other circumstances, its ravages have ceased, and the country has recovered its usual healthiness.* In the West

* Facts of the same kind have been witnessed in all the Ionian

India Islands and on the Gold Coast, the unhealthy year is a matter of calculation, though, I believe, far from precise; founded on experience of its recurrence, independent of any peculiarities of season.

2. Other striking facts, bearing on the mysterious origin of malaria, present themselves in connexion with situation.

In some places, marshy grounds, as is well known, are the seat of agues and of remittent-fevers; in other places this is not the case. The Pontine marshes are a remarkable example of the former; the low and marshy grounds on the south-west coast of Ceylon, between Negombo and Galle, are not a less remarkable example of the latter.

In some situations the production of malaria appears to be associated with profusion of vegetable matter undergoing decomposition; but not always. In the interior of Ceylon, in some of the hilly districts, where forest is abundant, the smell of vegetable matter decomposing is strong and disagreeable, and yet the country is exempt from malaria fevers.

In other situations the reverse appears to be the

Islands, especially in Santa Maura, Zante, and Cephalonia. Our troops in the garrison of Santa Maura suffer more from fever than in any other of the islands; the ratio of deaths annually there, per 1000 mean strength, appears to have been 37.6 from fever alone, during a period of twenty years; yet in 1832 the reverse happened; in all the other islands they suffered more; that year, in Santa Maura, the ratio of mortality, from all diseases, was reduced to sixteen, and this without any obvious cause; in 1828 it was as high as 170, chiefly from fever.

case : there is no apparent source of malaria in decomposing vegetable matter ; the air is free from any unpleasant smell : the climate, as far as sensation is concerned, is agreeable ; the country, like an English park, abounding in herds of deer and in wild animals ; and yet it is most unwholesome,—it is without human inhabitants, and the passing traveller is often the victim of fever. Of this description there are extensive desert tracts in Ceylon, especially in the eastern part of the island, between the sea-coast and the mountains.*

The reverse, too, is the case in a still more remarkable manner in some of the Ionian Islands. There it is not uncommon for remittent and intermittent-fevers to break out in places remarkable for aridity and want of water, and almost destitute of vegetation. Parts of the mountainous district of Zante are of this description ; the little island of Meganisi is so in an extreme degree, as is also the still smaller island of Vido ;—these, the latter two, are almost barren rocks. And in the Ionian Islands, and in the islands and shores of the Mediterranean generally, and also in Ceylon, the severest form of fever, that of

---

* Many parts of Ceylon, between the mountains of the interior and the sea-coast, now desert, overgrown with jungle and forest ; or, as in some situations above mentioned, only agreeably varied with clumps of trees, formerly were populous and cultivated, as is clearly proved by the works of man which are to be met with, some of them of vast dimensions—as the tanks of Candelay and Minery—one about twenty-one miles in circumference—the other about twelve—and the ruins of great cities of proportionable magnitude in the country adjoining.

the remittent kind, is most rife in the hottest weather, when the ground is most parched, and the circumstances are least favourable to the decay of vegetable matter.

3. Were particular instances of the prevalency of
remittent and intermittent-fevers limited to small
spots, collected, and the reverse—instances of partial
and very limited exemption,—the mystery of the origin of malaria would be increased. Of a party of
men, occupying two rooms in a small barrack-build-
ing, divided by a narrow passage, in Via, I have
known the inmates of one room to be attacked in a
large proportion, whilst those in the other entirely
escaped, although the aspect of the two rooms was
similar : the only difference between them which I
could ascertain was, that there was a tank under the
one and not under the other ; but this was a constant
circumstance, whilst the occurrence of the fever was
sudden and unexpected, and, considered altogether,
extraordinary and inexplicable. Farther, I have
known a detachment, stationed at the little fort
Alexandria, in the midst of the lagoon of Santa Maura,
retain their health during the sickly season, when
fever was prevailing in the adjoining fort of Santa
Maura, at the extremity of the lagoon, and on one
side exposed to the sea-breezes. By reference to
authors, there would be no difficulty in multiplying
such instances.

From what has been stated, and from all that has

come to my knowledge relative to malaria, it appears to me to be proved that we are entirely ignorant, both of the nature of this agent or agency, and of its causes. In relation to its causes or sources, confining the attention to the Ionian Islands, I believe I am fully borne out by facts in expressing the following negative conclusions :—

1st, That they are independent of luxuriant vegetation, which is proved by the instances of Meganisi, Cerigo, &c.

2dly, That they are independent of the decomposition of vegetable matter, which is proved by the same islands, and by Paxo.

3dly, That they are not constituted by the sun's rays acting on a moist surface nor on under-ground moisture, the power of the sun being much the same every year ; the under-ground moisture being, in all the islands mentioned, very scanty, and, there is reason to believe, very little subject to variation of quantity from year to year ; and farther, there being no constant relation between hot summers and rainy winters and malaria; or *vice versa*, which is a well established fact.

Lastly, That they are independent of the mixing of fresh and salt-water, and of the alternate inundation and exposure to the sun and air of muddy surfaces, there being hardly any appreciable tides in the Mediterranean, and the shores of the Ionian Islands being remarkably clean and free from mud.*

* Since the above was written, I have read Major Tulloch's valu-

Although entirely ignorant, as I believe we are, of the true nature of malaria, we have learnt by experience many of the circumstances which prove its operation, and some of the best means of avoiding its effects. It seems to be principally active by night, or when the sun is below the horizon—those who are exposed to the night air being most subject to the fever which it produces. The evidence in proof of this is very strong. In the Ionian Islands, and in most parts of the Mediterranean, where the hot dry weather of summer sets in after the snows have disappeared from the mountains, the inhabitants, especially the working class, are much in the habit of sleeping in the open air, partly for the sake of coolness and avoiding the torment of insects, which abound in their dirty dwellings, and partly for the purpose of protecting their garden and field-crops from nightly depredations. These people are particularly subject to the fevers under consideration, in a much greater degree than the higher ranks who sleep in their beds under cover. And amongst our troops, there is a similar difference between the common soldiers and the officers. From 1821 to 1834, inclusive, the 51st regiment lost eighty-one men from remittent-fever, and only one officer, who was carried off the first summer. According to the returns in

able Report on the Sickness among the Troops in Western Africa, St Helena, the Cape of Good Hope, and the Mauritius, in which are many remarkable facts recorded, similar to those I have described, and confirmatory of the conclusions arrived at.

the Statistical Report on our Army, drawn up by Major Tulloch, the mortality from fever in the Ionian Islands amongst the soldiers, during a period of twenty years, was thirteen yearly per thousand ; whilst amongst the officers, during a period of seventeen years, inclusive, estimating their aggregate strength at 2506, the total mortality from fever was only ten !* The common soldiers, like the peasantry, are much exposed to the night air—the officers little ; the former on duty on guard,—and independent of this, which is unavoidable, many of them, from the crowded state of the barracks, and from the rooms being infested with fleas and bugs, are tempted to come out and sleep in the open air :—I am speaking of what the barracks were, and of the habits of the soldiery during the period referred to. In Italy, especially in the Roman states, and in the vicinity of Rome, the harvest is gathered in by labourers who come from a distance for the purpose, and who, during the period of harvest, sleep exposed at night ; and fever (*la periodica*), every year more or less, prevails amongst them, and is often very destructive ;

---

* It appears, from this officer's reports, that the aggregate strength of officers in the Ionian Islands for seventeen years, viz. from 1820 to 1836, inclusive, was, as stated above, 2506 ; according to which the average yearly strength was 147 ; and that the total deaths from fevers during the same period were 10 ; consequently the average annual deaths were .588, or 5. per 1000, instead of 13, as amongst the men—an estimate in which there can hardly be any fallacy—as the fevers which prove fatal are rapidly so, commonly before the fourteenth day, not giving time for removal, as in the instances of protracted diseases, and for return to this country on sick leave.

whilst amongst the factors of the great landed proprietors, who live on the estates, we are assured that
those who avoid exposure to the night air escape
fever and enjoy good health.* In Ceylon, during
the period of the rebellion, which broke out in October 1817, and was not subdued till October of the
following year, our troops were tolerably exempt from
fevers as long as they were chiefly employed by day,
and no longer; as soon as they were employed more
by night than by day, particularly in convoys and the
relieving of posts, fever became very prevalent and
terribly destructive. The natives of that island, no
doubt warned by experience, carefully avoid the
night air, and in the interior, commonly have a fire
in the sleeping rooms. Many other facts of a like
kind might be mentioned illustrative of the agency
of malaria at night, and of the good effect of avoiding,
or of protection from, the night air. As the subject
is very important, I shall adduce a few additional
instances.

The temple of Kattragam, in Ceylon, is situated
in one of the most unwholesome districts of that
island, and which, there is reason to believe, has been
converted into a desert by the destructive effects of
fever. It is a place of pilgrimage, and a large number of the pilgrims are reported to be swept off

---

* Some interesting details on this subject are to be found in a dis-
sertation, " Sull' origine delle intermittenti di Roma e sua Campagna,"
by the experienced Dr Giacomo Folchi, senior physician of the great
hospital S. Spirito.

annually by disease Yet the officiating priest, a Brahmin, has resided there many years during the worst season, and with impunity. When I visited the temple, I found him in good health, active and energetic, though of the sparest form. The only precaution, I could learn, which he took to guard against fever, was sleeping in an inner room, without windows, having a fire in the middle of it, on the floor, —behind which, on leopards' skins, he lay at night; so that the outer air, before it could reach him, must pass through or over the fire.

The following passage from the Rev. Mr White's work on Spain, entitled, " Letters from Spain, by Don Leucadio Doblado," descriptive of the exemption from fever in the instance of the bakers of a town adjoining to Seville, some years ago, when the yellow fever raged in that city, and which they daily visited, leaving it before night, offers a striking example in point, as well as a strong argument that the fever was not contagious, as supposed by the author, but merely a severe form of remittent-fever, similar to that which has repeatedly appeared in Gibraltar and in other parts of the south of Europe.

" Alcalá de Guadaíra, is a town containing a population of two thousand inhabitants. and standing on a hilly spot to the north-east of Seville. The greatest part of the bread consumed in this city comes daily from Alcalá, where the abundant and placid stream of the Guadaíra invites to the construction of water-mills. Many of the inhabitants being bakers,

and having no market but Seville, were under the
necessity of repairing thither during the infection.
It is not with us, as in England, where every trades-
man practically knows the advantages of the division
of labour, and is at liberty to consult his own convenience in the sale of his articles.   The bakers, the
butchers, the gardeners, and the farmers, are here
obliged to sell in separate markets, where they generally spend the whole day waiting for customers.
Owing to this regulation of the police, about sixty
men, and double that number of mules, leave Alcalá
every day with the dawn, and stand till the evening,
in two rows, enclosed with iron railings, at the Plaza
del Pan.   The constant communication with people
from all parts of the town, and so long an exposure
to the atmosphere of an infected place, might have
been supposed powerful enough to communicate the
disease.   We certainly were in daily apprehension of
its appearance at Alcalá.   So little, however, can we
calculate the effects of unknown causes, that of the
people that thus braved the contagion, only one, who
passed a night in Seville, caught the disease and
died.   All the others, no less than the rest of the
village, continued to enjoy the usual degree of health,
which probably, owing to its airy situation, is excellent at all times."

What has been witnessed at Gibraltar, at different
times, when the garrison of that fortress has been
visited by endemic remittent-fever, is very similar to,
and even perhaps more remarkable than, the pre-

ceding. The troops that have been encamped on the low neutral ground, within gun-shot of the town teeming with sickness, have remained healthy,—and individuals, I have been informed, in a large number of instances, freely communicated with the town with impunity, provided their visits were made by day, and that they slept out of its atmosphere by night.

Dr Allan, in his account of the remittent-fever of the African Islands, viz., Madagascar and the surrounding islands, including the Seychelle group, adduces some facts equally strong of exemption from this most destructive malady, by avoiding sleeping on shore at night. " It is deserving of notice (he remarks), that all who slept on board ship escaped: every victim seen or heard of, had passed one night on shore; and no instance of recovery was known in those who were taken on board affected." He adds, " The writer had a vessel of a hundred tons moored within the reef at Fowl Point (on the east coast of Madagascar) under his charge, mainly for the purpose of protection from sickness. Such as remained in her all night were quite healthy; but no one slept on shore with impunity. The same occurred everywhere else." * This fever, like that of Gibraltar, and even more strictly, was limited to one attack; the fortunate few who escaped, were considered safe from any return of the disease. The natives, like the

* Observations on some of the Predominant Diseases of the African Islands. By J. B. Allan, M.D., in Ed. Monthly Journal of Med. Science for August 1841.

Cingalese, it would appear, endeavour to protect themselves from its cause by avoiding the night air, and having fires in their sleeping-rooms. Dr Allan, speaking of the little faith the Madagascans have in their own remedies, remarks:—" Their grand object is, when compelled to domicile in the low countries, to prevent attack. For this purpose, believing that the cause of all the evil is a *Tanghuin* (an indigenous vegetable poison) in the atmosphere, and that this poison can only be destroyed by fire, as it rises from the earth during the night, every house has in the centre of each apartment a raised box of sand, on which wood is kept smouldering after sun-set."

Next to the avoidance of the night air, in regard to prevention, is perhaps the due attention to clothing ; indeed the two have frequently been coupled together in degree of importance. Thus Dr Folchi, in his treatise already quoted, when comparing the condition of the peasantry engaged in the labours of the harvest, and a prey to fever from lying out, with that of their superintendents, remarks,—" It is a well known fact that some of the latter, inhabiting spots the most insalubrious that are in the Roman territory, have kept their health perfectly good for many years, by the precaution of retiring to their houses in the early evening, closing the windows, and warming the apartment ; not going out in the morning, until the sun is high, and then protected by a good cloak.

The imprudence of sleeping out is frequently combined with that of throwing off part of the clothing, for the temporary gratification of coolness, without consideration of consequences, especially in the hottest weather. Our soldiers are particularly thoughtless in this respect. When heated and perspiring on fatigue, or other duty, as soon as they are at liberty, they will throw off their coat, and perhaps their shirt; and, for the sake of coolness, expose themselves to the wind; and, often half-undressed, they will quit the guard-room or the barrack, where they are unable to sleep on account of the close oppressive heat, and seek repose in the open air. The effect, it is easily conceived, may be injurious, and favourable to the operation of malaria. In the Ionian Islands, the night air is commonly dry during the period of drought and heat; no dew forms; the difference between the moist and dry thermometer, according to my observations, varies, with the land-winds, from twelve to twenty degrees; and, consequently, the degree of evaporation is considerable from a perspiring surface, and the cooling effect is in proportion.

Whether there is any virtue in flannel as a means of protection against the effects of malaria, as has been advocated by some respectable authors, it is not easy to determine. There are objections to flannel for the use of the labouring class and the soldiery, not perhaps undeserving of attention, especially as regards its cost, comparatively little strength, and little fitness for washing. Another objection is its heating quality, and the temptation thoughtless men have, when heated, to throw it off at the very moment it is most wanted. On these accounts, I am of opinion that, for under-clothing, as for shirts, coarse soft cotton is preferable to flannel. In the Mediterranean, I have carefully watched, comparatively, the health of regiments, two of which wore flannel shirts and two cotton or coarse linen. Little difference was perceptible between them on the score of health; but, on the whole, it appeared to me that the wearers of the cotton-shirts had rather an advantage over the wearers of the flannel-shirts.

It is commonly supposed that persons fasting are most susceptible of the agency of malaria; and, from general observation, I am inclined to believe the opinion is well founded; and perhaps the comparative exemption of officers from fever, may be partly owing to their fast being earlier broken than that of the men, and to the principal meal, dinner, being taken by them at a later hour. The meal-hours of the common soldiers are indeed very unfavourable to health, especially where malaria prevails. They rise early— with the early dawn; are often exercised before sunrise, without eating; they breakfast at seven or eight; dine at one; and, having no regular meal after one, they too commonly fast till the following morning; so that both early and late they are exposed to the air when it is unwholesome, with an empty stomach, favourable to the contraction of disease from the influence of malaria. It is a good practice, and generally followed in the East, to take a cup of strong coffee on rising, breakfasting about two hours later, after taking exercise. And, were the practice followed in our army, and were an evening meal provided for the men, enforced in the regulations, it can hardly be doubted that the effects would be excellent, both directly and indirectly;—directly, in checking the disposition to be influenced by malaria, and indirectly by diminishing the temptation to resort of an evening to the canteen and wine-shop, and commit excess in drinking.

Diet, too, in relation to prevention, as well as the time of eating, there is reason to believe, is of some importance; and that that kind of diet is best adapted to enable the constitution to resist malaria, which is most conducive to general vigorous health, and of which animal food and fresh meat, with good bread, form a considerable part, living rather above than below par, during the unhealthy season, and using sound wine after dinner or supper, in moderation. Abstemiousness, perhaps, is even more injurious than slight excess in eating and drinking; but as there is little disposition to undue abstemiousness, it is sufficient to give the hint that, when malaria is dreaded, the drink should not be water alone, nor the diet be composed chiefly of vegetables. By some authors too much stress has been laid on intemperate habits, in connexion with the fatal effects of the remittent fevers of hot climates. It is not uncommon to hear it said, that, in the West Indies, and on the western coast of Africa, the dreadful mortality that occasionally occurs there, is more owing to the intemperance of the sufferers, than to the intensity of malaria. The mere circumstance of the periodical nature of the disease, the habits of the individuals being the same, is a sufficient refutation of this allegation. That intemperance is injurious to general health, is most certain, and conducive to organic changes, likely to terminate in serious disease, especially of the brain and liver; but experience does not seem to prove that it at all conduces to attacks of the fevers in question. I am more disposed to the contrary conclusion, partly from witnessing that persons of apparently the best constitutions, seem to be most susceptible of the malaria influence; and partly from observing, in fatal cases, on post mortem examination, how comparatively rare are the organic complications;—conveying to me the idea that the existence of tubercles in the lungs, or of serious organic lesion of any other viscus, may act as a protection against malaria, and secure the constitution against its influence.

As the range of malaria is often extremely limited, the most certain method of avoiding its effects is by leaving the spot where it has shown itself. Sometimes a removal of a few hundred yards may suffice to give security, as has been witnessed at Gibraltar; and so remarkably at Foul Point, on the coast of Madagascar, in the instance already referred to, described by Dr Allan; and commonly a situation can be found within a few miles, which, either from difference of elevation, or of exposure, or separation by water, is likely to have an untainted atmosphere. The importance of change of place, when destructive fevers prevail, cannot be too much insisted on. Remedial means, and means of prevention, are all uncertain. Removal is the only measure that can be calculated on with any confidence; and persons in command, on whom the distribution of large bodies of men may depend, whether in the field or in garrison, have much to answer for, who do not carry into effect this principle of security to the utmost limit that prudence permits. How many thousands of lives have been sacrificed in our West Indian possessions to tenacity of position!

CHAPTER XI.

ON THE FEVERS OF MALTA.

Kinds of Fever to which Malta is subject. Tables in illustration. Remarks on the Nomenclature of Fevers. Notice of the different
kinds affecting the British Troops and the Inhabitants. Further
Observations and Reflections on Malaria.

FEVERS are far less frequent and destructive in Malta
than in the Ionian Islands, and equally so amongst
our troops and the native population. It is commonly said that intermittent and remittent-fevers
are almost unknown there, and that, when they do
appear, they are of foreign origin, and have been
imported. This is not correct: it is proved by incon-
testible facts, that both these fevers occasionally occur
in the island, and indeed every year, though commonly to a very limited extent. The fevers of Malta
may, I believe, generally, be considered similar in
species to those of the Ionian Islands, differing more
in degree of intensity than in kind. In illustration,
I shall introduce two Tables, one relating to the
fevers treated in our military hospitals, the subjects
of which were British soldiers; the other, giving the
number of deaths amongst the natives, referred to

this order of diseases. The period included in both is very limited, in one to seven years, in the other to three. In the Appendix to Major Tulloch's work, already quoted, more extensive returns will be found, and which may be consulted with some advantage. I have been induced so to restrict myself, in point of time, for the sake of precision. During the seven years comprised in the first Table, I was stationed in Malta, and had an opportunity of becoming acquainted with the fevers as they occurred, and of marking their peculiarities. Another reason induced me to limit the Table of the Mortality from fever in the native population, namely, that previous to 1832, the general result only was given,—the species of the fatal fever was not assigned; it was then first attempted at my suggestion.

TABLE, SHOWING THE NUMBER OF ADMISSIONS, FROM FEVER, AND DEATHS AMONGST THE TROOPS IN MALTA, FROM 1827 TO 1835, INCLUSIVE.

Years, . .	1828.		1829.		1830.		1831.		1832.		1833.		1834.	
Strength, . .	2132		2287		2299		2056		2045		2124		2192	
Species of Fever.	Adm.	Died.	Adm.	Died.	Adm.	Died.	Adm.	Died.	Adm.	Died.	Adm.	Died.	Adm.	Died.
Feb. Quot. Inter.,	50	..	89	..	2	1	..	..	18	..	8	..	..	..
.. Tertiana, .	3	..	1	..	..	..	2	..	1	..	..	..	2	..
.. Remittens, .	3	1	1	..	1	..⁵	..	..	181	..	30	3	150	10
.. Cont. Com.,	250	5	164	1	185	5	334	7	213	..	240	1	441	4
.. Synochus, .	11	1	..	..	..	..	..	..	..	..	..	..	..	..

TABLE OF DEATHS FROM FEVER IN THE ISLAND OF MALTA, EXCLUSIVE OF THE BRITISH FORCE, FROM 1ST JANUARY 1832 TO 31ST DECEMBER 1834.

Species of Fever.	January	February	March	April	May	June	July	August	September	October	November	December	Total		Years.	Population, exclusive of British Force.	Total Mortality.
Febris intermittens,	...	...	...	1	2	...	...	...	...	1	...	...	4		1832	102,654	2468
remittens biliosa,	...	3	...	4	1	3	2	4	2	3	2	2	26				
putrida,	1	2	1	...	1	...	1	2	...	1	1	...	6				
nervosa,	1	2	4	4	6	5	4	5	1	1	1	2	22				
typhoida,	5	1	3	1	1	9	5	6	6	9	2	7	31				
lenta,	4	4	8	8	7	6	3	2	4	9	2	1	75				
com. synocha,	1	...	4	1	...	...	3	2	4	4	...	...	26				
	12	12	20	19	18	23	15	19	13	19	8	12	190				
Febris intermittens,	...	...	1	...	...	...	1	...	...	...	...	...	2		1833	102,798	3173
remittens biliosa,	4	1	4	3	1	5	4	3	2	1	1	3	32				
putrida,	...	...	...	...	...	...	...	1	...	1	...	...	2				
nervosa,	...	1	2	2	2	1	1	4	2	3	3	2	23				
typhoida,	...	1	2	4	3	2	3	2	2	4	...	8	31				
lenta,	7	1	8	4	4	8	6	7	5	7	3	15	75				
com. synocha,	7	1	1	8	6	...	5	3	1	7	5	4	48				
	18	5	18	21	16	16	17	20	12	23	12	32	213				
Febris intermittens,	...	1	...	...	1	...	...	...	...	...	...	...	2		1834	103,378	2732
remittens biliosa,	...	1	5	7	1	2	...	5	1	2	2	4	29				
putrida,	...	...	1	...	...	...	...	...	...	...	...	1	4				
nervosa,	...	4	5	6	1	3	4	3	7	1	7	7	52				
typhoida,	...	6	18	7	14	5	5	10	5	5	4	3	80				
lenta,	...	13	9	6	4	8	9	6	5	3	6	5	80				
com. synocha,	...	9	...	...	...	...	...	...	...	...	...	...	17				
	26	34	38	26	21	18	19	24	18	11	19	20	264				

Relative to the nomenclature adopted in the returns from which these Tables are formed, there is, as commonly happens in this very difficult matter, a certain vagueness depending on a variety of circumstances, as the special views of the individuals naming the diseases; the schools in which they have studied; and the description of fevers to which they had been previously most accustomed.

These remarks are generally less applicable to the military medical officers than to the native practitioners; yet they are applicable even to the former: thus the fever which, in 1828, was returned by one regimental surgeon as synochus, I have reason to believe would have been considered by most others as the common continued fever of the Mediterranean; and other like instances might be given.

The naming of diseases by the native practitioners, in fatal cases, is commonly carelessly done, and is little to be relied on as designating the true nature of the complaint. A post-mortem examination is rarely undertaken, and the disease, it is presumed, is usually named from some leading symptom or circumstance, of which, in many instances, the medical man is merely informed by the friends,—a practitioner being required whether he has attended during the illness or not, to sign a certificate of the death, to be transmitted to the police-office; and from the aggregate of these certificates, the yearly return of deaths is formed.

In casting the eye over the first Table, the disparity of number of the cases of fever, in different years, especially of the intermittent and remittent kind, can hardly fail to attract attention.

The instances of intermittent-fever, in 1828 and 1829, were chiefly confined to the Royal Fusileers, who had just before arrived from the Ionian Islands,* and in 1832 to the Royal Highlanders, shortly after coming from Gibraltar; the one regiment, in Cephalonia, had before suffered considerably from remittent-fever, and the other also from the same disease, in the severe form of yellow-fever. It was in Florian that the disease showed itself in the barracks, the situation of which is marked in the plan of Valetta and its suburbs, inserted in the map annexed. On neither occasion did it appear amongst the natives.

During the years 1832, 1833, 1834, remittent-fever was unusually prevalent for Malta. In 1832, it was principally confined to the 42d regiment, or Royal Highlanders, stationed in Florian. Though distinctly of the remittent type, the fever was very mild, of short duration, almost ephemeral, and hardly requiring any medical treatment. The next year the cases of the disease returned as remittent-fever, occurred in the 42d and in the 7th or Royal Fusi-

* In the general return of the sick of the garrison of Malta, the majority of the cases of intermittent-fever, for the years 1828–29, are given as of the quotidian type; but, according to the report of the able assistant-surgeon of the regiment, the late Mr O'Brien, more were of the tertian form, especially in spring, and in summer and autumn irregular.

leers, the former quartered in Cottonera, the latter
in Florian. They were also of a mild character; the
fatal cases were not genuine instances of remittent-
fever; they proved, on post-mortem examination, to
be examples of phlegmasiæ, in one instance affecting the brain, pus being found in the ventricles; in
another, the lungs, these organs having been found
extensively hepatized; and in the third, the intestines, which were severely ulcerated, both the small
and large, complicated with inflammation and ulceration of the larynx and kidneys. In 1834, the disease appeared in the regiments stationed in Lower
St Elmo barracks, in Valetta,—the extreme point
of the city towards the sea. The fever of this year
was unusually severe and fatal, and strongly marked.
As it was in some respects peculiar, I shall briefly
describe it.

At the commencement of the disease, the prominent symptoms were sudden, and great prostration of
strength, often attended, or immediately preceded by
rigors; a quick and small pulse; pains in the head,
in the region of the spine, and in the lower extremities, at first moderate, soon augmenting, and often
followed by soreness of throat, and some difficulty of
swallowing, and in many instances by quick respiration and cough; and very generally by pain at the pit
of the stomach, occasionally with vomiting, attended
with cramps of the muscles of the legs. The bowels
were generally confined; the secretion of urine
scanty; the skin cool, or very little above the natural

temperature; the tongue loaded, complete anorexia, considerable thirst. The rigors which introduced the disease occasionally recurred; and almost invariably there was an exacerbation towards night, often followed by sweating. About the fifth day, in a considerable number of instances, the skin became yellow, and often intensely so, accompanied with a deficiency of bile in the alvine evacuations. Delirium rarely occurred during any stage of the disease; the spirits were commonly dull and low; and there was often a want of sleep for many nights in sequence. A favourable change in the disease was commonly indicated by a papular eruption about the mouth, and, in a few cases, a bleeding from the nose appeared to be critical. If the patient survived the ninth day, he commonly recovered. The worst cases, and a large proportion of those which proved fatal, were attended with suppression of urine;—however, this was not invariably a fatal symptom. Bloody evacuations at stool were not uncommon, and they were always of bad omen. The convalescence, in the majority of cases, was more rapid than might have been expected; and there was little tendency to relapse, and none to pass into the intermittent form of fever.

In all the fatal cases, the bodies were subjected to a post-mortem examination. The appearances discovered were generally very similar. In most instances, the air-passages, and the primæ viæ bore marks either of inflammation or of venous congestion; and of the latter, especially the lower part of the ileum. The vessels of the brain were almost always in a state of morbid congestion. The spleen and kidneys bore no evident marks of disease. The gall-bladder, in many instances, was distended with a fluid which had no longer the character of bile [pale, albuminous, and deficient in mucus]—at the same time that the colouring matter of the bile abounded in the blood, and tinged most of the tissues of the body,—indeed all of them were more or less jaundiced, excepting commonly the gall-ducts and gall-bladder, and the stomach and intestines. In the fatal cases, which were preceded by suppression of urine, I examined the blood after death, and detected in it a notable quantity of urea.

On the treatment of the disease, a very few remarks may suffice. That method appeared to be most successful, which was of the mildest kind, and chiefly directed to the relief of symptoms, keeping in mind the pathology of the disease (if I may venture to say so), as indicated by the morbid anatomy of it: such as the abstraction of twelve or sixteen ounces of blood in the early stage; the application of leeches, in moderation, to the epigastrium, when the seat of pain and of apparent irritation; and the use of mild aperients, especially of castor-oil. When the disease first broke out, cynanche being then very commonly conjoined with it, at its commencement, with affection of the respiratory organs, I suggested the use of tartarized antimony. In many instances it appeared to be beneficial. If, however, it was continued above two or three days, or not given with discretion, it seemed to be injurious, and often to be followed by increased prostration of strength. Calomel was given, in many instances, both alone and combined with opium. Generally, as well as I could observe, the result was not in favour of its efficacy.

On the origin of this fever, I shall offer a few remarks, as it is a striking example of the mystery belonging to the subject. When the disease was most prevalent, as in the early part of the summer, it was reported that it was contagious; that it had been imported from Gibraltar, by the 53d regiment. Neither of these notions was borne out by any evidence; and fortunately the idea of importation was very easily proved to be erroneous, as the regiment in question arrived in Malta in good health, no fever of the kind having prevailed in the garrison it left for a considerable time before its departure ; and the identical fever having shown itself in the 73d regiment, before the arrival of the 53d, just before the former embarked for Corfu, on the 12th of April.

As regarded the question of contagion, in this instance, there being no reason, no proof of any kind, that the fever spread from man to man, that those who came in contact with the sick were liable to contract it, it was considered necessary, on principle, to view it as non-contagious. And, accordingly, it was treated as such. No unusual precautions were taken to guard against its extension, such as would have been necessary had it been considered contagious; and, in confirmation of the justness of the conclusion, I may remark it did not spread, but ceased spontaneously with change of weather, and *that* both in summer and autumn. In the first instance, when it was most severe, it was arrested apparently by the great heat of the season; and, in the latter, when it recurred in a milder form, on the breaking up of the summer, after the autumnal rains, it was stopped apparently by the heavy rains and the cool weather which occurred towards the end of the autumnal period.*

In the absence of contagion, it appeared necessary to refer the disease to malaria, with which origin the distinctly remittent character of the fever was in

---

* In every country the question of the contagious or non-contagious character of a disease is important, but especially in the Mediterranean, where quarantine is enforced. There especially it is necessary to act decidedly on principle; and, after weighing the arguments for and against, to come to a positive conclusion as the ground of action. If the conclusion is that contagion prevails, a system of seclusion, connected with terror, must be entered on, commonly and almost unavoidably highly injurious to the sick; and great hardships are immediately experienced in regard to foreign relations. In the case of Malta, the island would have been declared in quarantine, with all the ports of Sicily, Italy, and of France and Austria, to the great detriment of commerce, and of the various interests therewith connected. Strong certificates, I recollect, were required to ward off the evil, in the instance under consideration, and to allay the apprehensions of the watchful consuls, who very properly are held responsible by their respective governments for giving due warning on the appearance of a contagious disease.

accordance. But the difficulty was to comprehend how any malaria could be generated in the barracks of Lower St Elmo, or in their neighbourhood. The locality hitherto had been remarkably healthy; the troops stationed there, for many years, had been particularly little liable to fever, and not at all to remittent-fever; nor was there any material alteration of circumstances this year to account for the change in the salubrity of the place. In consequence of the construction of a new drain and sewer, the barrack-yard was even cleaner and drier than usual.

Three circumstances, however, it was supposed by some persons were to blame, viz., a partial paving of the floor of the barrack; a cleaning out, in the beginning of spring, of the great water-tank adjoining; and the dirty state of the ditch of Upper St Elmo, opening on one side into the barrack-yard of Lower St Elmo.

After careful examination and dispassionate consideration of the subject at the time, I was disposed to attach but little importance to any of the attributed causes; for the state of the ditch was much the same as it had been for several years,—not, indeed, so clean as it might have been, and as it ought to have been, but far from being very filthy; indeed, Sir Howard Elphinstone, who then commanded, in the temporary absence of the governor, Sir Frederick Ponsonby, and who inspected it himself, remarked that few farm-yards in England could be found in which there were not greater accumulations of fermenting and decomposing animal and vegetable matter. Secondly, As regards the cleaning out of the tank ; before it was undertaken I was consulted ; I examined the deposit that had collected, and finding it to be almost entirely free from any vegetable or animal matter, I reported accordingly that I could not consider it injurious. The tank, it may be remarked, was emptied on account of salt-water having entered it,—and the occasion was taken to remove some deposit, a part of which was spread over a small portion of the ditch, with a view to its cultivation. Lastly, As regards the paving of the floors of the barrack-rooms, experience, widely extended in Malta, seems to show that this operation can be performed to a much larger extent than in the instance in question, without any injury to the health of the inmates of the building, the floors of which are undergoing repair ; and, accordingly, I believe that no competent judge laid any stress on this circumstance, in connexion with the exciting cause.

The true cause of the disease, or the source of the malaria, supposing that to be the cause, must be confessed, I believe, to be entirely hid, and to afford another instance, in addition to the many on record, of the occurrence of malaria in a mysterious manner, independent of animal and vegetable decomposition. In harmony with this, though the fever was prevalent in some rooms of the barrack more than in others, it was not confined to any particular rooms, and though the artillery-men in the Upper St Elmo

barracks were exempt from it, situated immediately
above the ditch, the inhabitants in the vicinity did
not entirely escape; and further, in accordance, it
may be remarked, that the disease prevailed apparently, independently of the direction of the wind,
and whether blowing from, or into the accused
ditch.

On the common continued fever of Malta, a very
few remarks may suffice. The first Table shows that
the number of cases so returned amongst the military
is large, in comparison with the other descriptions of
fever, and though subject to fluctuations from year
to year, it is so in a much less degree than the others.
The character of this fever is very similar to that of
the same denomination in the Ionian Islands; like
it, however, and indeed every other fever, exhibiting
occasionally some variations, difficult to define and
describe, and occasionally some complications depending, it may be inferred, on peculiar atmospheric influences: thus, when remittent-fever prevailed amongst
the regiments in Lower St Elmo, in 1834, as already
described, the cases of continued fever which occurred
in the other regiments stationed in Cottonera and in
Floriana, showed a tendency to the remittent type.
When this fever proved fatal, it was commonly in
consequence of the inflammation of some important
organ; and many of the fatal cases might be considered as misnamed,—a conclusion fully warranted by
the results of the post-mortem examinations.

The fevers which occur amongst the native population, I believe, might be restricted to a smaller number of species than those assigned in the second Table; in truth, the names of these diseases, as I have before remarked of the diseases generally, are too often vaguely and hypothetically given, so that, for medical statistical purposes, not much reliance can be placed in them. This much, however, is certain, that both intermittent and remittent-fevers are not at all uncommon; but, as amongst our troops, the mild continued form is far more frequent.

All the remarks that I have made respecting malaria, or the cause of intermittent and remittent-fever in the Ionian Islands, are emphatically applicable in Malta. There especially this cause is enveloped in mystery. It would be difficult to name a spot any where on the surface of the globe, of the same extent, more naturally arid, or where there is less animal or vegetable matter undergoing decay, or where there is a greater absence of stagnant water or of marsh. Much has been said of the shallows at the head of the great harbour, and of the Quarantine harbour; and their noxious influences have, I believe, been greatly exaggerated. In both situations, it is true, the smell is often offensive; often there is a distinct smell of sulphuretted hydrogen, and on stirring the dark clay there forming the bottom, bubbles of air may be seen to ascend, and hence probably they have been considered as sources of malaria. The condition, however, of these shallows is constant; it seems, therefore, not logical to refer to

them, diseases remarkably inconstant of occurrence.
Moreover, I never could, in a satisfactory manner,
trace fever to these localities. During the whole time
I was in Malta, I never knew an instance of intermittent or remittent-fever originating at Fort Ma-
nuel, which is adjoining one of the shallows in question ; and this is the more worthy of remark, as there
is a military guard placed at the head of the cause-
way, passing through the shallow, connecting the fort
with the shore. Every year many cases of intermittent-
fever are admitted into the Civil Hospital ; but they
do not come from Valetta and its neighbourhood, but
chiefly from north-western parts of the island where
there is some rich land in cultivation at a distance
from any village, the labourers on which, during
their temporary sojourn there, lead a hard life, very
like that of the peasantry in the Roman states, already alluded to, employed in the cultivation of the
Campagna and the Maremme.

Dr M'Culloch, in his Essay on Malaria, page 229,
makes a singular statement relative to the insalubrity of a particular spot in Malta; his words are,
" That nearly a whole regiment was not only incapa-
citated in Malta in one night, and with the loss also
of great numbers, but rendered nearly useless through
the whole war, by persisting in occupying a village
which the natives had abandoned, and against the
most pressing remonstrances." Dr M'Culloch does
not state whence he obtained this information. During my residence in the island, I made careful in-

quiry on the subject, but without any success ; no one knew of any such event. Probably trusting to his memory, it deceived him ; he referred to Malta some occurrence of the kind, which had taken place elsewhere. His ingenious work contains too many loose statements,—by which its value is almost entirely undermined.

The subject of malaria hitherto has been commonly considered in a vague and hypothetical manner ; idle rumours and reports have too frequently been substituted for well authenticated facts ;—truth and falsehood have become mixed ; in a large number of instances, it is difficult to distinguish between them ; and the consequence is, that the subject as matter of inquiry is become almost inextricable, at least to those who would wish to weigh conflicting evidence, and form their opinions from the details to be found in books.

A conviction of our ignorance is a good preparatory state of mind for the discovery of truth. This, it appears to me, is the principal progress hitherto made in the investigation of malaria. We find that we are completely ignorant of its true nature ; whether it is a ponderable or etherial substance ; simple or compound ; whether generated in the atmosphere, or produced from the soil, or emanating from the bowels of the earth ; and that all the hypotheses yet advanced to account for its origin, are imperfect, founded on a very limited and partial survey of facts.

That it is a substance, *sui generis*, I think, can hardly be doubted; the ordinary exciting causes of disease, connected with vicissitudes of temperature and of atmospheric humidity, such as affect our senses and influence animal temperature, being pretty regular in operation, widely acting, limited to no particular region; and in many instances least remarkable, as in tropical countries, where the effects of malaria are most severe and conspicuous. It can hardly, too, be doubted that it is extremely subtle; that if ponderable, it acts in extremely minute quantities; and if imponderable and etherial, it possesses properties peculiar to itself, and which, for their discovery, may require new instruments and new methods of research.

The progress of physical science in modern times holds out the highest encouragement. There are many living who remember the philosophers to whom we are indebted for pneumatic chemistry, previous to whose labours water was considered an element, atmospheric air was considered an element. Within a few years we have witnessed two new substances, possessed of energetic properties—iodine and bromine—brought to light, which exist in excessively minute quantities in the waters of the ocean, and which we may be sure never would have been brought to light, except by processes of concentration. Could analagous processes be brought to the aid of atmospheric chemistry, it is impossible to say what new substances might not be discovered in the aërial ocean.

That it must contain, in however minute quantity, portions of every thing gaseous and volatile, is manifest to reason ; but how few of them have been detected. And that it must contain also a variety of substances in the solid form, in impalpable powder, is highly probable; the matter of blight wafted by the wind ; the spray of the sea carried inland very many miles by the storm ; dust falling in showers over a vast extent of surface, are facts in favour of it, without taking into account meteoric stones, the history of which is not less mysterious than that of malaria, and the existence of which, though marked by properties so manifest and striking, was so long disbelieved, merely because in opposition to current ideas and commonplace knowledge.

The analogies of nature may be considered in favour of different species of malaria. Certain epidemic diseases, the probable effects of atmospheric influences, are also in favour of their existence, and especially what is known of that most remarkable and terrible of all diseases—cholera.

This view of the subject it may be well to keep in mind, as it imparts to it peculiar interest and importance, and gives additional motive to engage in the careful investigation of it.

CHAPTER XII.

ON THE CLIMATE OF THE MEDITERRANEAN, IN RELATION TO PULMONARY CONSUMPTION.

Popular Opinion that the Climate of the Mediterranean is less productive of Pulmonary Disease than that of Great Britain. Opposite results of recent Statistical Inquiries. These results scrutinized. Comparison of Cavalry and Infantry Soldier as regards
circumstances affecting Health. Evidence derived from the
Troops serving at home and in the Mediterranean. Proportional
prevalency of Phthisis amongst the native Maltese. Tables in
illustration. Deduction in favour of the Climate of Malta. Problem of the greater Liability of British Troops to Phthisis in
Malta than in the Ionian Islands. Returns of Fatal Cases in
illustration. Circumstances likely to conduce to the greater
Liability in Malta. Remarks on its Climate, with Suggestions
for Invalids proposing to winter there. Reflections on the Formation of Tubercle in the Lung, and on the Means of Prevention.

THIS is an inquiry of much importance and of some
difficulty. The popular opinion is, that the climate
of the Mediterranean is more favourable than our
own to a healthy condition of the lungs. The result
of the latest statistical research, on the contrary, is,
that this conclusion is not well founded; and that
pulmonary complaints generally, and pulmonary consumption especially, is at least as common and as
fatal there as at home ; indeed, Major Tulloch, in his

Statistical Report already quoted, expresses himself even more strongly on the subject: he says, " It is beyond a doubt, that except in the Ionian Islands, the liability of troops to consumption in the Mediterranean stations is even greater than in the United Kingdom." *   And the conclusion to which he has come respecting other pulmonary complaints, is similar.

The results of his estimates, from whence his deductions were made, are the following :—

1st, *Relative to Consumption.*

Stations.	Aggregate Strength of Seven Years, from 1830 to 1836, inclusive.	Total attacked by Consumption these Seven Years.	Ratio per 1000 of Mean Strength, attacked annually.
United Kingdom, . .	43,163	286	6.6
Gibraltar, . . .	22,868	187	8.2
Malta, ...	15,031	101	6.7
Ionian Islands, . .	24,401	129	5.3

2d, *Relative to Inflammation of the Lungs and Pleura.*

Stations.	Aggregate Strength of Seven Years, from 1830 to 1836, inclusive.	Total Died of these Diseases in the same Period.	Ratio per 1000 of Force attacked annually.	Ratio per 1000 of Force Died annually.
Great Britain, .	43,163	37	17	.9
Gibraltar, . .	22,868	13	29	.6
Malta, . .	15,031	28	30	1.8
Ionian Islands, .	24,401	30	23	9

* Report, p. 63.

It may be right to add Major Tulloch's remarks :—

" Here, then, we find that inflammatory affections of the lungs are nearly twice as prevalent in the Mediterranean as among the same number of troops in the United Kingdom, and that in the mild climate of Malta they are also twice as fatal.

" These facts, combined with a careful examination of the abstracts in the Appendix, lead to the inference that residence in the Mediterranean, though so often recommended to patients labouring under pulmonary affections, is by no means likely to be attended with beneficial results : in some cases, no doubt, change of air, change of scene, and the sea-voyage, may have benefited a patient, and led to a partial recovery ; but the same would, in all probability, have taken place wherever he had been sent, it being by no means likely that any beneficial influence can be exerted by the climate itself, when a body of selected soldiers, subject to no severe duty and exposed to no hardship, lose annually a larger proportion of their number by consumption than in the United Kingdom. This inference, however adverse to generally received opinions, is strikingly corroborated by the prevalence of consumption and other pulmonary affections among the civil inhabitants of Malta, as shown in Appendix, No. III. of this Report."

These conclusions. it appears to me, in justice to the subject, ought to be questioned and carefully scrutinized, and not admitted as truths, excepting on demonstration, or, what is equivalent, being found proof against valid objection,—a procedure, I am confident, the author himself cannot but approve.

The subject, perhaps, may be conveniently divided for discussion under two heads : 1*st*, The comparative liability of our troops to consumption and other pulmonary diseases; and 2*dly*, The comparative liability of the natives to the same complaints.

Major Tulloch seems, from the foregoing observations, to have taken the admissions into hospital, on account of pulmonary diseases, as a criterion of the tendency to these diseases. For a long period,— supposing the same regulations to be observed regarding admissions,—this mode of estimation may be deserving of confidence ; but I am doubtful that it is for so short a period as that of seven years, and especially those seven referred to,—viz., from 1830 to 1836, inclusive,—which were more than usually productive of pulmonary diseases,—an epidemic catarrh having prevailed, during the period, at each of the stations.

I am disposed to think that the mortality from any disease affecting a vital organ, such as the lungs, is a better criterion of the disposition of the constitution to be impressed by it and to receive it,—especially pneumonia and tubercular phthisis,—which hardly come under the denomination of epidemic diseases, and more especially phthisis, which, sooner or later, there is good reason to believe, is always fatal.

The two following Tables show the total deaths from all diseases of the chest, amongst a portion of the army serving at home, and another portion serving in the Mediterranean, for a period of seven years.

I.—DEATHS from all Diseases of the Chest among the Dragoon Guards and Dragoons serving at Home, among the Foot Guards, and the Household Cavalry, and the Depôts of Corps serving in the West Indies, from 1st January 1830 to 31st March 1837.

Year.	Description of Force.											
	Dragoon Guards, and Dragoons.			Foot Guards.			Household Cavalry.			Depots of Corps serving in the West Indies.		
	Strength.	Deaths.	Deaths per 1000.	Strength.	Deaths.	Deaths per 1000.	Strength.	Deaths.	Deaths per 1000.	Strength.	Deaths.	Deaths per 1000.
1830,	6402	37		5010	63		1138	9		2551	23	
1831,	6018	48		4589	67		1155	7		2952	25	
1832,	6408	46		4959	73		1218	9		3511	27	
1833,	6379	64	7.7	4962	59	14.1	1202	13	8	4794	47	9.6
1834,	6261	39		4852	62		1198	11		3346	30	
1835,	5902	47		4524	58		1217	9		3462	44	
1836¼,	7241	62		5642	105		1521	11		2921	30	

II.—DEATHS from all Diseases of the Chest, in the Mediterranean Stations, from 1830 to 1836, inclusive.

Year.	Station.								
	Gibraltar.			Malta.			Ionian Islands.		
	Strength.	Deaths.	Deaths per 1000.	Strength.	Deaths.	Deaths per 1000.	Strength.	Deaths.	Deaths per 1000.
1830,	3707	23		2299	10		4646	28	
1831,	3480	18		2056	22		3388	14	
1832,	3526	26		2045	8		3254	14	
1833,	3053	24	7.	2124	19	7.4	3257	15	5
1834,	3034	13		2198	19		3284	14	
1835,	2988	31		2123	18		3274	18	
1836,	3080	32		2186	16		3298	21	

The results contained in these Tables appear to show that pulmonary diseases are less fatal amongst our troops in Gibraltar, Malta, and the Ionian Islands, than in Great Britain; the lowest mortality in either description of forces serving at home, namely, that of the dragoon-guards and dragoons, being a little higher than the highest in the Mediterranean; and the highest at home, that of the foot-guards, being nearly double.

Now, unless there are circumstances connected with the troops serving at home, which, independent of climate, render them more susceptible of pulmonary diseases, the unavoidable inference, it appears to me, is, as regards this class of men, that the Mediterranean climate is less productive of pulmonary diseases, and à fortiori* of phthisis, than the climate of Great Britain. Excepting in the instance of the Foot Guards, I am not aware of any such circumstances existing. The cavalry may be considered as the least disposed of any description of troops to contract pulmonary diseases. Their recruits are generally a better description of young men than those of the infantry. They are better clad; they have more regular, and less fatiguing exercise; they have less night-duty; their average age is greater; and they

---

* It appears from the Tables of deaths given by Major Tulloch, that, of the total mortality in the dragoon-guards, and dragoons, and the household cavalry, serving at home, the large proportion of forty per cent. is caused by phthisis pulmonalis and only 21.6 per cent. in the troops serving in Malta.

have a greater facility of invaliding than troops on foreign stations. It may not be amiss to dilate a little on some of those particulars.

That the recruiting of the cavalry is carried on in a more severe manner, and a superior description of men obtained, are notorious. They are selected chiefly from the country, from the agricultural class, whilst the majority of the recruits for the infantry are from towns. The superiority of the one over the other, is perhaps tolerably well indicated by the ratio of rejection of those who enlist. It appears that, of the country recruits, the rejected are to the approved, on medical examination, in about the ratio of twenty-five to one hundred; and of town-recruits, in the ratio of about seventy-seven to a hundred. * In some cavalry regiments, it is understood that there is even a fastidiousness of selection. I have heard of one into which none but farmers' sons were admitted, and each was required to have a certificate of good character from the clergyman of his parish.

Their being better clad, too, is equally notorious, especially in the dragoon-guards and the household cavalry. Indeed from their kind of clothing, they are more likely to experience inconvenience from the excess of heat than from chills and coldness ; and, in this respect, are strongly contrasted with the troops of the line, who, a good part of the year, wear white

* This estimate is for the year 1837, at three recruiting districts, Dublin, Edinburgh, and London.—*Vide* Mr Marshall's useful work " On the Enlisting, Discharging, and Pensioning of Soldiers," p. 71.

trowsers, without drawers, better fitted to carry off warmth than to confine it.

As regards exercise and fatigue on duty, the dif-ference between the cavalry and infantry is strongly marked, and that both when in quarters and in the field. The one, having the care of his horse, has much to do, requiring only moderate bodily exertion, such a degree as is conducive to health; and, when on active service, being carried, he is spared exces-sive exhausting fatigue. The other, when in quarters, has more idle time, more time for drinking and dis-sipation. Even on march the exertion required of him is great, having to carry, when in heavy march-ing order, not less than fifty pounds weight. The pressure the soldier of the line is exposed to is well marked in the frame of the veteran. If stripped, there is no difficulty in distinguishing between the chest of the old cavalry and the old infantry soldier; the former is well expanded, and convex in front; the latter has a crushed, contracted, peculiar ap-pearance, especially its upper portion, which is more or less bent in. This remark is offered as the result of pretty extensive experience; after having examined, in the course of five years uninterrupt-edly, about ten thousand invalids in the manner just mentioned.

I have said that the average age of the cavalry is greater than that of the infantry. The full period of service in the former is twenty-four years; in the latter twenty-one; the proportion of men annually invalided in the cavalry, is less than in the infantry,* sufficient proof that the statement above made is correct. What the exact difference of the average age of the two descriptions of troops, at any particular time, has been, I am ignorant; but, from tables given by Major Tulloch, it would appear that the proportion of men between the age of thirty-three and forty, in the cavalry serving at home, from the 1st January 1830 to 31st March 1837, compared with the foot guards for the same period, was as 193 per 1000 for the former, to 168 per 1000 for the latter. And probably in the army generally, the difference is greater, as it is likely that less favour is shown to men in the line, in regard to making up a full period of service ; and farther, as the latter are subject to strict examination, both on returning from, and preparatory to going on, foreign service. I rather dwell on this subject of age, because I believe it to be an important element in the problem under consideration. That certain ages are more prone to pulmonary consumption is unquestionable. The following Table, drawn up from the necrological registers of the general hospital at Fort Pitt, from the 27th July 1826, to the 23d December 1839, during which period the total deaths amounted to 1092 from all diseases, may be deserving of insertion, for the purpose of reference and illustration. It has been thought proper to include also the cases of chronic

---

* According to Major Tulloch's estimate for four years, viz. from 1830 to 1833 inclusive, the ratio per 1000, is, in the household cavalry, as 18., and in the foot-guards, as 36.4!

catarrh and of hæmoptysis, as the great majority of these proved eventually to be instances of tubercular phthisis, as was ascertained by post-mortem examination.

RETURN of Fatal Cases of Phthisis pulmonalis, Catarrhus chronicus, and Hæmoptysis, which have occurred in the General Hospital, from 27th of July 1826 to 22d December 1839.

Ages.	Phthisis pulmonalis. No. of Cases.	Catarrhus chronicus. No. of Cases.	Hæmoptysis. No. of Cases.
17	1	...	...
18	7	3	...
19	8	1	...
20	14	3	1
21	22	1	...
22	19	3	...
23	22	5	...
24	36	4	2
25	21	4	...
26	27	4	...
27	24	5	...
28	21	1	...
29	19	4	1
30	24	4	...
31	8	3	...
32	22	2	...
33	19	3	...
34	13	2	...
35	10	1	...
36	11	3	...
37	3	3	...
38	7	1	...
39	8	3	...
40	10	1	...
41	5	...	...
42	7	3	...
43	1	1	...
44	3	...	...
45	3	...	1
46	...	1	...
47	2	...	...
48	3	...	...
49	3	...	...
50	1	...	...
55	2	...	...
60	...	1	...
70	...	1	...
	406 *	71 †	5

* Age unknown in six cases.   † Age unknown in two cases.

The last circumstance to which I shall call the attention, is the greater facility of invaliding at home than
abroad. The troops of the line, on home service,
part with their inefficient men twice yearly, namely,
at the time of the half-yearly inspections, and the
Guards at shorter intervals, commonly monthly. On
foreign service, although the inspections are half-
yearly, the men then brought forward, considered
unfit, are commonly detained many months; hitherto
invalids from the Mediterranean stations have been
sent home more commonly once than twice annually.*
An unavoidable difference, in relation to the mortality as returned, is consequent on this; a larger
proportion of the cases of phthisis, occurring in the
troops serving in the United Kingdom, die amongst
their friends, after having been discharged the service, than in the corps serving abroad; thereby augmenting the proportional mortality from this disease

* The arrivals from the Mediterranean, at Chatham, are given in
subjoined Table for nine years, omitting the ships of war which have
occasionally brought home a few invalids, but rarely bad cases, especially consumptive.

Years.	From Corfu.	From Malta.	From Gibraltar.
1831	1	2	4
1832	2	2	3
1833	1	1	...
1834	1	2	1
1835	1	1	1
1836	1	1	1
1837	1	...	1
1838	1	2	2
1839	1	1	2

in the returns of the latter.   The following Table shows the number of fatal cases amongst the invalids, furnished by different stations at home and abroad, whose ages have been given in the preceding Table. It is formed from the records of the General Hospital, and may be depended on for accuracy: it is inserted, as bearing on the preceding remarks ; and it may be added, in relation to the last of these remarks, that a large proportion of the men who die in the General Hospital of phthisis, are carried off within a month or two from their disembarkation.

RETURN of the Number of Cases of Phthisis pulmonalis, Catarrhus chronicus, and Haemoptysis, with the Stations at which the Disease was contracted, which have proved fatal in the General Hospital, Fort Pitt, from the 27th July 1826 to the 31st December 1839.

Diseases.	Great Britain.	Ireland.	Canada.	Nova Scotia.	Newfoundland.	East Indies.	Ceylon.	West Indies, including Jamaica, Bermuda, and Leeward Isles.	West Coast of Africa.	Cape of Good Hope.	New South Wales, including Van Diemen's Land.	Mauritius.	Portugal.	Gibraltar.	Malta.	Ionian Islands.	Unknown.	Total.
No. of Invalids arrived from following Stations, during the period,	9298	53	1216	646	384	5884	430	2716	348	361	473	417	208	1188	798	870	389	25709
Phthisis pulmonalis,	138	18	36	13	3	30	4	76	2	6	3	8	2	20	19	11	27	416
Catarrhus chronicus,	21	4	9	2	...	6	3	9	...	1	1	...	...	7	1	1	7	72
Haemoptysis,	...	...	1	...	...	...	...	2	...	...	...	...	...	1	...	...	2	6
Total,	159	22	46	15	3	36	7	87	2	7	4	8	2	28	20	12	36	494

To conclude :—As the statistical facts show that pulmonary complaints are more fatal amongst our troops serving at home than in the Mediterranean; and as all the circumstances, independent of climate, so far as I am acquainted with them, affecting the question, appear to be in favour of the troops serving at home, especially the cavalry, I am not only not able to adopt the opinion referred to, that the climate of the Mediterranean is more productive of diseases of the chest than our own climate, but am obliged to fall back on the old and hitherto generally received opinion of an opposite nature.

Let us next consider the comparative liability of the natives of these southern regions to pulmonary complaints, especially phthisis.

Of the three stations under consideration, Malta is the only one of which we have any returns showing the yearly mortality amongst the civil population from different diseases. It has been already mentioned how these returns are formed. Major Tulloch has referred to them in confirmation of his conclusion before alluded to. He remarks—" Nor is the fatal influence of diseases of the lungs (in Malta) confined to the troops alone; it extends, in a corresponding degree, to the inhabitants. A reference to Abstract, No. III. of Appendix, shows that the deaths from these diseases, among the population of all ages, in the course of thirteen years, from 1822 to 1834, inclusive, have been as follows :—

Diseases.	Jan.	Feb.	Mar.	Apr.	May.	June	July.	Aug.	Sept.	Oct.	Nov.	Dec.	Total
Inflammation of Lungs,	75	58	73	73	55	29	10	19	25	27	31	48	523
Pleurisy, ...	15	7	11	7	12	3	7	6	3	4	6	11	92
Spitting of Blood, .	13	10	20	7	4	13	4	8	7	10	13	9	118
Phthisis pulmonalis,	115	94	115	122	147	91	110	110	103	129	105	122	1363
Consumption,* . . .	238	177	205	179	202	223	294	249	258	301	233	227	2786
Catarrh, ...	110	118	128	102	71	66	60	64	53	70	83	131	1056
Asthma, ...	80	73	74	53	46	31	38	30	19	34	43	66	587
Hooping-Cough, . .	30	23	18	14	16	11	8	3	7	2	2	5	139
Total, . .	676	560	644	557	553	467	531	489	475	577	516	619	6664

The author proceeds :—" This total of 6664 deaths in thirteen years shows the mortality to have been 513 annually, which, upon an average population of 100,000 of all ages, is about $5\frac{1}{8}$ per thousand of the strength, being scarcely one per thousand less than among the troops, notwithstanding the night exposure of the latter in the course of their military duties."

He adds :—" Though the climate of this island has been supposed favourable to diseases of the lungs, its inhabitants appear to suffer from them nearly as much as those of high northern latitudes ; for the returns of Sweden show that there were only 14,087 deaths from this class of diseases out of the whole population in one year, being in the ratio of $5\frac{6}{10}$ per thousand, or within a fraction the same as in Malta."

From my professional knowledge of Malta and of

* " The deaths reported by the Maltese medical practitioners, under the head of consumption, as distinguished from pthisis pulmonalis, are understood, in many instances, to have referred to that class of cases more generally designated *marasmus*."

its medical concerns, I have no hesitation in saying, that in this statement I believe Major Tulloch has greatly overrated the proportion of deaths from pulmonary diseases. He has, no doubt, been misled by the term consumption: as used by the native practitioners, it was commonly employed to express marasmus, or wasting and loss of strength, without cough and other pectoral symptoms; and consequently the whole number, so returned, amounting to 2786, require to be deducted from the total, 6664, reducing it thereby to 3878, which, instead of being in the ratio of $5\frac{1}{8}$ per 1000, is a little less than 3 per 1000, namely, 2.98.

In consequence of the official situations which I held in Malta, especially as President of the Medical Committee, which, under the local government, superintended the medical concerns of the island, my attention was directed to the forms of the monthly returns of mortality; and, seeing how open to misconception the term "consumption" was, as used in the old forms, I proposed its omission altogether, with some other alterations, which were adopted and used afterwards by the police physician.

The following Table, drawn up from the monthly returns of mortality, after the new form was brought into use, will convey, I believe, a more correct idea of the fatality of pulmonary diseases:—

TABLE showing the Deaths from Pulmonary Diseases, in Malta, from 1831 to 1834, inclusive.

Year, ...	1831.	1832.	1833.	1834.
Population, ...	102,830	104,263	104,056	103,926
Deaths from all Diseases, . .	2581	2476	3173	2732
Pneumonia, ...	53	56	58	56
Pleuritis, ...	3	5	8	12
Hæmoptysis, ...	10	12	12	13
Phthisis pulmonalis, ...	113	99	178	150
Catarrhus, ...	44	41	101	83
Asthma, ...	56	45	57	38
Pertussis, ...	...	118	13	8
Total, ...	279	376	427	360

From which it appears that, during these four years, in three of which one or more pulmonary diseases were unusually prevalent and fatal, the average annual mortality from all of them was in the ratio of 3.8 per 1000 of the population, and that pulmonary consumption alone constituted only about 37 per cent. of these diseases, and of the total deaths not quite 5 per cent.

In 1829 certain questions were submitted to the Medical Committee in Malta by the Secretary of Government, proposed by the Royal College of Physicians of London, in reply to the first of which, viz.—" What proportion do the annual deaths bear to the population ? " the following information was given :—

TABLE showing the Population of Malta, and Mortality, from 1824 to 1828, inclusive.

Year.	Population.	Deaths.	Ages of those who died.					
			Infants under 8.	Children from 8 to 15.	Young Persons from 15 to 28.	Persons from 28 to 50.	From 50 to 70.	From 70 upwards.
1824,	96,404	2345	1125	80	158	231	372	379
1825,	97,627	2612	1276	82	179	293	398	384
1826,	98,739	2277	1090	62	152	330	370	373
1827,	99,549	2434	1180	60	160	260	385	384
1828,	100,949	2592	1260	79	178	291	390	394

During the period of five years there died annually 550 of dentition, 280 of diarrhœa, 200 of marasmus, 170 of nervous complaints, 150 of debility, 130 of dysentery, 120 of apoplexy, 120 of miscarriage, 100 of phthsis pulmonalis.

From which, I may remark, it appears that, of the principal fatal complaints, pulmonary consumption is returned as the least fatal, and in a considerably less degree, than in the following years (excepting one), included in the table preceding the last, which were unusually unhealthy, and, as before observed, rife in pulmonary complaints. This document I have thought it right to notice, as it is strongly illustrative of the point at issue ; and that the particulars may have due weight, I may mention that the members of the committee by whom it was drawn up were the most experienced medical men in the island, being the physician and senior surgeon of the Civil Hospital and the police physician.

I shall insert another document, bearing on the same point—a return of the medical cases treated in 1834 at the public dispensary, which was established the year before by government, at my suggestion, to relieve the Civil Hospital, then in danger of being crowded to excess.

RETURN of the Number of Persons who received Medical Aid at the Dispensary in Valetta during the Year 1834.

Diseases.	City.					Country.					Total.
	Men.	Women.	Boys.	Girls.	Total.	Men.	Women.	Boys.	Girls.	Total.	
Alienatio,	..	3	..	..	3	..	..	..	..	..	
Amenorrhœa,	..	159	..	..	159	..	49	..	..	49	
Angina,	2	5	2	..	9	2	5	1	..	8	
Anorexia,	5	9	..	1	15	4	44	..	2	50	
Aphonia,	4	5	1	..	10	5	5	..	..	10	Of City.
Aphtæ,	..	3	1	..	4	..	1	..	..	1	2238
Astenia,	..	..	..	..	..	1	..	..	..	1	
Asthma,	2	8	2	1	13	18	8	5	4	29	
Bronchitis,	177	283	34	32	526	136	210	30	25	401	
Cephalalgia,	2	2	1	..	5	4	2	..	..	6	
Colica,	11	25	14	7	57	11	36	4	6	57	
Convulsio,	8	26	5	5	44	1	13	1	2	17	
Dentitio,	..	..	16	11	27	..	..	11	11	22	
Diarrhœa,	52	72	26	35	185	21	58	26	29	134	
Dysenteria,	13	25	10	11	59	10	18	7	9	44	
Dyspepsia,	1	1	..	..	2	..	..	..	..	..	
Enteritis,	..	2	..	..	2	..	..	..	..	..	
Epilepsia,	2	2	..	..	4	2	2	1	..	5	
Exanthemata,	2	1	1	1	5	1	2	..	..	3	
Febris,	58	185	39	41	323	512	104	28	23	667	Of Country.
Gastrocismus,	140	401	11	26	578	199	358	9	10	576	2228
Hœmatimisis,	..	..	..	..	..	..	1	..	..	1	
Hœmaturia,	3	..	..	1	4	..	..	1	..	1	
Hepatitis,	..	..	..	..	..	..	1	..	..	1	
Hydrops,	4	5	..	..	9	1	19	1	..	21	
Hypochondria,	..	2	..	..	2	..	.½	..	..	..	
Icterus,	4	3	2	..	9	2	5	..	..	7	
Menorrhagia,	..	28	..	..	28	..	12	..	..	12	
Ostitis,	..	1	..	..	1	..	3	..	..	3	
Palpitatio,	2	9	8	2	21	4	5	..	..	9	
Paralysis,	2	6	..	..	8	5	8	..	1	14	
Phthisis,	8	11	1	..	20	3	6	..	..	9	
Pleuritis,	4	10	..	..	14	3	2	..	..	5	
Pyrosis,	6	11	18	15	50	2	2	9	11	24	
Rheuma,	16	26	..	..	42	10	30	..	1	41	
Total,	528	1329	192	189	2238	950	1009	135	134	2228	4466

The small proportion of pulmonary diseases in this return, with the exception of bronchitis or acute catarrh, which prevailed during the winter season, is very remarkable ; and, in my opinion, strongly indicative of the little prevalency of tubercular phthisis in Malta,—a disease peculiarly suitable to dispensary practice, especially in a mild climate, and amongst a poor population. And, it appears to me, that the records of the Civil Hospital are in favour of the same conclusion. The following Table, showing the amount of pulmonary diseases, treated in this hospital during three years, is taken from Dr Hennen's Sketches of the Medical Topography of the Mediterranean.

Summary View of the Admissions and Deaths from Pulmonary Complaints in the Civil Hospital in Malta, from 1821 to 1823 inclusive.

Diseases.	Males.						Females.						Remarks.
	1821.		1822.		1823.		1821.		1822.		1823.		
	Admitted.	Died.	Admitted.	Died.	Admitted.	Died.	Admitted.	Died.	Admitted.	Died.	Admitted.	Died.	
Cough and Catarrh,	99	25	90	14	90	22	71	14	69	10	53	8	Total Admissions,
Consumption,* . .	4	2	..	..	3	2	9	6	6	5	5	3	723; deaths 180; proportional mortality 1 in 4.16
Hæmoptysis, . . .	12	1	8	2	15	1	6	..	5	..	9	1	
Pleuritis, ...	19	..	19	2	14	..	10	..	13	12	17	1	
Phthisis pul., . .	4	4	1	0	7	5	7	4	7	5	11	6	
Pulmonic, ...	7	4	9	4	4	3	5	4	6	5	9	5	
Total, . . .	145	36	127	22	133	33	108	28	106	37	104	24	

* This term, as before remarked, is used by the Maltese-medical men to express disease with wasting, without cough.

The total admissions, *i. e.* of patients of every description during the above period, with the number of deaths, were as follows :— *

Years.	Treated.	Died.
1821	3350	353
1822	3193	385
1823	3162	395

Showing, with the preceding Table, that of 1133 deaths out of the total treated, viz. 9705, only 173 were instances of pulmonary diseases, which is in the small proportion of about 15 per cent.

After giving the subject all the consideration in my power, the inference in relation to the native population appears to me unavoidable, that they suffer comparatively little from pulmonary diseases, and especially from pulmonary consumption, very much less than our troops in that island, and also than the civil population of Great Britain. Now, as they are generally very poor, and ill fed, and ill clad, in these particulars they may be considered as in the way of predisposition to phthisis. May not, then, their comparative exemption be fairly attributed to climate? And, I may add, that the rareness of scrofulous complaints in Malta, which are so often con-

* These numbers are taken from the books of the hospital ; and I am indebted for them to Mr Montanaro, the zealous and able purveyor of the establishment.

nected with the phthisical diathesis, is in favour of this conclusion.*

From the Table given, page 281, it appears that the mortality from pulmonary consumption amongst our troops in the Ionian Islands, was less than in Malta, in the ratio of 5.3 to 6.7 for 1000 of the strength. It may be worth while, and not uninteresting to inquire, Is this difference the result of climate, or of other circumstances independent of climate?

Two questions may be proposed in connexion with this inquiry, 1st, Whether the ages and period of service of the men forming the regiments in Malta, might not, in part, give rise to the difference; and, 2dly, Whether it might not be partly owing to a greater mortality from fever in the Ionian Islands, and removal thereby of a certain number of men with tubercles in the lungs, in the early stage, who in Malta would have lived till they became the victims of phthisis?

In relation to the first question, the following tabular view of the fatal cases of phthisis, which occurred in Malta, during a period of nine years, may be of use. I had it drawn up from documents in the

* This conclusion, I may add, is confirmed in a satisfactory manner, by the results of the post-mortem examinations made by my talented friend Dr Charles Galland, professor of anatomy in the university of Malta, results of much value, and which, I trust, he will publish in detail. During thirteen months, viz. from December 1840, to the end of December of the following year, he examined 615 bodies, without exercising any selection, fatal cases of various diseases; of which number he found that seventy-seven only were owing to tubercular disease, thirty-four females, forty-three males.

office of the principal medical officer; and it may be considered quite correct, excepting the column of duration of disease, the time specified in which was the time the men were in hospital, reckoning commonly from the last admission; i e. the period they were last under treatment, on account of phthisis.

TABLE of Deaths from Phthisis pulmonalis, in Regiments serving in Malta, as they appear in the Returns from 1822 to 1830, inclusive.

Strength.		Year.	Regiment.	Age.	Duration of Disease.	Service in the Mediterranean.	
Annual Average.	Corps.				No. of Days.	Years.	Months.
2480	Royal Art., 127 18th Foot, 634 80th ... 622 85th ... 650	1822	18th Foot, 80th ... 85th ... 85th ...	25 26 28 25	106 75 111 23	1 1 0 1	6 0 11 4
2234	Royal Art., 124 18th Foot, 591 80th ... 605 85th ... 629	1823	Royal Art., 18th Foot, 18th ... 80th ... 80th ... 80th ... 80th ...	32 22 31 22 28 31 24	14 112 73 112 85 61 183	1 2 2 1 1 1 2	0 0 8 10 11 11 2
1928	Royal Art., 127 18th Foot, 588 80th ... 600 85th ... 624 95th ... 574	1824	Royal Art., 18th ... 18th ... 80th ... 80th ... 80th ... 85th ... 95th ...	32 31 34* 30 19 30 42 32†	92 56 ... 115 16 244 30 ..	3 3 ... 2 0 3 0 ...	5 0 ... 11 2 3 7 ...
2036	Royal Art., 114 80th Foot, 568 85th ... 514 95th ... 533	1825	Royal Art., 18th Foot, 80th ... 80th ...	29 32 26 28	49 244 86 372	3 7 3 3	0 0 2 10
2618	Royal Art., 109 80th Foot, 513 85th ... 539 95th ... 510 Rifles, 2 Bat. 554	1826	Royal Art., 80th Rifles, 95th ... 95th ... Rifles.	34 28 20 24 27	113 213 150 365 46	4 5 2 2 0	6 0 0 0 2

* Left behind on his regiment proceeding to Corfu, period of servitude and duration of disease not given.

† Arrived from England by Surry transport; died the following day.

Table of Deaths from Phthisis pulmonalis, &c.—(*continued.*)

Strength.		Year.	Regiments.	Age.	Duration of Disease.	Service in the Mediterranean.	
Annual Average.	Corps.				No. of Days.	Years.	Months.
1774	Royal Art., 154	1827	Rifles.	22	53	0	8¼
	80th Foot, 577		85th Foot,	26	125	5	6
	95th ... 536		95th ...	22	55	3	3
	Rifles, . 559		95th ...	22	73	3	3
			Rifles,	21	64	1	0
2667	Royal Art., 159	1828					
	7th Fusil., 502		Rifles,	40	211	1	0
	80th Foot, 339		95th ...	22	4	4	2
	95th ... 542		Rifles,	29	57	2	0
	Rifles, . 540		Rifles,	23	80	1	6
2291	Royal Art., 153	1829	Royal Art.,	38	56	3	0
	7th Foot, 515		7th Foot,	31	40	3	10
	85th ... 551		7th ...	29	53	4	2
	95th ... 827		85th ...	32	65	7	3
	Rifles, 541		85th ...	28	83	7	4
			95th ...	24	50	4	11¼*
2400	Royal Art. 155	1830	95th ...	32	82	5	2
	7th Foot, 514		95th ...	24	123	1	9
	73d ... 529		7th Foot,	26	60	5	3½
	85th ... 532		7th ...	27	50	5	5
	Rifles, 542		95th ...	23	153	5	8†

From this it appears that, of the forty-eight men returned as having died of phthisis, the average age was twenty-eight, and that only three individuals were above the age of thirty-four; and further, that their average period of service in the Mediterranean, was under three years (2.8 years), and the average duration of their disease was 102 days. These results considered, and that regiments commonly proceed from Malta to the Ionian Islands, it appears not

* The Fusileers were three years previously in the Ionian Islands.
† Left behind when the regiment proceeded to Corfu.

improbable that the first question should be answered in the affirmative. On so difficult and obscure a subject, however, it would be unwise to speak with any degree of confidence. Incidentally, I would remark, it is obvious that some of the men who died of phthisis, must have laboured under the disease in its advanced stage, before they left England, and were probably injudiciously sent out, with the hope that they might derive benefit from change of climate,— a practice greatly to be reprobated, at least in the army, and which was too common a few years ago, before the stethoscope had come into common use, in aid of diagnosis in pulmonary complaints, and when the knowledge of these complaints was comparatively rude and little advanced. This reflection, however, is applicable to all the Mediterranean stations, but I believe in a greater degree to Malta than to Gibraltar and the Ionian Islands, on account of its reputation for superior mildness.

Relative to the second question, whether or no the greater mortality from fever in the Ionian Islands than in Malta, may not be concerned in diminishing the number of deaths from phthisis in the former, in the manner alluded to, I shall give a statement of the results of the post-mortem examinations in our military hospitals in the Ionian Islands, at which I was present, from August 1824 to February 1828, and in the conducting of which, in every instance, special attention was paid to the state of the lungs.

The following is a list of the fatal cases examined,

of which I took notes at the time.   The names of the
diseases are given, as they were assigned and returned
by the respective medical officers of regiments, by
whom they were treated.

Disease.				No. of Fatal Cases of each.
Febris intermittens,	.	.	.	5
... remittens,	.	.	.	38
... com. cont.,	.	.	.	9
Phthisis pulmonalis,	.	.	.	9
Pneumonia,	.	.	.	8
Gastritis,	.	.	.	1
Asthma,	.	.	.	1
Catarrhus acutus,	.	.	.	2
Dysenteria,	.	.	.	5
Lumbar abscess,	.	.	.	1
Psoass abcess,	.	.	.	1
Rheumatismus acutus,	.	.	.	1
Enteritis,	.	.	.	1
Diarrhœa,	.	.	.	1
Anasarca,	.	.	.	1
Apoplexia,	.	.	.	1
Enteritis,	.	.	.	1
Ascites,	.	.	.	1
Hæmoptysis,	.	.	.	1
Erysipelas,	.	.	.	1
Total,				90

Of the total number examined, the lungs were
found diseased in 33 instances (36.6 per cent.); in
17 with tubercles (19 per cent.); in 16 without
tubercles (17.7 per cent.),—according to the detail
in the following Table—

TABLE.

No.	Age.	Disease, as returned.	State of Lungs.
1	26	Feb. intermit.	Lungs partially hepatized.
2	20	...	Abscess in lung with partial hepatization, without tubercles.
3	39	Feb. remittens.	Excavations ; minute tubercles in progress.
4	30	...	Cavities and vomicæ ; melanotic tubercles.
5	22	Feb. continens.	Lung partially hepatized.
6	35	...	Ditto, ditto.
7	23	Phthisis pul.	Tubercles and vomicæ.
8	36	...	Softening tubercles.
9	24	...	Cavities and tubercles.
10	23	...	Ditto, ditto.
11	53	...	Abscesses; hepatization ; gangrene of lungs.
12	21	...	Vomicæ and tubercles.
13	35	...	Ditto, ditto.
14	...	...	Tubercles and vomicæ.
15	19	...	Ditto, ditto.
16	20	Catarrhus ch.	Granular tubercles, very numerous.
17	28	...	Tubercles and small vomicæ.
18	41	Asthma.	Vomicæ and tubercles.
19	22	Dysenteria.	Tubercles and cavities.
20	29	Pneumonia.	Empyema.
21	28	...	Tubercles and vomicæ.
22	14	...	Lungs partially hepatized.
23	42	...	Lung hepatized.
24	24	...	Ditto, ditto.
25	25	...	Ditto, ditto.
26	42	...	Ditto, ditto.
27	36	...	Partial hepatization of lung.
28	39	...	Partial hepatization ; death from bursting of an aneurism into trachea.
29	28	Hæmoptysis.	Left lung hepatized ; an aneurism of the aorta had burst into it.
30	23	Psoas. abscess.	Tubercles with partial hepatization.
31	20	Gastritis.	Inferior lobe of left lung hepatized.
32	28	Enteritis.	Perforation of ileum ; tubercles and minute vomicæ in right lung.
33	27	Anasarca.	Two abscesses in right lung.

Thus, it appears that in two of the fatal cases of fever, tubercles were found in the lungs, and that of the total number, of the average age 28.8, in which these bodies were found, nine only were returned as phthisis pulmonalis.

This result seems, in some degree, to favour the conclusion implied in the answer in the affirmative of the question under consideration; but in fairness, it is right to compare the results of a similar inquiry instituted in Malta,—results, as we shall presently see, which lead to an opposite inference.

During the period I was stationed in Malta, namely, from March 1828 to April 1835, I made notes of 218 fatal cases which were subjected to a post-mortem examination in our military hospitals. The following is a list of them as they were returned :—

Disease.	Total Cases of each, which occurred Yearly.								
	1828.	1829.	1830.	1831.	1832.	1833.	1834.	1835.	Total.
Febris remit., . .	1	...	...	2	...	1	7	...	11
... Com. cont., .	5	...	3	4	2	3	7	...	24
Dysenteria, . .	4	5	11	7	5	1	3	...	36
Diarrhœa, . .	3	2	2	...	1	1	...	...	9
Enteritis, . .	1	...	...	...	...	...	...	...	1
Peritonitis, . .	...	1	...	...	...	2	...	...	3
Hepatitis, . .	1	3	1	1	2	1	...	...	9
Pneumonia, . .	...	...	...	...	3	3	2	2	10
Rheumatismus acutus,	1	...	...	1	...	...	...	...	2
Icterus, . . .	...	...	1	...	...	...	1	...	2
Colica, . . .	...	...	...	...	...	...	1	...	1
Obstipatio, . .	1	...	...	...	...	...	...	...	1
Cholera, . . .	...	...	...	2	...	...	...	...	2
Dyspepsia, . .	...	...	...	...	...	1	...	...	1
Hæmatemisis, . .	...	...	...	...	...	1	...	...	1
Morbus cordis, . .	1	...	...	...	...	...	...	1	2
Mania, . . .	...	...	...	1	...	...	...	1	2
Amentia, . .	...	...	...	1	1	...	...	...	2
Delirium tremens, .	...	...	1	...	...	...	3	...	4
Apoplexia, . .	1	...	1	3	1	...	1	...	7
Paralysis, . .	1	...	...	...	...	1	...	...	2
Pulmonary apoplexy,	3	...	1	...	...	...	...	...	4
Carry forward,	23	11	21	22	15	15	25	4	136

TABLE—(*continued.*)

Disease.	Total Cases of each, which occurred Yearly.								
	1828.	1829.	1830.	1831.	1832.	1833.	1834.	1835.	Total.
Brought forward,	23	11	21	22	15	15	25	4	136
Hæmoptysis,	1	...	...	...	...	...	...	...	1
Phthisis pul.,	2	4	5	12.	3	1	12	1	40
Catarrhus chr.,	...	1	...	2	2	1	2	3	11
... acutus,	...	...	...	...	...	...	4	...	4
Debilitas,	...	...	1	...	...	...	...	...	1
Ascites,	...	...	1	...	...	1	...	...	2
Anasarca,	...	...	...	...	2	...	...	...	2
Abscessus,	...	...	1	...	...	...	...	...	1
Erysipelas,	...	...	...	...	1	...	...	...	1
Œdema glottidis,	...	...	...	...	...	1	...	...	1
Dyspnæa,	...	...	...	...	...	...	1	...	1
Contusio,	...	...	...	...	...	1	...	...	1
Fractura,	2	...	1	1	1	1	1	...	7
Amputatio,	1	...	...	...	...	...	1	1	3
Vulnus,	...	3	...	1	...	...	...	...	4
Aneurisma,	...	1	...	...	...	...	...	...	1
Variola,	...	...	1	...	...	...	...	...	1
Total,	29	20	31	38	24	21	46	9	218

Of this total number examined, the lungs were found diseased in 114 instances (the average age of whom was 29.4), which is in the ratio of 52.2 per cent. : of these, 67 (30.7 per cent.) had tubercles ; 47 (21.6 per cent.) were without tubercles, according to the detail in the following Table—

TABLE.

No.	Year.	Age.	Disease, as returned.	State of Lungs.
1	1828	22	Phthisis pul.	Tubercles ; small vomicæ.
2	...	23	...	Tubercles ; a few small vomicæ.
3	...	36	Hæmoptysis.	Tubercles ; vomicæ.
4	...	27	Pul. apoplexy.	Blood extravasated into lungs ; no tubercles.
5	...	32	...	Ditto, ditto.
6	...	32	...	Ditto, ditto.
7	...	29	Obstipatio.	Tubercles ; vomicæ.
8	1829	25	Phthisis pul.	Tubercles ; vomicæ ; hydrothorax.
9	...	24	...	Tubercles ; vomicæ.
10	...	23	...	Large cavities ; tubercles.
11	...	22	Dysenteria.	Tubercles ; minute vomicæ.
12	1830	27	Phthisis pul.	Large cavities ; tubercles.
13	...	43	...	Cavities ; tubercles.
14	...	22	...	Ditto, ditto.
15	...	28	Dysenteria.	Two small clusters of granular tubercles in superior lobe of right lung.
16	...	26	Variola.	Partial hepatization of lung.
17	...	37	...	Ditto, ditto.
18	1831	26	Phthisis pul.	Vomicæ ; tubercles.
19	...	32	...	Ditto, ditto.
20	...	22	....	Ditto, ditto.
21	...	28	...	Ditto, ditto.
22	...	33	...	Ditto, ditto.
23	...	31	...	Ditto, ditto.
24	...	30	...	Ditto, ditto.
25	...	31	...	Ditto, ditto.
26	...	36	...	Ditto, ditto.
27	...	21	...	Ditto, ditto.
28	...	23	...	Ditto, ditto.
29	...	46	Catarrhus ch.	Ditto, ditto.
30	...	26	...	Granular tubercles in left lung.
31	...	34	Pneumonia.	Partial hepatization of lungs.
32	...	26	...	Similar.
33	...	33	...	Right lung hepatized.
34	...	34	...	Right and part of left lung hepatized.
35	...	36	...	Partial hepatization of lungs.
36	...	24	...	Small abscesses ; no tubercles.; pneumathorax.
37	...	30	...	Partial hepatization of lung.
38	..	27	...	10 Pints of serum in left pleura ; no tubercles.
39	...		...	Tubercles ; hepatization ; empyema.
40	...	36	...	Right lung hepatized.
41	...	37	...	Both lungs much hepatized.
42	...	24	Mania.	Small abscesses ; partial hepatization.
43	...	24	Frac. of Cran.	A few granular tubercles.

TABLE—(*continued.*)

No.	Year.	Age.	Diseases, as returned.	State of Lungs.
44	1831	28	Hepatitis ch.	Partial hepatization; effusion into pleura.
45	...	26	Chol. Morbus.	Similar.
46	...	26	Dysenteria.	Tubercles; small vomicæ.
47	...	24	Febris con.	Granular tubercles; minute abscesses.
48	...	24	...	Left lung hepatized.
49	...	45	...	Lungs hepatized.
50	1832	29	Phthisis pul.	Cavities; tubercles.
51	...	38	...	Ditto, ditto.
52	...	29	...	Ditto, ditto.
53	...	25	Catarrhus ch.	Cavity in right lung; tubercles; pneumathorax with empyema.
54	...	30	...	Abscess of liver communicating with lung and pleura; in latter much fetid air and fluid.
55	...	21	Pneumonia.	A small cavity in left lung; many tubercles; 6 pints of purulent fluid in left pleura.
56	...	30	...	$3\frac{1}{2}$ Pints of pus in pericardium; $2\frac{1}{2}$ in left pleura.
57	...	28	...	Lungs partially hepatized; 39 oz. of purulent fluid in right pleura.
58	...	27	Dysenteria.	A small vomica and two or three clusters of granular tubercles in superior lobe of each lung.
59	...	28	Febris.	Hepatization of right lung.
60	...	27	Amentia.	Abscess and gangrene of lung.
61	...	30	Anasarca.	Partial hepatization of lungs.
62	...	49	...	$3\frac{1}{4}$ Pints of serum in pleura; partial melanosis of lungs.
63	...	48	Hepatitis chr.	Gangrene of inferior lobe of right lung.
64	...	26	...	Abscess in lung and liver freely communicating.
65	...	27	Phthisis pul.	Tubercles and cavities.
66	...	24	...	Ditto, ditto.
67	...	35	...	Ditto, ditto.
68	...	32	...	Ditto, ditto.
69	...	25	...	Ditto, ditto.
70	...	30	...	Tubercles; cavities; pneumathorax.
71	...	29	...	Tubercles; cavities.
72	...	27	...	Tubercles; cavities; hydrothorax.
73	...	28	...	Tubercles; cavities.
74	...	23	...	Ditto, ditto.
75	...	27	...	Tubercles and cavities; three pints of turbid serum in right pleura.
76	...	'27	Pneumonia.	Pus in bronchia (bronchitis).
77	...	27	...	Hepatization of superior lobe of left lung.
78	...	47	...	Blood extravasated into substance of lung.
79	...	28	...	Slight hepatization of lungs, with hypertrophy of heart.

TABLE—(*continued.*)

No.	Year.	Age.	Disease, as returned.	State of Lungs.
80	1833	28	Catarrhus ch.	Tubercles and cavities.
81	...	32	Dyspepsia.	Hepatization of right lung.
82	...	26	Febris con.	Ditto, ditto.
83	...	27	...	Two clusters of granular tubercles in left lung; hepatization of right lung.
84	1834	27	Phthisis pul.	Cavities; tubercles.
85	...	22	...	Ditto, ditto.
86	...	32	...	Ditto, ditto.
87	...	27	...	Ditto, ditto.
88	...	41	...	Ditto, ditto.
89	...	24	...	Ditto, ditto.
90	...	30	...	Ditto, ditto.
91	...	30	...	Ditto, ditto.
92	...	27	...	Ditto, ditto.
93	...	27	...	Cavities; tubercles; empyema; pneumathorax.
94	...	24	...	Ditto, ditto.
95	...	29	...	Cavities; tubercles.
96	...	28	Catarrhus ch.	Ditto, ditto.
97	...	30	...	Ditto, ditto.
98	...	28	Catarrhus ac.	Blood in bronchia and lungs from ruptured aneurism.
99	...	25	...	Lymph on pleura (perforation of ileum; peritoneal inflammation.)
100	...	...	Pneumonia.	Partial hepatization; small abscesses.
101	...	27	...	Tubercles; cavities; pneumathorax.
102	...	42	...	Blood extravasated into lungs from ruptured aneurism.
103	...	40	Delirium trem.	Partial hepatization of lungs.
104	...	44	...	Bronchia very red, as if inflamed.
105	...	28	Febris con.	Partial hepatization of lung.
106	...	16	...	Œdema of lungs.
107	1835	29	Phthisis pul.	Tubercles and cavities.
108	...	29	Catarrhus ch.	Ditto, ditto.
109	...	32	...	Ditto, ditto.
110	...	32	...	Ditto, ditto.
111	...	26	Pneumonia.	Partial hepatization of lungs.
112	...	32	...	Ditto, ditto.
113	...	35	Mania.	Hepatization of left lung.

Thus it appears that, of the total number of cases in which tubercles were found, namely 67,* 46 were

* This is a large proportion, viz. 30.7 per cent.; and yet not so large as I have found to exist amongst the fatal cases in the General Hospital

returned as phthisis pulmonalis ; whilst, in the Ionian Islands, of 17 with tubercles, 9 only were returned

at Fort Pitt, in which the invalids, as already mentioned, are received from all our foreign, as well as home stations ; there the proportion I have found to be as high as 61.7 per cent., as shown in the subjoined Table, formed from the careful perusal of 1205 detailed fatal cases, and chiefly from my own notes, exclusive of a period of nine years, viz. from 1826 to 1834.

RESULTS of the Examination of the Lungs in 1205 fatal cases, in the General Hospital, Fort Pitt.

Years.	Phthisis.	Misnamed Phthisis.	Chronic Catarrh and Haemoptysis, with cavities and tubercles.	Other Diseases, with cavities and tubercles.	Other Diseases, with cavities.	Other Diseases, with tubercles.	Diseases without cavities or tubercles, including misnamed Phthisis.	Total.
1821	6	..	2	3	..	2	17	30
1822	18	1	4	6	..	7	25	60
1823	14	..	1	1	..	4	21	41
1826	11	..	..	3	2	6	38	60
1827	31	1	1	6	..	8	54	100
1828	34	..	4	5	..	7	36	86
1829	31	1	4	9	..	8	23	75
1830	16	1	5	17	..	3	22	63
1831	25	..	5	9	2	10	26	77
1832	23	..	4	10	1	14	19	71
1833	37	1	4	11	..	9	19	80
1834	36	1	2	5	1	7	25	76
1835	18	1	1	9	2	..	11	41
1836	24	..	..	4	..	12	22	62
1837	38	3	11	15	..	4	34	102
1838	18	..	14	6	3	13	31	85
1839	35	1	6	12	..	5	38	96
	415	11	68	121	11	119	461	1205

34.4 per cent.   38.2 per cent.

61.7 per cent.

The proportional number of instances in which Dr Galland has detected tubercles in the lungs in the bodies of natives of Malta, examined in the Civil Hospital, has been very much smaller, in the ratio, on the whole, of about 19.6 per cent.; farther, in confirmation of the conclusion, that the climate of that island is comparatively little favourable to the formation of these bodies,—at least in the instance of the native inhabitants.

For the sake of comparison, and as valuable data, I shall give the

under the head of this disease. The greater prevalence of tubercles in the lungs in Malta amongst our troops than in the Ionian Islands, shown by these returns, can hardly be considered otherwise than strongly in favour of the conclusion, that phthisis also is really more prevalent in the former than in the latter.

results of his inquiries on this most important subject, in the three following Tables, for which I am indebted to him.

TABLE I.—In reference to Age and Sex.

Sex.	Age.	No. of Bodies examined.	Instances of the presence of Tubercles.	Instances of their presence in the Lungs.	Instances where they proved fatal.	Instances where fatal in the Lungs.	Instances of Ulceration of the Larynx, with Tubercles in the Lungs.
MALES.	0 to 10	59	7	6	6	4	..
	10 20	27	7	6	6	4	1
	20 30	35	16	15	13	13	5
	30 40	33	7	7	5	4	2
	40 50	24	5	4	5	3	1
	50 60	46	6	6	3	3	..
	60 80	82	6	6	3	3	..
	80 100	10	..	..	..	..	..
	Of all Ages,	316	54	50	41	34	9
FEMALES.	0 to 10	53	7	6	6	4	..
	10 20	24	15	12	14	8	5
	20 30	32	19	19	19	17	7
	30 40	31	10	9	8	7	2
	40 50	29	6	5	4	3	1
	50 60	34	3	3	2	1	1
	60 80	80	7	7	4	3	..
	80 100	16	..	..	..	..	..
	Of all Ages,	299	67	61	57	43	16
	Total,	615	121	111	98	77	25

Mean age of the 316 Males, = 41.3 }
299 Females, = 42.6 } Mean age of the 615 = 41.95.

TABLE II.—In Reference to Residence.

Number of Bodies examined.				Instances of Tubercular Deposit.			
Sex.	Town.	Country.	Total.	Sex.	Town.	Country.	Total.
Male, .	107	209	316	Male, .	26	28	54
Female,	90	209	299	Female,	22	45	67
	197	418	615		48	73	121

Should the results now brought forward accord with further and more extended observations of the like kind, may they not be adduced as strong evidence of

NOTE (*continued.*)

TABLE III.—In Reference to the Obvious Diseases.

In such as were instances of Tubercles.		Same obvious Diseases in others.		Other obvious Diseases.	
Phthisis pulmonalis in	11 } 32	7 {	4	Hæmoptysis in., . . .	1
.. tubercularis, .	19		2	Trachitis, ...	1
.. trachealis, . .	2		1	Croup, ...	1
				Hydrothorax, ...	23
Pneumonia acuta, .	} 21	27 {	13	Dysenteria, ...	42
.. chronica, .			14	Enteritis, ...	5
				Colitis, ...	1
				.. chronica, . . .	2
				Peritonitis, ...	1
Bronchitis, ...	1 } 9	29 {	4	Gastroentero meningitis,	1
.. chronica, .	8		25	Gastroencephalitis, .	3
				Gastroenteritis chronica,	1
				Cystitis acuta, . . .	3 } 4
Pleuritis, ...	2	2		.. chronica, . . .	1
Marasmus, ...	1	30		Splenitis, ...	2
Debilitas, ...	1	..		Febris synochus, . . .	1
				.. nervosa, . . .	2
				.. putechialis, . .	2
Diarrhœa, ...	20 } 25	133 {	122	Petechiæ, ...	2
.. chronica,. .	5		11	Febris intermit. perniciosa,	3
				.. icteroydes, . .	3
Gastro enteritis, . . .	1 } 2	13 {	10	Anasarca, ...	19
Gastritis chronica, . .	1		3	Ischuria, ...	1 } 2
				Strictura urethræ,. . .	1
				Eclampsia, ...	6
Hepatitis chronica, . .	1	5		Concussio, ...	5
Ascites, ...	1	9		Myalitis chronica, . .	1
Peritonitis puerperalis,	1	1		Tetanus, ...	5
				Dentitio, ...	11
				Tumores, ...	1
Metritis, ...	1 } 2	6 {	2	Phlegmon, ...	3
.. chronica, . .	1		4	Abscessus lumbaris, . .	1
				Fractura, ...	9
Apoplexy, ...	2	25		Gangrena, ...	19
Cephalagia chronica, .	1	..		Cancer, ...	7
Meningitis, ...	1	2		Tabes, ...	1
Encephalitis, ...	1	..		Syphilis consc. . . .	1
Hypertrophia cordis, .	2	3		Delirium tremens, . .	1
Rheumatismus chronicus.	1	..		Gangrena senilis, . .	1
Scrofula, ...	3	4		Caries, ...	1
				Rubiola, ...	1
				Ambustio, ...	1
Ulcers, ...	2 } 3	5 {	3	Opthalmia acuta, . . .	1 } 3
.. chronic, . . .	1		2	.. chronica, . .	2
				Gastritis, ...	1
Abscessus, ...	3	4		Gastro hepatitis, . . .	1
Contusio, ...	1	..		Effects of insolation, .	1
Herpes, ...	1	..		Sudden death, ...	1
Typhus, ...	1	6		Leucoma, ...	1
Rachitis, ...	1	..		Colica Verminosa, . .	1
Total, . . . 121		287		Total, . . . 207	

the rapid formation of tubercles in one situation, and
of their probable dispersion in another; and also, that
in some seasons their production and development is
greater and quicker than in others?

It is difficult to conceive, and very improbable, that
the difference of age of the troops in the two stations,
should be mainly concerned in so great a difference
of the tubercular diathesis as that exhibited; especially as I believe it may be fairly taken for granted
that the average age of the troops in the Ionian
Islands, was at least below thirty. It is also very
improbable that the tubercles which were discovered
in Malta, pre-existed in every instance in the individuals before they left their native country. As it
appears to be demonstrated by the researches of MM.
Lombard, and Papavoine, that tubercles are extremely
uncommon in the lungs of children who die within
the first year from their birth, and are very common
in those cut off after reaching their third year, it follows that no long period of time, at least in early
life, is requisite for their development; and many
considerations lead to the same conclusion, in relation
to a more advanced period, and especially the fact of
a large number of soldiers falling victims to the disease before their twentieth year, who, we know, only
a few months before, had been carefully examined
by medical officers, and pronounced to be in good
health and fit for military service.*

* It may, perhaps, be said, that though such recruits as those
alluded to were apparently healthy on enlistment, yet tubercles ex-

It is a question of high interest, how are our troops in Malta so subject to tubercles and tubercular phthisis? This is matter for speculation. The natives, it would appear, are comparatively, in a great measure, exempt; and the English residents are, I believe, equally so. During the whole time I was in the island, I recollect only a single individual a victim to phthisis; and his habits of life were careless and unfavourable to health. This marked difference is somewhat analogous to what is witnessed at home in the Foot-Guards, compared with the Household Cavalry, the station of both of which is commonly London. It may be asked, are the circumstances and habits of life of the troops in Malta at all similar to those of the Foot-Guards in London? I am of opinion that they are. In Malta, the troops are collected in Valetta and its suburbs, and, excepting a small party detached to Gozo, they never quit the city,—the regiments merely exchange barracks yearly. The opportunities and facilities for dissipation in Valetta are probably as great as in our own metropolis. Wine and spirits are extremely cheap, —tempting to excess; and the large number of loose women, belonging to a proportionally excessive population, needy in the extreme and abject, lead to excesses of another kind, and consequent disease. That dissipation, by injuring the general health and

isted in their lungs; and in very many cases such, it is likely, really happened: the proportional extent remains to be ascertained, and on that the argument must rest.

debilitating the constitution, conduces to tubercular disease, can hardly be doubted; at the same time, the degree of its influence is not easily appreciated. In another respect, the condition of the troops in Malta and the Foot-Guards in London is very similar, —that of severe sentinel duty, and much exposure on this duty to the night air,—to the wind and to currents of air,—and, at the same time, to vicissitudes of temperature much greater than might be expected, considering the character of the climate,—the guard-rooms, during the summer and autumnal months, being commonly oppressively hot, inducing perspiration, which is suddenly suppressed in passing into the open air.

Nowhere, in the Mediterranean, is the Sirocco wind more powerfully felt than in Malta. During the summer and autumn, when its temperature exceeds 80°, it is decidedly relaxing and weakening: and so far it may conduce, with other causes, to the production of tubercles in constitutions such as ours.*

---

* Dr Hennen, in his Medical Topography of the Mediterranean, has some speculations on the climate of Malta in connexion with phthisis, which, on account of his authority, may be deserving of incidental notice. He considers the air of Malta "exsiccated in the highest degree from the general aridity of the soil," accompanied with great rarefaction from deficiency of moisture. This is unsound doctrine, theoretically viewed; and the statement is not in accordance with facts. With the Sirocco wind, at all seasons, even in the hottest, and when the surface is most parched, the atmosphere is moist; and then, as regards comparative rareness, it is most rare; the particles of the gaseous constituents being farthest asunder, owing to the large quantity of aqueous vapour interposed.

I entered on this subject with the remark, that it is matter for speculation. With what I have advanced I am but little satisfied; and, I fear, it would be a waste of time to indulge further in conjecture; what is obscure is not likely to be elucidated, excepting by a very extensive collection of facts, in all parts of the globe, carefully made (so that we may be sure they are not improperly so called), and then rigorously examined.

Now that facility of communication with Malta is greatly increased in consequence of steam navigation, we are becoming more and more interested in the nature of its climate in relation to invalids. There is no question respecting its summer climate;* even were it wholesome, its great heat would render it disagreeable. Of its spring and winter climate, I think favourably, especially for those who are in delicate health, who are likely to be benefited by a mild atmosphere, and are in easy circumstances, so as to be able to command good accommodations, and to use horse or carriage-exercise, as may be thought most advisable. During the last few years, and especially since the visit of the Queen-Dowager, the influx of strangers has been great; and this has given rise

* The high temperature of Malta, in the hot months of summer, extended experience has shown to aggravate greatly the symptoms, and to accelerate the progress, of consumption. In a preceding note, p. 313, the proportion of deaths from this disease, in 615 fatal cases, has been given, the result of Dr Galland's inquiries, amounting to seventy-seven. Of this number, nearly two-thirds were carried off during the warmer months, confirming strongly the injurious effects

to the improvement of the hotels and lodging-houses, and their increase, insuring comfort to the invalid immediately on his arrival. The best time to proceed there, is in the latter end of October or beginning of November: it is good for the voyage; the climate of the Mediterranean then is generally delicious. The chief objections to Malta, as a winter-residence, are—the strong winds to which it is subject, and the common description of dwelling-houses, better fitted for its summer than for its winter climate; but these are comparatively of little importance to that class to whom alone I consider it suitable; who, as before observed, have the means of engaging warm comfortable apartments, and of using carriages. Many invalids, happily so situated, I have known benefited by passing the winter there.

Whether the climate of Malta is fit for those who

of heat in the advanced stage of this malady. In each month, the fatal cases, the subjects of his examination, were as follows, viz., in

December 1840, ...	7
January 1841, ...	3
February, ...	3
March, ...	6
April, ...	5
May, ...	4
June, ...	10
July, ...	9
August, ...	6
September, ...	9
October, ...	3
November, ...	7
December, ...	5
Total,	77

are decidedly labouring under pulmonary consumption, is a distinct question, and not easily answered. When the disease *is decided, it is advanced*, and is incurable. On this point the best judges are agreed; and the removal then of a patient from home, especially to a distant country, is of very doubtful propriety, and can hardly be recommended, merely with a view of affording temporary relief and palliating symptoms—all that appears to be practicable in that stage, and which may commonly be effected with less risk by the use of medicine and the regulation of diet and of temperature. If the disease *be not advanced*, its nature is almost always *doubtful;* it may not be tubercular phthisis, but chronic bronchitis, or some obscure affection of the lungs, coming under the vague designation of asthma. If either of these, I am of opinion that the winter climate of Malta may be very serviceable to the invalid. But if tubercles do exist, and are even in their early stage, I am not warranted to say that the same might be expected. What description of climate is best for those who have tubercles in this stage, with a view to their removal (if that be possible), is a very important problem, which, I fear, it must be confessed, is yet unsolved. Whatever conduces to the general health and to vigour of constitution, seems to be the best check to the tubercular diathesis. This seems to be proved by the comparative exemption from phthisis of those who follow occupations which are carried on entirely or principally in the open air, requiring a good deal of muscular exertion, and who are not confined to one spot,—as fishermen, water-men,* and butchers. The analogy of what is witnessed in animals, in sheep, and rabbits, is very strong on this point. When we consider the invigorating effect of a very cold dry atmosphere,—the excellent health enjoyed by the arctic voyagers and travellers when breathing air many degrees below zero,—and the robust health and fine forms commonly witnessed in the peasantry of the higher Alps,—it seems probable that a very cold and dry atmosphere is most likely to have the effect desired, and that more good may be expected from wintering in Canada than in Malta or Madeira, and that the Grand St Bernard is better fitted, as a summer station, for the consumptive patient in the earliest stage of the disease, than Albano or the baths of Lucca. And certain physiological and pathological considerations are rather in favour of this view: the more an organ is exercised, commonly—provided the exertion made is not excessive—the stronger and more vigorous that organ is rendered. The most common situation of tubercles is in accordance with this; it is towards the summit of the lungs, where the motion to which the lungs are subjected is trifling indeed, in comparison with their in-

* I have been informed that the Thames water-men are a very healthy class of men, and particularly little liable to pulmonary complaints, notwithstanding the atmospheric vicissitudes to which they are exposed; and it is worthy of remark that they seldom wear flannel. Requiring for their calling great good health and strength, they are careful of themselves, marry early, are sober, and live well.

ferior margin contiguous to the diaphragm, where
the extent of movement is obviously great.*　These
remarks, however, are entirely conjectural, and deserving of no attention, excepting in connexion with
inquiry, by which alone, conducted in a philosophical
spirit, this and many other problems connected with
this fatal, most important, and mysterious malady,
can be resolved.†

---

　* *Vide* Sir James Clark's valuable work on Pulmonary Consumption, p. 300, where this point is noticed after Dr Carswell, in connexion with the important subject of strengthening by exercising the
lungs.

　† Since writing the above, I have learnt, on good authority, that
pulmonary consumption and diseases of the lungs generally, are of
uncommon occurrence in the elevated country of Armenia, particularly in the town of Erzeroum, standing nearly 6000 feet above the
sea, where the winter is almost as long and as severe as within the
arctic regions,—the thermometer not unfrequently falling many
degrees below zero of Fahrenheit's scale; and where the summer-heat
is comparatively high, often ascending to 80°, combined with much
dryness of atmosphere.

CHAPTER XIII.

OBSERVATIONS ON QUARANTINE.

Supposed Importance and Object of Quarantine. Notice of the effects
of the Measures which have been considered necessary for its
Inforcement. Reflections on the existing System. Farther inquiries necessary to decide on many important Points. Foundations of existing System of doubtful Soundness. Question of the
Contagion of Plague. Considerations for and against the Doctrine. Recent Facts seemingly Demonstrative of Contagion.
Remarks on the time the Disease may be latent. On the questionable Propriety of the Classification of Substances into susceptible and non-susceptible. Reasons for considering all Substances
susceptible, excepting those which have the Power of destroying
Contagion. Other objections to the present System of Quarantine. Desiderata in Relation to farther Inquiry. Prospects of
a successful Termination, and of a Revision of the Quarantine
Laws. Facts in favour of both. Advantages likely to result
from the adoption of a milder and more efficient System.

THE importance of the subject of Quarantine in its
various influences, as affecting national prosperity,
the general welfare, and the interests of individuals,
can hardly be duly appreciated, excepting by those
who have witnessed and felt them in the Mediterranean,—in the ports of which the quarantine

system was first introduced, and to which, with a small part of eastern Europe, it has, till very lately, been almost entirely confined.

The great object of quarantine has always ostensibly been to afford protection from contagious and infectious diseases, but more especially the former, and particularly the plague, by preventing its importation, on the supposition that it is purely contagious, that it now never arises *de novo*, but is propagated, in uninterrupted succession, from one person to another; occasionally with great facility and rapidity, appearing in its devastating epidemic form terrifying nations ; occasionally, and it is supposed not uncommonly, in a very different manner,—as a sporadic disease, exciting no attention, and known only to medical men.

To effect this object various regulations have been enacted.   Sanatary codes have been framed, founded on the above mentioned conclusion of propagation by contact ; and, on the other conclusions, 1*st*, That certain articles are capable of receiving, and retaining, and conveying, the contagious matter, and that certain other articles are destitute of the power— forming the two classes of substances, the susceptible and the non-susceptible ; and, 2*dly*, That the contagion can lie hid or dormant, in the living system, only a certain time.

In carrying the system into effect, the necessity of it, for the preservation of life, having been considered absolutely necessary, the greatest rigour of forms has commonly been observed ; no regard has been shown to personal liberty; no regard has been shown to property; no regard to the interests of commerce, or of international intercourse.

When a country is proclaimed in quarantine, persons arriving from that country are taken into a lazaretto, are strictly guarded, and are subject to the punishment of death, if they leave their place of confinement before the expiration of the specified period. The ships are received into a quarantine harbour, or are surrounded by guard-boats; their cargoes are landed, and the articles variously treated ; the susceptible articles are unpacked, and either exposed for a certain time to the air, or are subjected to fumigation.

Such is a very brief outline of the quarantine system, which, with various modifications on the part of different governments, has been in activity in the Mediterranean, exclusive of the countries under Mohammedan rule, now upwards of four centuries.*

Reflecting on the vast interests involved, especially in the commercial relations of nations, it were natural to infer that the subject, in its different branches, has been most deliberately considered, most carefully investigated by unbiassed and competent men,—that nothing has been taken for granted,—that facts have been diligently collected,—evidence rigorously examined,—and that the preceding conclusions, which

* In 1423, a lazaretto, to prevent the introduction of plague, was established in Venice.—*Daru* ii., 318.

constitute in principle the foundations of the quarantine system, have been proved to be true in a demonstrative manner, or as nearly so as the nature of the subject permits ; and, consequently, that no serious objection can be made to the system,—that men's minds are at rest respecting it, and that all are reconciled to it, to its rigours, and to the annoyances and losses involved, from a firm conviction of its necessity.

This is what might be expected ; but how different is the reality. I believe it must be confessed that quite the reverse of all that has been supposed has taken place ; that fear and panic have legislated, and not reason and judgment, and, consequently, that there has been no deliberate inquiry,—no examination of evidence,—no determination of facts,—and no establishment of principles from facts on the scientific inductive plan ; and, therefore, as a further inevitable consequence, no confidence has been felt in the measures of quarantine amongst reflecting persons, and no satisfaction,—they have engendered doubts, and suspicions, and fears,—they have been viewed by many as irrational, arbitrary, and tyrannical.

To show that this is not an overcharged picture, I shall give an extract from a pamphlet which has recently appeared, the substance of which was submitted to the British Association of Science, assembled at Newcastle in August 1838, and which we owe to the pen of an individual high in the confidence of the late ministry, and who made his observations when employed by her Majesty's government in instituting inquiries relative to the commerce of the East.

Dr Bowring prefaces his remarks by observing, " The question is of consummate importance. The theory upon which quarantine regulations are founded is, in its consequences, of such enormous cost, is creative of such innumerable vexations, impediments, and miseries, that their infliction can only be justified or tolerated by a strong necessity,—a necessity founded on accurate observation, and sustained by undoubted and incontrovertible facts."

He proceeds,—" When honoured by a mission from her Majesty's government to inquire into the present state and probable future development of our commercial relations in the East, my attention was naturally and necessarily called to those regulations which impede the free transit of merchants and merchandise, which levy enormous contributions upon commerce, which subject travellers to visitations and arrests, the most capricious and the most despotic, and which have created, in almost every state, tribunals holding unchecked and irresponsible authority over persons and property, exercising that authority in arbitrary waywardness, and allowing the sufferer no appeal against injury, no redress for wrong."

He adds,—" The pecuniary cost may be estimated by millions of pounds sterling, in delays, demurrage, loss of interest, deterioration of merchandise, increased expenses, fluctuations of markets, and other calculable elements;* but the sacrifice of happiness, the weariness, the wasted time, the annoyance, the sufferings inflicted by quarantine legislation,—these admit of no calculation—they exceed all measure. Nothing but their being a security against danger the most alarming—nothing but their being undoubted protections for the public health, could warrant their infliction; and the result of my experience is not only that they are useless for the ends they profess to accomplish, but that they are absolutely pernicious; that they increase the evils against which they are designed to guard, and add to the miseries which it is their avowed object to modify or remove."†

Considering how the system of quarantine has grown up, how long it has been endured, how deeply rooted it is in the fears and ignorance of the populace, and how little the attention of governments has been paid to it, with a view to abide by the results of honest inquiry, it cannot be expected that any great change can suddenly be made, or that any material reform can soon be expected Public attention must be directed to the subject; public interest must be

* In his speech in the House of Commons, delivered on the 15th of March last, moving for farther inquiry, so much wanted on the subject of quarantine, Dr Bowring states that he believes that the losses from quarantine in the Mediterranean alone, are not less than two or three millions sterling a-year.—*Hansard's Parl. Debates.*

† " Observations on the Oriental Plague, and on Quarantine as a means of arresting its progress, addressed to the British Association of Science, assembled at Newcastle, in August 1838." By John Bowring.

excited; the subject must be discussed and agitated; and, probably, in process of time, an impression will be made, truth will prevail, and the system will be either entirely abolished; or, if at all necessary, will be so modified by the wisdom of sound experience, as to be rendered as efficacious as possible, and at the same time as little vexatious to individuals, and as little injurious as possible to the ordinary interests of society.   With this feeling, I enter upon the topic, as a duty, to endeavour to contribute the little I may have in my power towards the attainment of the end proposed.   Like Dr Bowring, I can speak from what I have myself witnessed of the evils of the present system; and, like him, I have come to the conclusion, that the system, in a sanatory point of view, is entirely a failure.   This opinion has not been hastily formed.   I have come to it after a ten years' residence in the Mediterranean, after many voyages backwards and forwards, and to the adjoining countries, and after having been four different times in quarantine, and constantly in the habit of considering quarantine questions.   I have alluded to the fundamental parts of the existing system.   It is these, in the first instance, which require to be carefully tested and probed; and on these I shall now proceed, and offer some remarks.

The first great question is, Is the oriental plague truly a contagious disease, incapable of arising *de novo*, capable of spreading only from individual to individual, by contact either directly of person, or through the medium of articles that have been touched by the diseased?

This fundamental question, I apprehend, cannot now be answered in a satisfactory manner. It can be determined only by future, very careful, and extended inquiry. The prevailing opinion, it is well known, is in the affirmative. It is the doctrine taught in the medical schools; it is the received doctrine, sanctioned by governments, and maintained by law, by the severest penalties. When I left this country for the Mediterranean, in 1824, I held the contagion of plague to be as clearly proved as that of small-pox. For a long time my belief remained firm; now I am undecided. This state of doubt has been produced by some strong evidence, recently published, in opposition to the doctrine of contagion, especially that contained in Dr Bowring's pamphlet—the substance of the experience of Dr Laidlaw, in Egypt, who, from a decided contagionist has become an anti-contagionist, in consequence of what he himself witnessed, in observing the course of the disease. Certain facts which came to my own knowledge had the same tendency to raise doubt in my mind. I shall mention two in particular. My first voyage to Malta was made in the brig Aurora, trading with Alexandria, the master of which, Mr Jackson, a very intelligent man, and in whose statement I place perfect reliance, assured me that, on the preceding voyage, on his return, a few days after leaving Alexandria, where the plague then prevailed, two of his crew were found labouring under the disease, in a well-marked form. Without delay he made for port; but, before he reached Alexandria, one of the men died. The body was buried at sea; all of the small crew assisted on the occasion, and gave their aid in lifting the corpse, as they did also after arrival in harbour, in carrying the other from his berth to the boat which conveyed him to the lazaretto, where he ultimately recovered. But the master did not stop for him; he forthwith proceeded on his voyage, but in fear that the disease would re-appear, and that he himself might be its next victim, every man on board having come in contact with the sick, but no one so much as himself, having dressed their buboes and been their chief attendant. His fears, however, were not realized; they all remained perfectly healthy.

Whilst the Russian fleet was in the Mediterranean, in 1828 or 1829, a Russian frigate arrived at Malta from Greece. During the voyage, a disease broke out amongst the crew, which, by the surgeon of the ship, was considered as fever; some of the cases proved fatal. At Malta, the circumstances appearing suspicious, minute inquiry was made into the character of the disease; the result of which was, the opinion, that the surgeon was mistaken, and that the disease was plague. The ship and crew were treated accordingly; the latter were landed and secluded in the lazaretto; the former was thoroughly fumigated. As no precautions had been taken to prevent communication with the sick during the voyage—as very

many had come in contact with them—it was presumed that the disease would spread amongst the
crew after landing; but not a single fresh case occurred; hence giving rise either to the inference, that
those experienced in the symptoms of plague may
mistake another disease for it; or to the conclusion,
if no mistake was made, that the disease was not
contagious, or only in a very slight degree.   Other
circumstances may be mentioned which tend to raise
doubt relative to the contagion of plague—and two
especially; first, the difficulty there always is in distinguishing between a contagious epidemic or endemic disease, and an endemic or epidemic disease, the
cause of which exists in the atmosphere, or in some
circumstance to which the population generally is
exposed; and, secondly, the course which the plague
has commonly been observed to run when it has
broken out amidst a dense population.   Dr Russel,
one of the ablest writers on this disease, describes it,
at its outbreak, as very fatal, and spreading slowly;
towards its height, as spreading rapidly, and fatal in
a somewhat less degree; and towards its decline, as
spreading very slowly, and being very little fatal.   He
adopted the doctrine of contagion, and supposed that
its contagion varied at different times, and that its
virulency was marked by the rapidity of the extension
of the disease, and *vice versa*, its mildness, and ultimately its effeteness, by the slow spreading of the
disease, terminating in its cessation.   The anti-con-
tagionists may say that this described course is rather

that of an endemic disease, destitute of contagion, than of a purely contagious malady. That there should be much similarity often between an epidemic or endemic disease, with and without contagion, seems to be almost a matter of necessity. Ingenuity can easily reconcile difficulties. Every disease that has ever been very prevalent has, in some place, or at some time or other, been considered contagious. Dysentery, pulmonary consumption, common catarrh, may be specially mentioned as having been so considered. Cholera morbus affords a memorable example of the difficulty in distinguishing between the two kinds of disease; a large proportion of the medical profession have come to the conclusion that it is contagious; whilst another section of the profession are satisfied that it is entirely free from contagion. These remarks are offered to show that doubt may be reasonable even respecting the contagion of plague; 1st, Whether it exists at all?* 2dly, If proved to have

---

* Since the above was written, some facts, well authenticated, which came to my knowledge whilst in Constantinople, have satisfied me of the reality of the contagion of this disease. I shall briefly relate them; for as they carried conviction to my mind, previously in doubt on the question, they may, perhaps, have a like effect on the minds of others—of such as have not yet come to a positive conclusion on the subject.

On the 8th of last June, a merchant vessel, belonging to Yazidjy Oglou Mehemet, arrived at Constantinople from Alexandria with several cases of plague on board amongst the passengers and crew. At this time, and for three years previously, the capital and its neighbourhood had been free from plague; indeed, it was in this month that free communication was, for the first time, permitted between Turkey and

existence, as to its character, and its qualities? On so important a subject nothing ought to be taken

Austria, by way of the Danube. Amongst the persons employed to carry into effect the sanatory measures considered necessary on this occasion, two require to be specially mentioned, viz., one Abdullah, a young man of nineteen, who from infancy had resided in Constantinople, and for the last two years had been employed as a guardiano; the other, Mehemet Hussein, a porter by trade, and who also from childhood (he was thirty-seven years of age) had lived in Constantinople. Abdullah, on the arrival of the infected vessel, was sent on board of her in perfect health, with the caution, not to touch any of the passengers. This caution he neglected, having, as he said, no fear of the disease; he assisted even in landing at the lazaretto some of the individuals labouring under it. On the 13th of the same month he was taken ill; on the 15th he expired. The symptoms of plague were decided, accompanied with a large bubo in the left groin. He was seen and examined, both by the director-general of quarantine, M. Robert; the director of the lazaretto, Cherif Mehemet Effendi de Ghes; and by the health officer, Dr Davout Oglou. The porter Mehemet Hussein was taken into the lazaretto to aid in removing the effects of the passengers and the merchandise from the infected vessel. On the 22d of June it was reported that he was labouring under plague. He was then seen by M. Robert and by Dr Davout Oglou, and was found to have the symptoms of plague, with a large bubo in the groin.

If these two cases be admitted as true cases of plague, and I must express myself satisfied that they were, there being no occasion for doubt, as far as I was able to judge, after careful inquiry, may they not be considered demonstrative that plague is contagious? May it not be concluded as a thing certain that, if these two men had not communicated with the persons and effects brought in the infected vessel, they, in common with the whole population of the city and its suburbs, amounting, it is estimated, to about 800,000 souls, would have remained free from the disease? Had plague broke out about the same time in Constantinople or its environs, or shortly after, then it might be inferred that the individuals in question might have had the disease independent of such communication; but, as the plague

for granted; analogies should be cautiously used—
there should be a constant watchfulness that they
do not lead astray.   For if plague has its peculiar contagious virus, it does not follow that it is
similar in any way to any other contagious virus.
All its properties may be perfectly distinct, *sui generis*,
and, in relation to propagation, as much so as any
animal or vegetable species; and, in relation to circumstances, not dissimilar; a certain range of temperature may be requisite for its activity; one degree
of atmospheric humidity may promote it, another
may check it; and, in consequence, under certain
circumstances, the disease may have the character of
being contagious; and, under others, of being non-
contagious.*

did not appear in a single instance amongst the population, and afterwards only in a solitary case, an individual just liberated from the
lazaretto, such a conclusion seems to be quite inadmissible.

A distinguished member of the Superior Council of Health of Constantinople, M. Pezzoni, has done me the honour of addressing a letter
to me, chiefly on those two cases, as proofs irrefragable of the contagious nature of plague, the circumstances connected with them being
such as, in his opinion, not to admit of their being considered of endemic origin—a conclusion in which I cannot but concur with him.
His letter is accompanied by declarations, signed by M. Robert, certi-
fying as to the facts of the cases in question, and which, with M. Pezzoni's letter, have been communicated to the Royal Medico-Chirur-
gical Society of London, and will probably appear in the next volume
of their Transactions, it being his express wish that all possible publicity should be given to it.   (*Vide* " Lancet," the No. for April 29.)

* It is curious to observe how opinion, always vague on the subject of the origin of the plague in different places, has varied at different times.   A rather amusing example of this vagueness is afforded
in some answers to queries from the Royal Society, by Paul Rycaut,

But, setting aside doubt relative to the contagious nature of plague—suppose it be taken for granted that a peculiar matter is generated in the disease, by which alone it is propagated, other great and fundamental questions remain open for discussion; 1*st*, Relative to the time that the disease, after infection, can lie hid in the system; 2*dly*, Relative to the de-

---

Esq., in 1668, the British consul at Smyrna, and who had been resident several years in Constantinople.

" Constantinople," he remarks, " hath been always greatly afflicted with the plague, especially in June, July, and August, more than any other part of the world, which is the reason that Hippocrates, born in the island of Coos, prescribes to the Grecian emperors so many rules against the contagion in their imperial city. And now, by reason of that principle of predestination, the contagion increases amongst the Turks, together with the heats, and no rules or remedies applied to prevent it; by which means the pestilence is become so universal, that, unless one dies of old age, or a violent death, the disease, if mortal, without further inquiry, is, for the most part, concluded to be pestilential.

" The reason that Constantinople is thus subject to the plague is attributed to divers causes. Some say that the multitude of slaves, brought yearly by the Black Sea, and their hard diet, beget this corruption. Others say, that the commonalty, being for the most part nourished in the summer-time by cucumbers and melons, drinking water upon them, and using no helps to correct the crudities, fall into malignant and pestilential fevers. But most physicians there conclude that the air of Constantinople is infected by the north-east winds, which blow commonly for three months, beginning about the summer solstice, arising from unwholesome marshes in Moscovy and Tartary, and passing over the Black Sea, a place known to abound with fogs and mists, do bring with them certain dispositions tending to corruption, which, working upon bodies prepared already by bad diet (as is said before), may well be judged to be the causes of this distemper."— *Birch's History of the Royal Society of London*, vol. ii., p. 287

scription of substances to which the matter of contagion can adhere, and by contact with which the
disease can be communicated.

Relative to the first question, so fundamental in
the system of quarantine, I am not aware that there
are any sufficiently precise data for determining it.
It is a question, in the abstract, involved in extreme
difficulty ; I apprehend the solution of it is really
attended with as much difficulty as the problem of
the contagious nature of the disease itself. The long
periods hitherto fixed on by authority for probation,
have commonly been arbitrary, and, in a sanatory
point of view, cannot be admitted to be deserving of
confidence.*

Concerning the second question, the susceptibility
and non-susceptibility of certain substances to become
the medium for conveying contagion, I have no hesitation in expressing my belief that the classification
is equally arbitrary and erroneous, and that this part
of the basis of the present system of quarantine
is faulty in the extreme, and subversive of all
the rest, were that quite perfect and free from all
objection.

Cotton, wool, silk, flax, hemp, leather, are placed

* Eight days recently have been considered as the extreme latent
period of the disease ; the researches of M. Bulard have led him to
this conclusion, and all analogy (taking for guidance the laws of the
contagions which have been most carefully studied) favour at least the
idea that the time between the receiving the matter of the contagion
into the system, and the production of the symptoms of the disease, is
probably short, not exceeding a very few days.

in the class of susceptible articles. Wood, metal, glass, are placed in the class of non-susceptible articles. Whilst you are detained in quarantine, you may deliver money to a person who comes to see you ; you may drink out of the same glass ; you may receive trays and baskets of provisions, and return them, with plates and glasses, without infraction of quarantine regulations—without bringing into quarantine the person into whose hands these articles have been placed. But should any one touch your glove or hat, or any part of your dress, or should you touch any part of his, he is immediately subject to quarantine of the same duration as yourself.* Why such distinctions have been made it is even difficult to conceive—they are so unscientific, so contrary to all the analogies of other contagious matters—and I may add, without exaggeration, so irrational. I have referred to authors for the grounds of the distinctions in vain ; I have referred to living authorities, those conversant with plague and the quarantine regulations, equally in vain. I have been told by the latter, vaguely and generally, that common experience has proved that one class of articles are susceptible, and

---

* I have known an individual placed in quarantine because the tassel of the cap on his head touched a line on which some of the clothes were airing belonging to a friend whom he came to visit ; although, aware of the danger of imprisonment, he immediately cast off his cap with the end of his walking-stick. This occurred in the lazaretto of Schupanick, close to Orsova on the Danube, on the Austrian frontier—a lazaretto where idle, useless forms merely are observed, and what is essential is neglected.

that those of the other class are not,—precise facts and data I have in vain asked for.

To be deserving of the designation of non-susceptible, in the sense used, substances ought to have positive active qualities rendering them so, by which the contagious matter is either repelled, or destroyed, or rendered inert. That the articles enumerated as instances, have no such qualities, must, I apprehend, be admitted by all who are competent to give an opinion on the subject ; they are the very substances which are selected for holding things the most delicate and perishable. Vaccine lymph on points of wood, in glass tubes, and between plates of glass, has been sent all over the globe—it has occasionally retained its efficacy, so conveyed, for several months, and after twice passing through the tropics. It would be wonderful in the extreme, then, that substances, not known to have any action on any other substance, should have a specific action on the matter of plague ; the strongest evidence would be required to prove it ; the bringing forward of vague assertion, in lieu of proof, is little better than an insult to common sense.*

* When plague is prevalent in a place, money, though considered a non-susceptible article, is passed through water or vinegar from the hands of those in quarantine, for the sake of greater security. When plague was in the lazaretto of Constantinople I witnessed the process. The money was placed in a wooden perforated ladle, dipt for an instant in water, and then delivered to the persons to whom due, not in quarantine. On returning to my lodgings, as a kind of test-experiment, I touched two surfaces of glass, one with an extremely minute quantity of saliva, the other with the cerumen of the ear, and allowed

Relative to the class of articles designated susceptible, I apprehend they must be admitted to be so,
in common with all other substances, which, as before mentioned, are merely negatively inert,—have
no active power incompatible with the preservation
of contagious matter. These articles are commonly
more or less spongy and porous, soft, compressible,
and abounding in air between their particles and
filaments,—as cotton, wool, &c.,—whether in the
raw or manufactured state. Whether this condition
has rendered them obnoxious to suspicion—and suspected they have been condemned—I know not; but
if so, the decision cannot be considered in accordance
with the principles of science, and with the best experience relative to the preservative powers of bodies.
Who, with even a smattering of chemical knowledge,
would think of selecting an article abounding in air
for the purpose of keeping any matter peculiarly
susceptible of change from the action of atmospheric
air, such as contagious matter is supposed to be?

the former to dry. The quantity of each was so small as hardly to be
visible to the naked eye, although very distinct under the microscope.
Both pieces of glass were immersed in water, and kept there about a
quarter of a minute, twice as long as the money in the instance mentioned. Again submitted to the microscope, the matter of the saliva
was found to be diminished, but only slightly, whilst that of the cerumen had undergone no sensible diminution. In a paper, read before
the Royal Society of Edinburgh, on the Classification of Substances,
with a View to the Prevention of Plague, I have given other instances
of the inefficacy of this method of immersion for removing adhering
animal matter, thereby rendering it probable that it can be of little
use as regards the removal or destruction of contagious matter.

The logical conclusion, reasoning on the subject as a matter of science, is, that if the substances pronounced to be non-susceptible are so in reality, those placed in the opposite class are, *à fortiori*, non-susceptible, on account of the superadded air which they contain. Compare cotton-wool, and wood, the one declared susceptible, the other non-susceptible; as they are very similar, chemically considered, and both in themselves inert, the remark just made is strongly applicable to them.

Perhaps the advocates of the established system of quarantine may set up a defence of the distinction of articles into susceptible and non-susceptible, on the result of the accumulated experience of lazarettoes. They may say, as in the instance of Malta, " here is an establishment which has been under observation more than a century; hundreds of persons annually, arriving from the Levant, have performed quarantine in it; the non-susceptible articles, as glass, porcelain, metals, &c., have been freely taken to and fro, without bad effect; there is no instance on record of the plague having been thus communicated."

The conclusion, I conceive, would not satisfy the rigid inquirer. It is probable, he would reply, " As I am convinced that the articles you refer to are inert in relation to animal matter, and, consequently, to the matter of plague; what you state as a fact of the non-transmission of the disease by them, appears to me proof that the disease was not transmissible through the medium of any substances, and it raises doubt in my mind that it is at all contagious." And this, it appears to me, is an argument which may be fairly used in support of the propriety of entertaining doubt on the subject, or, at least, of the disease being easily propagated through the medium of inanimate substances. But, even granted that the statement of the advocates of the present system alluded to, and their reasoning upon it were conclusive and satisfactory, I believe the same applicable to some of the articles which have been esteemed most susceptible, especially raw cotton, which is annually imported in such large quantities into Europe from the Levant, especially from Egypt, and often at the period of the prevalency of plague. Now, what is the result of experience in lazarettoes relative to it? It is entirely negative; there is no instance on record of plague having been communicated by it; there is no instance of the men employed in the lazarettoes in unpacking, and airing, and re-packing the bales of cotton, having contracted the disease. I have, as far as my opportunities permitted, made diligent inquiry on this point, and the result has been as I have stated; and, a short time before his death, I was assured by the late Sir Frederick Ponsonby, who, as governor of Malta, had ample means of instituting inquiry on the subject, that the information he had obtained was to the same effect; and, I believe, that no lazaretto in the Mediterranean was passed over by him in search of evidence on a matter which he justly considered as of the first importance.

Besides these objections to the present established system of quarantine, fundamentally considered, there are others, not, perhaps, undeserving of notice.

Admitting the disease to be contagious, passing by all objection to the groundless distinction of articles into susceptible and non-susceptible, can lazarettoes be considered secure, and capable of insulating contagion, when, though surrounded by walls, they are open to the atmosphere, and more or less exposed to the winds? There is nothing to prevent light substances, as fibres of cotton, bits of paper, or feathers, from being blown from the enclosure of a lazaretto into the adjoining country or town. There is nothing to prevent flies and musquitoes from passing direct, even from those labouring under plague, and, on the principle of contagion, infecting the population. A musquito can pump up with its proboscis hundreds of the red particles of blood, with their proportional quantity of serum and lymph, as is indicated by its coagulation and appearance under the microscope; and there is reason to infer, that if the contagion of the plague is contained in the blood, a single particle may be as efficient in propagating it as an indefinite number.*

---

* In the lazaretto already alluded to, near Orsova, on the Austrian frontier, all the windows on one side of the building, in which travellers are received, open into a garden of small dimensions. The windows are protected with iron bars and an iron grating, well fitted for a prison; but when open, flies, musquitoes, and other insects which abound there have free access, so that, in less than a minute, they can pass from a person in one apartment to a person in another, and

The severest penalties, the greatest vigilance, have not, in any country, prevented contraband trade. Malta has frequently been placed in quarantine with Sicily, notwithstanding which it is understood that the contraband trade between the two countries has been continued. This of itself is sufficient to vitiate the whole system of quarantine, and to render all its regulations nugatory.*

spread contagion from the diseased to the sound, supposing cases of plague to be shut up in the building (the objects for which it is designed), and the disease contagious. Imagine a sanatory establishment, placed in a hollow, subject to malaria, in which are hundreds of winged inoculators, defying iron bars and grating, constantly flying from room to room, and some idea may be formed of this lazaretto.

* The following remarks of Sir Charles Napier, from his work on the Ionian Islands, although not made in relation to any question about quarantine, are forcibly applicable to the subject, and strongly show how inadequate are the means at present employed to prevent infraction of the quarantine laws.

"In Cefalonia there are about twelve ports. Of these, that of Argostoli was alone left open for general commerce; Lixuri under some slight restriction; and St Eufemia for the importation of cattle; all the rest I found closed. A 'shut port' is a port where one man is paid by government to dwell, and prevent smuggling and clandestine landings; he receives about L.26 a-year. He is generally a smuggler, or winks at smuggling 'for a consideration.' But smuggler or not smuggler, he must sleep, and when he sleeps others smuggle. On one single occasion, in Cefalonia, a man dared to give the government information on this ticklish subject; the goods were seized in consequence, and his throat was cut in a week after. I never knew of any other instance of information given from a closed port, and, I imagine, the fate of this man will serve as a hint to all officious guardians of shut ports for the next century.

The difficulty, I may say the impossibility, of preventing smuggling, and, consequently, the infraction of the sanatory regulations, must be known to every one acquainted with the Mediterranean and its

Have other diseases, decidedly infectious and contagious, been excluded by means of quarantine? If they have, it is a satisfactory proof of the efficacy of quarantine, and *vice versa*. They have not been excluded. In Malta, during the period I was there, I witnessed small-pox, measles, scarlet-fever, hooping-cough, amongst the people; and excepting small-pox, on one occasion, none of them could be traced to their source: how they were introduced, or whether they arose *de novo*, could not be ascertained.

It has been asserted, and I believe truly, that the plague never appeared amongst the crew of any

shores. In an account of Greece and of the Ionian Islands, by a German traveller, published about sixteen years ago, the author states, that he left his vessel, was landed on a wild part of the shore of Santa Maura, without a thought about health-offices, walked many miles through the country, and was received on board again off Sappho's Leap, close to which a boat was waiting for him. In excursions amongst the islands, I have frequently landed where inclination led, and, excepting on one occasion, without being called to account. It is true, a guardiano accompanied us, but that made no difference, excepting as to propriety. Last summer, in Constantinople, two English gentlemen, whom I met at table, described how they had landed, without receiving pratique, slept in Pera, and how, the following morning, they met by appointment the master of the vessel in which they arrived, and with him proceeded in his boat to the health-office, and formally received pratique. Dr Bowring, in his speech already referred to, spoke of a communication he had had from a well-known traveller on the northern coast of Africa, who said,—" There is a perpetual violation of the quarantine on the southern coast of Spain. Of the persons who visit the Barbary coast, great numbers never think of entering the Spanish lazaretto. Would I be such a fool as to subject myself to imprisonment for weeks because I have been in Africa for a few days? I never did enter a lazaretto—I never will." By paying a small fee, it is stated, that he escaped the annoyance.

British ship of war in the Levant;* but small-pox
has frequently. The disease which carried off 1172
of the inhabitants of Malta was imported in the
Asia, bearing the flag of Sir Pultney Malcolm, on
her return from the Archipelago, and after going
through the regular course of quarantine; and not
long after, it appeared in H.M.S. Tyne, on her return

* Since the above was written, two instances have come to my
knowledge of plague appearing in ships of war,—one in the steamer
Acheron, in 1839; the other in H.M. frigate Castor, in 1841. The
former, coming direct from Alexandria, at a time that plague prevailed there, lost two of her crew during the voyage, who died of the
disease. They had been employed as servants, and had made the
beds of the passengers, many in number ; yet the latter all escaped,
as did also the surgeon, who felt the pulse of the plague patients, and
touched them freely, without using any precautions. The Castor, at
a time plague was known to be rife in Syria, especially in the towns
on the coast, received on board the crew of the Zebra, as a measure
of necessity, that ship having suffered shipwreck near Kaiffa. This
was on the 22d February, and between that day and the 27th, thirteen
men were attacked with plague, of whom one only belonged to the
Castor ; nine of them died. The disease did not spread farther,
although a large number of the men of both crews must have communicated, directly or indirectly, with the infected. These particulars are extracted from an account of the occurrence contained in a
Malta newspaper, and, I believe, are to be depended on for correctness. They are in accordance with a statement made to the Admi-
ralty by Sir Wm. Burnett, published in the British and Foreign Med.
Review, the Number for January. In this statement it is mentioned
that, "in order to prevent the diffusion of the malady, eleven men
were selected to attend wholly on the infected persons. Not one of
these was attacked by the disease, nor were any of the Castor's people,
except an artificer who had been landed, and lived with the Zebra's
men at Kaiffa, though there were at least twenty-four persons, including four medical officers, fully exposed to the contagion, during its
continuance on board the Castor."

from the coast of Syria. Are not these circumstances, at the same time, likely to encourage doubt as to the contagious nature of plague, and to destroy confidence in the preventive power of quarantine, should it be contagious?

For a quarantine system to be efficacious, supposing it to be required, it ought to be conducted in an exact manner, with perfect consistency and perfect justice, with the sole object of preserving the public health.

But how differently is it commonly conducted? how often is it abused? how often are gross inconsistencies practised? as if it were entirely out of the pale of reason, and common sense, and common justice.

Can we be surprised at its inconsistencies in the Mediterranean, after what was witnessed in this country when cholera prevailed? when towns seaward were placed in quarantine, not landward, as if a dry surface were incompatible with the transmission of contagion?

In the quarantine establishments of the Mediterranean, it is the last port which commonly fixes the attention of the authorities. England, for example, is in quarantine with Malta; France is not. Two parties may leave England at the same time,—one through France, embarking at Marseilles, and may arrive in a fortnight from the time of starting; the other may proceed the whole way by sea, in a sailing-vessel, and may be a month on the voyage. On their arrival they will find their friends at liberty; having come by the shortest and quickest route, they escape quarantine, to which the slow voyagers will be subjected.*

Dr Bowring, in his able pamphlet already referred to, considers quarantine establishments as "for the most part instruments, and terrible instruments, of diplomacy and state policy." This, I believe, in too many instances, is unquestionably true. In illustration, I may relate what I myself witnessed, during a voyage which I made with a sick friend and his father, from Corfu to Malta, where my friend died in quarantine, and from whence we proceeded to Naples, touching at several places on the Sicilian coast, and at the Lipari Isles, on our way. We first visited Girgenti; no difficulty was there made to our landing, Malta being at that time in " *pra-*

---

* The inconsistencies of quarantine, as at present conducted in the different States of Europe, are almost endless; a volume might be filled with examples of them, and our own country is not an exception. I shall mention one instance only, in addition to the above, the last that has come to my knowledge. On leaving Constantinople to return to England by land, my heavy baggage was sent by sea. The vessel conveying it took her departure on the same day as that on which I set out, and arrived about a fortnight after me. Having come by land, the baggage I brought with me was subjected to no detention, whilst that which came by sea was subjected, in common with the cargo of the vessel, to a quarantine of forty days,—and this although, on quitting Constantinople, we had a clean bill of health. It is true that the baggage brought with me was in quarantine at Orsova, on entering the Austrian territories, ten days, but that was merely an idle form; the greater part of my wearing-apparel was not even exposed to the air whilst there.

tique" with Sicily; we went some miles into the interior, saw the sulphur-mines, and spent the night in the town, at an hotel. We next proceeded to Syracuse, and were received in the same manner there. Catania was the next port which we entered; there our reception was totally different; our landing was prohibited; our little vessel was surrounded by guard-boats, sentries were placed on the adjoining pier, and they threatened to fire on us if we attempted to land. After a delay of two days, the ship's crew were permitted to go on shore, but not the passengers, in consequence, it was stated, of a telegraphic communication with Messina to that effect. On the third day, a messenger, whom we had commissioned to go to Syracuse for the intervention of our vice-consul, there being no consular office at Catania, returned with a letter to the authorities, in which he held himself responsible for our conduct, if permitted to land. This, then, sufficed: we accordingly landed, and immediately proceeded to ascend Etna, and returned to Catania the following day. The weather was unfavourable; our journey to the mountain was rapid, and was the cause of suspicion; our guide was summoned before the police, in the dead of night, and most minutely questioned; it was maintained that, in such weather, we could not have ascended the mountain, as we stated; that was impossible; we must have gone, therefore, elsewhere; that we were practising concealment and deceit, and must be plotting mischief; and they threatened to have us also before them. The following day we re-embarked, and went round to Palermo, where we landed without molestation or any objection. The treatment we experienced at Catania, it was hinted to us, arose out of the fears of the authorities that one of the party.was Lord Dundonald (then Lord Cochrane), who, at that time, was in the Mediterranean, on his way to Greece, and whom we had left in the harbour of Malta.

In connexion with this voyage, I may notice an incident, exemplifying the very lax manner in which the quarantine regulations are occasionally carried into effect, entirely subversive of all confidence in the system, supposing it to be planned on unobjectionable principles. At the island of Lipari, on landing at the Sanità, the first person who received us was the British vice-consul, a native of the place,—and he immediately shook hands with us and entered into conversation. Presently, the inspector of health was seen approaching; the sight of him acted like a repelling force on the vice-consul; who instantly retired to the proper distance, and expressed all proper horror of touching our persons or papers whilst the forms of examination of the letters, held at arm's-length by means of iron tongs, were going through, preliminary to the granting of *pratique*,—and which, being granted, he again shook hands and offered his congratulations.

I have now gone over some of the grounds of objection to the quarantine system, as at present established . there would be no difficulty in stating others ; as, I am confident, the more minutely the system is examined, the more faulty and objectionable it will be found to be, and fully warranting the conclusion of Dr Bowring, already quoted, viz., that the regulations of quarantine are not only useless for the ends they profess to accomplish, but are absolutely pernicious, increasing the evils against which they are designed to guard, and adding to the miseries which it is their avowed object to modify or remove.

Dr Bowring concludes his pamphlet with some remarks, by way of suggestion, in the propriety of which I fully accord ; and believing that, if acted on, the consequences may be most beneficial, I shall transcribe them, to increase the chance of their publicity.   His words are :—" I shall have done some service, if I have succeeded in awakening your attention to a subject of paramount importance, and which, it appears to me, cannot be allowed to rest in its present state of uncertainty,—an uncertainty unsatisfactory to science, dishonourable to inquiring philosophy, and greatly injurious to the commercial interests of the nation.   On such a subject, it would become a government like ours to take the initiative of inquiry,—to send a commission into the Levant, in order thoroughly to investigate the whole question, and to ascertain, by an extended, minute, searching, and unprejudiced inquest, whether these sanatory regulations, which are so costly, so capricious, so vexatious, and so despotic, are demanded by a due regard to the general health and to the public interests; whether quarantines are really useful, or only inefficient, or whether they are not pernicious; whether the contagiousness of plague is of a highly perilous and communicable character, or whether it requires for its propagation conditions rarely combined, and such as may be provided against by civilization and good police? And as other countries have also a deep concern in the solution of these interesting questions,—as our own sanatory legislation could scarcely be changed, unless the governments of Europe were willing to concur in some general modification,—it would be highly desirable that the leading commercial powers should be invited to carry on a contemporaneous, if not a united inquiry, which might either serve to justify the existing state of things, or lead to improvements friendly to economy, to trade, to knowledge, and to happiness."

Should such inquiry ever be instituted, and for the interests of mankind it is ardently hoped that it will be, and at no distant period, it is hardly necessary to observe, that the individuals employed ought to be men of the highest character for moral integrity, for resolution and firmness of mind; for intellectual capacity, and for medical knowledge; free, as much as possible, from all bias, and unconnected officially with any quarantine establishment. All these qualifications, I apprehend, will be requisite for the objects in view: resolution to search diligently; firmness of mind to throw aside vain terrors and despise clamour; perfect integrity to resist individual influence and interests; and intellectual capacity and medical knowledge to investigate the many difficult questions involved in the inquiry. Were a commission composed of men of this description formed, sent into the Levant, provided with ample powers, and authorized to collect evidence on oath, it is highly probable that, in two or three years, they would be enabled to draw up a report which might be a basis for legislation; or, at all events, for farther and extended inquiry, with diminished difficulties, and increased chances of final success.

That the result of inquiry would finally be successful, I think can hardly be doubted. There are many circumstances encouraging such expectation, and that equally whether the plague be decided to be a contagious disease or not. Thus, if decided in the affirmative, little difficulty can be expected in coming to a useful practical conclusion relative to the properties of the so called susceptible and non-susceptible articles, and thereby removing one very defective part of the existing system.

Farther, if a specific plague virus be admitted to exist, and to be the sole cause of the propagation of the disease, it is highly probable that, by studying its nature and properties, some simple means may be discovered of destroying it, or of rendering it permanently inert, without risk of injury to merchan-

dise, applicable to letters, and indeed of universal
applicability. The plague, it is said, is commonly
arrested by the summer heats. It is asserted that it
has never passed from Upper Egypt into the climate
of higher temperature of Nubia. It is doubtful
whether it has ever appeared within the tropics.*
Would not this seem to show that a certain temperature is incompatible with its existence or activity, if
contagious? The results of the experiments of the
late Dr Henry on the action of heat on the contagious matters of certain diseases, went far to prove
that they were deprived of their power of specific
action by a moderate temperature, under two hundred degrees of Fahrenheit, which exercises no injurious effect on the most delicate fabrics, and can be
borne even by man with impunity, for a sufficient

* Minute inquiry is wanted on the effect of heat on the plague. If
it be a fact that the disease is commonly arrested in Syria and Egypt,
by the higher temperature of summer, it is desirable to learn both
what is the exact degree of heat that appears to be requisite, and the
degree of dryness of the atmosphere accompanying it. When the
plague prevailed in Malta and in the Ionian Islands, in 1813, it was
most severe, and widely spread after mid-summer. It endured the
uninterrupted heats of July, August, and September, as well as of
June. Last year, in Syria, the disease ran into the summer; and it
also re-appeared in Egypt during the summer. From documents
lately published, it appears certain that plague has, at different times,
broken out in several districts of western India, bordering on the
tropic, viz. between the parallels of 22° and 27° north latitude. Its
origin there, as in Egypt, is obscure.—*Vide* for much interesting information on the subject, Dr Frederick Forbes' Treatise " On the
Nature and History of Plague, as observed in the North-Western
Provinces of India."—*Edinburgh*, 1841.

time, if advisable for the clothes on his person to be disinfected. And, as heat is unconfinable and can penetrate through all bodies, it would probably be equally applicable to unpacked bales of goods, to books, to unopened letters, and, in brief, to every description of property.* Moreover, if plague be proved to be propagated by contagion, and never to arise *de novo*, it is highly probable that the laws of its propagation may be discovered by a careful collection of facts, and that it will appear that it is only under certain circumstances that the contagious matter can act, and that there is no reason to dread its being propagated abroad, when it is not endemic or epidemic at home; that is to say, for the sake of an example, we need not fear its introduction into Malta from Alexandria, when it is not prevalent in the latter city, although a few cases of it may, from time to time, occur there. In some of the islands of the Archipelago, as Hydra, Ipsara, and Syra, before the establishment of the kingdom of Greece, quarantine was, I believe, conducted in accordance with some view of this kind. They were in free intercourse with all the adjoining countries, so long as the disease was not officially declared to be rife—with Con-

---

* Temperature differing only a very few degrees may act very differently on the contagious matter of plague. Ice cannot exist at 33ⁿ; nor water, under ordinary atmospheric pressure at 212° Fahrenheit: —so, perhaps, of contagion; at 85° it may be active; at 86° inert. Moreover, the state of the atmosphere, in relation to humidity, may have a powerful influence on it. A moist atmosphere may favour its activity; a contrary state may have an opposite effect.

stantinople, Smyrna, Alexandria, Tripoli, and all the
intermediate ports, amongst one or other of which
plague was supposed to linger. Quarantine was established only for those coming from a place where the
disease, at that very time, was actually prevalent
and severe. And it is asserted that this occasional
quarantine was found sufficient, and that there was
no instance on record of the disease having been
imported, or of its breaking out in either of the
islands mentioned,* although engaged in active trade.
The same, as before stated, is asserted of our ships of
war, and also of the ships trading to Turkey, which
belonged to the Old Levant Company. If it be true
that plague never reached the crews of either, it is
strongly confirmatory of the conclusion that favouring
circumstances are required for its extension, and that
precautions far from rigorous are sufficient to prevent its spreading.†   The same, too, it is said, may

---

* Some of the most strenuous contagionists have maintained that
three conditions conjoined are essential to the propagation of plague ;
1st, The presence of contagion ; 2dly, A habit of body favourable to
receive it ; and, 3dly, A congenial state of atmosphere. A wide survey
of facts has led to this conclusion—a conclusion which, by the non-
contagionists, must be considered an hypothesis to reconcile with the
doctrine of contagion the facts they can bring forward against it.

† The exceptions mentioned in the foot-note, page 346, do not mi-
litate against the above conclusion. In both the instances mentioned,
of plague having been introduced on board ship, no sanatory precautions whatever appear to have been taken to exclude it. The two
vessels freely communicated with the shore, plague then prevailing.
Commonly in ships of war, hitherto, as in the ships which belonged
to the Old Levant Company, the commanders instituted a quarantine
in any port in which there was danger of contracting the disease.

be deduced from the experience of opulent Turks. I was informed by a gentleman who had been long resident in Constantinople, and was attached to our embassy there as interpreter, * and was well acquainted with the habits of the people, that the influential men, and men in office, never interrupted business on account of plague, and gave audience to all who applied to them, as freely when plague prevailed as in the most healthy seasons, and he believed with impunity. As there are responsible persons employed by our government,—consuls or vice-consuls,—in all the principal ports of the Levant, there ought to be no difficulty in knowing, with sufficient preciseness, what is the state of health of the inhabitants at all times; and, if it should be decided that a modified system of quarantine is necessary on emergencies, as on the appearance of plague, in its virulent spreading form, it can be adopted with ease for a limited time, as long as the emergency lasts, according to the plan said to have been followed with apparent success at Syra, and some other of the Greek islands.

Indulging in the hope that, were careful inquiry made on the subject of plague, conducted by competent persons, the result might be a revision of the laws of quarantine, and the rendering them far less severe, and at the same time increasing their efficiency, I shall mention a few facts, in addition to those already brought forward, tending to confirm

* The late Mr Wood; he died of plague.

this favourable view. And, first, relative to the degree of activity of the contagion, taking it for granted that the disease is contagious.

That its activity commonly is not great, appears to be proved by many facts. During the last summer, at Constantinople, when the plague was introduced into the lazaretto, of the fifty porters employed there in landing the effects of the passengers, and the merchandise of the infected vessel already mentioned, one only, the individual already named, contracted the disease.

During the spring and early summer of last year, at Beirout, on the coast of Syria, many remarkable instances occurred of escape from plague, after communication with the infected, which have come to my knowledge through an able report of Dr Robertson, Deputy Inspector-general of hospitals, employed on Particular service in Turkey, transmitted to the Foreign Office. I shall introduce here only one of the many he has brought forward, and shall give the relation in his own words.

" The Mohammedan inhabitants, impatient of guardians being placed over the houses in which there were cases of plague, and also indignant that the bodies of the dead were taken into the lazaretto, to be buried with lime, assembled one day in great numbers, seized a body which was being conveyed to the lazaretto ; and, to show their contempt for all sanatory regulations, embraced the dead body and rubbed themselves with the coverings of it. The mob also dispersed all the guardians that were over the infected houses, and from that day (the 17th May), there was no longer even the semblance of quarantine in Beirout.   I never heard (Dr Robertson adds, writing on the 26th July, when the plague was on the decline all over Syria), that any of the persons concerned in this affair suffered in their health."*

There are very many instances, well authenticated (I have already mentioned some), of individuals who have attended on patients labouring under plague, who have freely touched them, without taking any precaution, and who have escaped the disease.   On the 20th of June, I visited the lazaretto of Koulely, in the neighbourhood of Constantinople, in company with M. Robert, to see the cases of plague, four in number, which were then under treatment, " a plague doctor" having the charge of them.   He was a Jew of the name of Abraham, about sixty years of age, who never had plague, though he had often attended and practised in plague hospitals.   Whilst we were present, he touched the patients with the greatest unconcern, and dressed a suppurating bubo, and other sores, using his fingers, without a forceps, to remove the dressing, and shortly after he took a pinch of snuff, without even washing his hands.

* In a letter addressed to me by Dr Robertson, in March last, on his return from Syria, through Egypt, which, with his permission, will be inserted in the Appendix, some farther particulars will be found, tending at least to show that plague is not always actively contagious, or a spreading disease.

There are also many instances of towns remaining free from plague, when freely communicating with other towns suffering under the disease. Constantinople, before quarantine was introduced, had been exempt, at intervals, for comparatively long periods, for three or four years; and, as I have been assured by good authority, even for eight years uninterruptedly.

The last time that plague occurred in Constantinople, was in 1838. At the same time it broke out in the Turkish towns on the Danube, with the exception of Widdin, one of the largest of them; that town, though it freely communicated with the others, I have been assured, entirely escaped the disease; and yet no precautions whatever had been taken to avert it.

In Syria, during the last spring and summer when plague prevailed in most of the towns and villages of that country, from Beirout eastward, I have been informed that it did not extend westward, although the nearest quarantine-station was Konia, where quarantine was so negligently conducted that it was the merest of forms.*

---

* My informant, coming from Syria, where, to the eastward of Beirout, plague was then prevailing, had to pass through Konia. On his arrival, he was admitted to the pasha, sat with him on the same couch, smoked a pipe, and had coffee with him, and then was placed in quarantine, in a tent outside the city, but with liberty to go where he pleased. The quarantine, in fact, was merely nominal. The city of great extent, was protected by two guardianos!

During four years that I was stationed in the
Ionian Islands, and seven in Malta, not a single case
of plague occurred in the lazarettoes of either, though
they were almost constantly receiving persons from
Egypt and the Levant, and several times when
plague was prevailing in one or the other.* But,
during the same time, other contagious diseases appeared. Twice I witnessed small-pox in Malta, imported in spite of quarantine.

Many other statements might be made, and additional facts given, confirmatory of the conclusion that
the activity of the contagion of plague is not commonly great, and rendering it probable that it may
be guarded against easily, more easily than most
other contagious diseases, especially small-pox.

Next, relative to merchandise and articles of dress
and furniture, &c., there seems to be good reason to

* In June last, some cases of plague occurred in the lazaretto of
Malta, traced to contagion, introduced in the crew of a vessel from
Alexandria. The cases were ten in number, nine belonging to the
crew, one of whom was landed labouring under the disease. The
tenth case was in the person of a Maltese boatman, who had communicated with the crew. A narrative of the occurrence has been published by Dr Gravagna, physician to the establishment, and adduced
by him in proof of the contagious nature of the disease. The manner
in which he concludes his reports, is sufficiently indicative of the rareness of such an event.

" Nei ragionamenti forse io avrei sbagliato, come pure sbagliano
quelli che opiniano differentemente da me. Ma nei fatti v'è la pura
verità nella sua più semplice esposizione. E quando un fatto non
giova a che accumulare cento? Il mio fatto oggi e uno. Il barcaj-
uolo Maltese Giovanni Cauchi communico una gente appestata ed
egli trasse la peste e morì."

believe that their power of retaining and conveying contagion has been greatly exaggerated. It is well known that, after plague as an epidemic has ceased, and traffic is renewed with activity in Turkish towns, that the dresses of those who have died of the disease are plentifully offered for sale, and readily purchased and worn without scruple, and that without a fresh outbreak of the disease. Could articles of dress retain the contagion of plague long, Constantinople, and indeed every eastern town, ought never to be free from plague, as every one, I fancy, must be convinced who has ever walked through the old-clothes bazaar of the city just mentioned, and witnessed the enormous quantities of articles of dress accumulated there, of all descriptions and conditions, and with the least possible attention to cleanliness, as the Turkish name of the quarter indicates.

Considerations arising out of the probable slight activity of the contagion of plague; the short time, it is probable, that it remains latent in the living system; the little aptitude that articles of merchandise, dress, and furniture seem to have to preserve the matter of contagion, are all in favour, I cannot but think, of the necessity for a revision of the laws of quarantine, with a fair prospect, as I have already observed, of their being greatly mitigated, and at the same time rendered efficient, to the great comfort of the traveller, the incalculable advantage of commerce, and the universal benefit of mankind.

Were reason and the results of experience followed in the institution of quarantine, independent of crooked political motives, altogether unworthy of right-minded governments, it can hardly be doubted that very mild measures of quarantine would suffice, were it only for the protection of health. It is probable that no restrictions would be found requisite in the importation of merchandise from the Levant, and that no quarantine would be required on persons coming from the Turkish dominions, provided they had a certificate of health from a board or council of health, or from the consular agents of the principal towns which lay in their way. Whilst I venture to offer this opinion as my belief, I should witness with regret any alteration in the existing quarantine laws, not preceded by inquiry. A searching inquiry into the whole subject is the first thing necessary. When that is made, and the results published, it may be presumed it will be easy to form regulations, on the principle of protecting the public health, with as little vexation as possible to individuals, with as little loss of time, and as economically as possible. So necessary is this inquiry, that there is no author lately who has written on the subject who has not advocated it, excepting, indeed, those who hold plague to be an endemic disease, destitute of contagious power, and quarantine consequently, however modified, totally useless.

Were an efficient sanatory system adopted, and that universally, I trust it is not too much to expect that plague might be ere long entirely extirpated.

And, when we consider the absence of the disease in this country for so many years, notwithstanding its vastly increased commercial intercourse with Turkey, Egypt, and the Barbary States;—when we consider how Italy for a long time has remained free from it, and also Sicily, and Spain, and Portugal, notwithstanding the extensive contraband trade which has been carried on with the two former; and lastly, when we reflect how certain other countries have escaped the disease, in which precautions have either been entirely neglected to exclude it, or have been only temporarily taken, there seems to be good ground of hope that measures may be discovered without difficulty to root it out entirely; and that the time may come when its existence will be merely matter of history, as in the instance of leprosy, which at one time was as much the terror of Europe.

In the quotations which I have made from Dr Bowring's pamphlet, the great evils of quarantine, though briefly, are strongly expressed, but not, in my opinion, in terms of any exaggeration. Were a new system to be adopted, consisting of sanatory restrictions, as mild as are compatible with the object in view, the advantages which would result from the change may in part be imagined, arising out of the removal of so many positive evils; but I believe only in part, inasmuch as the bad consequences of the present system are, I apprehend, even greater than they at first sight appear, and, not least, in the paralyzing influence they exert on the people, and the handle they afford to crush national liberty, and accustom men to arbitrary rule, and to depress those energies on which the prosperity of nations seems mainly to depend.

Sicily may be adduced as an example, for no other country is under greater subjection to the system, in all its manifold evils.   And what is its present condition? With the finest climate, with a generally excellent soil, fitted now, as it was formerly, to be the granary of an empire, fitted for producing a vast amount of the richest produce, in fruits, oil, and wine, and silk—it is, considering the mass of the people, one of the poorest, as well as one of the least enlightened countries of Europe; without manufactories of any importance; the sciences and the fine arts neglected; the useful arts in a rude state; its agriculture that of the middle ages; and its limited commerce chiefly in the hands of foreigners.   How much exactly of this low state of things is owing to sanatory regulations, and the restrictions exercised under their cloak, it may be difficult to determine with precision, but that a large proportion is mainly attributable to it in its direct operation and indirect influences, can hardly be questioned.   In ancient times there was a constant intercourse between Greece and Sicily, arising out of mutual interests.   Now, there is far less intercourse between them than there is between the most remote region that can be mentioned and England.   Although Corfu is only about three hundred miles from the eastern coast of the island, when we touched at Girgenti, in a government schooner, bearing the Ionian flag, that flag was not recognised— it was the first time it had been seen in the Sicilian waters. Nor is such interruption of intercourse surprising, when it is considered that a ship direct to Sicily from the Ionian Islands would have to remain idle in quarantine about a month,—the crew, at the mercy of suspicious authorities, liable to be subjected to great vexations, and to sustain severe losses.

The shores of Turkey in Europe afford another example of the same kind, illustrating, I apprehend, the baneful effects of quarantine on civilization and improvement. Having for many years been in uninterrupted quarantine with the adjoining countries, the mariner passes them by as prohibited regions ; or, if compelled by a storm to take refuge in their ports, he weighs anchor as soon as he can with safety ; no friendly intercourse is ventured on with the natives ; contact is carefully avoided : the quarantine system is rigorously observed : or if not, at the end of the voyage, the penalty is incurred, or a false oath is taken, and the system abused.

For the evils of this system, in some detail, I would refer the reader to a little work of Dr Chervin, addressed to the French Chamber of Deputies, under the title of " Pétition addressée à la Chambre des Députés sur la nécessité d'une prompte réforme dans notre système sanitaire," an able production, worthy of the high reputation of the author, and every way deserving of attention, especially for the particulars it gives of the abuses of the sanatory system, the dreadful evils resulting from it, and the irrational, unscientific manner in which it has been instituted.

CHAPTER XIV.

ON THE SMALL-POX OF 1830-31, IN MALTA.

How introduced.   Progress of the Disease, its Extent and Mortality.
Tables in illustration.   Remarks founded on the Numerical Results.   Conjecture that Warm Air freely circulating in the
Apartments may be · beneficial in the Treatment of the Disease.
Influence of Sex, Age, Vaccination.   Tables in illustration.
Return of Small-Pox amongst the Men, Wives, and Children of
the British Troops.   Remarks on the Results in Proof of the Protecting Power of Vaccination.   Some Peculiarities of the Disease
noticed.   Remarks on Chicken-Pox, in relation to the question
of its identity with Small-Pox.   Observations on the degree of
Credit due to the Tables illustrating the Disease, and on the
manner of forming them.

I AM induced to treat of this subject, partly on account of the interest imparted to it by the late prevalency of small-pox in many parts of England and
Scotland, and the shaken confidence, as it has been
reported, in the efficacy of vaccination; and partly
with the hope that the information collected amongst
so limited a population as that of Malta, and so much
under observation in consequence, may be useful as a
contribution to the statistics of the disease.

In the former chapter, allusion has been made to
the manner in which small-pox was introduced into

the island. As the instance is an instructive one, it may be right to describe it more particularly.

It was mentioned that the disease was imported in H.M.S. Asia; this is an undoubted fact. The Asia, bearing the flag of Vice-Admiral Sir Pultney Malcolm, came into the harbour of Malta on the 18th of February 1830, from Napoli de Romania; on the following day, it was reported that a Greek boy was labouring under symptoms of small-pox; on the 20th, he was removed to the lazaretto, where he died on the 2d of March. On the 4th of March, after a quarantine of fifteen days, the Asia was allowed "*pratique*," her surgeon having signed the following certificate :—" That there was no contagious disease on board; that there were only fourteen men on the sick-list, and these were afflicted with chronic complaints or trifling accidents." On the 9th of March, it was officially reported that another case of small-pox had occurred in the Asia, in the person of a marine, who had sickened on the evening of the 5th. This man was landed and placed in a house apart, near the naval hospital, and under charge of its surgeon, with instructions that he should be carefully secluded.* These instructions, however, it is understood, were not observed with the requisite rigour. There is reason to believe that persons went to and

* These particulars are from an official letter on the subject, from the superintendent of quarantine to the acting secretary to government, of which I was favoured with a copy by order of the lieutenant-governor, with permission to use it.

fro from the house, and that the linen of the patient
was taken to the adjoining village of Zabbar to be
washed; and it was asserted (I never heard it con-
tradicted), that it was in this village that the disease
first broke out amongst the native population, and
that the first family in which it appeared was that of
the washerwoman who had received the infected
linen.

The disease spread with a gradually increasing
rapidity until the month of July; in that month,
1464 persons were attacked. In the following
month, there was a slight abatement, 1325 fresh
cases occurred. From that time, it slowly and gradually subsided, until August of the following year,
when, according to the official reports, it ceased
entirely.

Some attempts were made, on the part of the
police, by order of the local government, to endeavour
to arrest its progress by separation of the infected;
but as they were manifestly unsuccessful, they were
not long continued; the disease was allowed to run
its course uninterruptedly, excepting by vaccination.*

From its first outbreak, in March 1830, to its cessation in August 1831, 8067 persons were attacked
in Malta; and from its first appearance to its cessation, in the adjoining island of Gozo, between April
of one year and May of the following, 2284 were
attacked; of whom 1172 died in Malta, and 351 in

* Between March 1830 and February 1831, 14,500 were vaccinated.

Gozo (making a total mortality of 1523 for the two islands), which is in the ratio of 1 in 6.8 of the number attacked in the former, and of 1 in 6.2 in the latter.

For the purpose of displaying the progress of the disease, and some other points of interest connected with it, I shall avail myself of the returns which were furnished to me at the time by order of the Lieutenant-Governor, who was pleased to direct that every facility should be afforded to collect information on so important a subject, and this was most freely given by the experienced police-physician, Dr Gravagna.

The first return I shall insert will show the progress of the disease in the numbers attacked, from its commencement to its termination, and in the different parts of the island,—Valetta, Floriana, Vittoriosa, Cospicua, Senglea, including the population of the city, and the casals or villages which follow, including that of the country. As a preliminary, I shall insert a table, showing the distribution of the population at that time, in the different districts.

District					Males and Females.
Valetta	.	.	.	.	} 28,342
Floriana	.	.	.	.	
Vittoriosa	.	.	.	.	4,784
Cospicua	.	.	.	.	10,079
Senglea	.	.	.	.	5,680
Zabbar	.	.	.	.	3,564
Zeitun	.	.	.	.	5,817
			Carry forward,		58,266

District.				Males and Females.
Brought forward,		.	.	58,266
Tarxien,	.	.	.	1,066
Luca,	.	.	.	1,450
Hasciah,	.	.	.	1,231
Gudia,	.	.	.	995
Cherchop,	.	.	.	} 592
Safi,	.	.	.	
Zurrico,	.	.	.	3,217
Crendi,	.	.	.	1,043
Micabiba,	.	.	.	924
Siggieui,	.	.	.	3,670
Zebbug,	.	.	.	5,052
Curmi,	.	.	.	4,662
Attard,	.	.	.	1,016
Lia,	.	.	.	1,236
Balzan,	.	.	.	613
Birchircara,	.	.	.	5,618
Nasciaro,	.	.	.	3,047
Musta,	.	.	.	3,577
Gargur,	.	.	.	1,209
Dingli,	.	.	.	535
Notabile,	.	.	.	} 5,342
Rabbato,	.	.	.	
		Total,		105,367

NUMERICAL RETURN OF THE PERSONS ATTACKED BY SMALL-POX IN THE ISLAND OF MALTA, FROM 16TH MARCH 1830, TO AUGUST 1831.

Months.	Total attacked.	Valetta.	Floriana.	Vittoriosa.	Cospicua.	Senglea.	Zabbar.	Zeitun.	Taxien.	Luca.	Haschih.	Gudia.	Chercop.	Safi.	Zurrico.	Crendi.	Micabiba.	Siggieui.	Zebbug.	Curmi.	Attard.	Lia.	Balzan.	Birchircara.	Nasciaro.	Musta.	Gargur.	Dingli.	Notabile.	Rabbato.	Pietà, Misida, Marsa, &c.	Military.
March,	26	5	1	8	2		8												1			1										
April,	110	11	1	28	35	1	11			1	1					1			4	12											4	
May,	266	40	8	18	91	15	12	6		1	1	1			4		1		2	59		2		2	2						1	1
June,	831	167	97	52	192	22	33	43	11	9	6	6	6		20	8		1	16	120	4	4		28	1	1	1	1			1	1
July,	1464	461	111	91	164	81	47	114	12	12	11	6	6		29	11	2	4	28	183	5	6	7	67	4	3	1			3	4	5
August,	1325	438	133	55	74	142	48	161	8	16	4	2	2		63	7	22	5	18	55	2	7	5	73	3	3		3	4	4	7	4
September,	1088	255	102	29	40	99	55	201	3	22	8	2			85	2	16	6	15	15	2	6	21	88	2	6	5	7	1	15	6	3
October,	942	140	35	7	38	109	47	129	6	26	2	6		2	69	2	14	7	50	11	7	26	17	94	7	9	4	9	3	45	8	5
November,	762	91	12	5	23	52	19	76	4	25	4	5	3	1	15	8	10	11	46	7	20	35	17	71	10	31	9	2	2	81	8	1
December,	482	25	5	1	2	23	11	14	3	12	5	3	6	3	5	3	6	26	46	4	26	20	3	44	31	42	3			79	16	
January,	345	19		1	4	7	6	12	6	6	1	4	4	5	5	8	7	32	37	2	18	8	2	15	39	50	1			35	6	1
February,	158	4	1	1		7		7		1	1					9	4	13	24		6	7		4	33	17			1	9	2	
March,	125	3					2	1	1		1	1				2	10	13	22			7		1	42	10				8		
April,	72	7						1								4	3	6	5		1	2		1	34	6						
May,	57	7		2	1		1	1									8	2	2			2		3	9	5						
June,	9	1						1														4			1							
July,	4																		1					1								
August,	1																															
Total	8067	1674	506	298	666	558	300	769	53	131	45	35	27	11	273	65	103	125	318	468	91	137	72	492	218	183	23	22	11	279	63	21

A careful examination of this return, with reference to the relative situation of the different villages, and the amount of the population of each, will show some peculiarities which could hardly be expected from a merely contagious disease, and tending to prove, as indeed is commonly admitted, that predisposition, or disposing circumstances, are requisite for its diffusion. Thus, although Birchircara is one of the nearest of the casals to the city, and a large number of its inhabitants are daily employed in the city, the disease was two months later in appearing there than in Valetta and its suburbs, and in two or three of the more distant villages. Notabile is another instance of the same kind in regard to the temporary exemption, whether compared with Valetta, with which it has daily intercourse, or with Rabbato, contiguous to it. It will be perceived further, that though, in many instances, the number attacked with variola, corresponds with the population, there are some exceptions; for example, Birchircara, Notabile, and some others; and also, there are a few exceptions to the regular increase and decline of the disease.

The next return I shall give will be that of the deaths, in which the same order of construction will be followed as in the first.

NUMERICAL RETURN OF DEATHS FROM SMALL-POX IN THE ISLAND OF MALTA, FROM MARCH 1830, TO AUGUST 1831.

Localities.

Months.	Military.	Pieta, Misida, &c.	Rabbato.	Notabile.	Dingli.	Gargur.	Musta.	Naxaro.	Birchircara.	Balzan.	Lia.	Attard.	Curmi.	Zebbug.	Sigêul.	Micabiba.	Crendi.	Zurrico.	Safi.	Chercop.	Gudia.	Hasciín.	Luca.	Tarxien.	Zeitun.	Zabbar.	Senglea.	Cospicua.	Vittoriosa.	Floriana.	Valetta.	Total Died.
March,																													1		1	2
April,													2					1								1		8	4	1		16
May,	1						1		3				6									1			1		1	11	3	1	3	29
June,			1		1		1	2	10				16	1	1		1	1					2	2	1	1	5	26	10	11	20	95
July,	1								18				30	3			2						2		5	5	7	24	11	15	62	185
August,	4		1	1			1	1	14	1			12	3	1	1	1	6				2	3		8	3	13	13	13	29	69	190
September,		1	2	1			1	1	22	1			5	1	1			8				1	2		16	8	21	14	13	23	38	173
October,	2	3	12	1	8		8		21	3	2		2	8	3			8					7		15	11	21	5	2	10	38	161
November,	1	5	9			1	7	2	15	3	5	2	3	10	2	1	2	2				1	1		9	2	16	2			17	136
December,		2	6				5	5	4	1	2	2	1	4	4	1	1									3	4		1		5	64
January,		1	3				10	6	1		4	1		5	4		1	1							1			1			1	46
February,			1				8	8						4		2									1		1				1	32
March,							2	5			2			1	2																2	18
April,								3				1		3																	1	15
May,							1				1																		1			7
June,																																1
July,											1																					1
August,																																1
Total,	9	12	35	3	9	1	39	33	109	9	17	6	77	44	19	5	8	27	..	..	..	5	17	2	57	34	89	104	59	90	260	1172

It might be expected from what is known of the nature of small-pox, and of the effects of the heating and cooling regimen in the treatment of the disease, that a very marked difference of proportional mortality would appear on comparing the number of fatal cases which occurred in the hot months, with those of the cool season,—comparing, for instance, the numbers attacked, and the deaths, in the months of June, July, August, September, October, with those of March, April, May, November, December, January, February; but, on making the calculation, this supposition is not borne out by the results,—the difference of proportional mortality is found to be but small, and that contrary to expectation, not in favour of the cool, but of the hot months. Thus, while 1 case in 6.6 proved fatal in the former, 1 in 7.1 was the proportion in the latter; and 1 in 7 in August, the hottest month. As the fact is clear and precise, may it not with propriety suggest doubt, whether the commonly received opinion is correct, that warm air is really injurious in this disease? Formerly, when the heating regimen referred to was popular, it was commonly combined with the use of stimulants, and a want of free air and proper ventilation ; these might have done the harm, and not the warmth by itself. Practically, it may be deserving of consideration, whether a mild, or even warm, temperature of air may not be as proper in variola as it has been found to be in measles, pre-supposing that the ventilation is good. We know, that in a large proportion of the deaths from small-pox, the fatal event is owing to inflammation of the lungs and larynx. I would not attach much weight to this; but, analogically viewed, it is in favour of the supposition, that cold air may have had an undue preference, and that bad effects and loss of life, the common results of errors in practice, may have been the consequence.

As regards locality, it might perhaps be expected that some regular difference would appear in the ratio of mortality, on comparison of the results in different situations; but this does not seem to be the case. The general rate has been mentioned as having been 1 in 6.8; in Valetta, it was 1 in 6.4; in Curmi, 1 in 6; in Birchircara, 1 in 4.5; in Zabbar, 1 in 8.8; in Rabbato, 1 in 7.9. Zabbar and Rabbato are both elevated, and are esteemed healthy situations: Curmi and Birchircara are both low, especially the former. The description of people inhabiting the two villages is very similar, consisting chiefly of the working class. Why the disease proved so much more fatal in the one than in the other, it is difficult to understand.

The next return which I shall give will relate to the circumstances of sex, age, and vaccination, and will also exhibit the number of cases of a second attack of variola.

Return of those attacked by Small-pox, included in the preceding Table, specifying the Sex, Age, &c.

| Months. | Sex. | | Age. | | | | Vaccinated, &c. | | | |
	Males.	Females.	Infants to 7 years.	8 Years to 14.	15 Years to 28.	Beyond 28 years.	Not vaccinated.	Supposed to have been vaccinated.	Well vaccinated.	Had before small-pox.
Mar.,	11	15	12	7	7	...	26	...	...	...
April,	58	52	42	30	38	...	91	17	...	2
May,	143	123	92	93	81	...	189	71	...	6
June,	440	391	268	274	285	4	557	243	9	22
July,	720	744	501	486	471	6	941	481	30	12
Aug.,	727	598	487	436	395	7	857	404	46	18
Sept.,	582	506	364	370	347	7	587	410	80	11
Oct.,	500	442	295	279	358	10	528	320	83	11
Nov.,	405	357	262	195	291	14	413	271	69	9
Dec.,	247	235	168	125	180	9	255	190	34	3
Jan.,	191	154	119	88	132	6	195	132	16	2
Feb.,	94	64	65	45	45	3	90	61	6	1
Mar.,	63	62	55	27	42	1	58	58	9	...
April,	38	34	27	16	29	...	29	41	2	...
May,	38	19	34	9	13	...	32	19	6	...
June,	4	5	5	2	2	...	9	...	...	...
July,	1	3	3	...	1	...	2	2	...	...
Aug.,	1	...	1	...	...	...	1	..	...	...
Total,	4263	3804	2800	2482	2717	68	4850	2720	390	97
Sex of each Age. { Males,	1490		1316.	1419	38					
Females,	1310		1166	1298	30					

Relative to sex, comparing the numbers of each sex attacked, as given in the above return, there is a preponderance on the side of the males, but probably not greater, or very little greater, than accords with the larger number of males born, and the consequent numerical preponderance of that sex in infancy, the age most subject to small-pox; compare, for instance, the male and female births in Malta, during the year 1830, as given in the official returns, —the former are stated to be 1888, the latter 1619. Now, had the numbers of the two sexes attacked been in the same proportion, they would have been as 4263 and 3671, between which and the actual numbers the difference, it will be perceived, is but slight.

This accordance is what might be anticipated, supposing the disease to be propagated solely by contagion; on the contrary, were it not contagious, did its production depend solely on atmospheric influences, a different result might be expected,—viz. that the proportion attacked of these most exposed, as the male sex, would be greater than that of the female sex. Perhaps, in weighing evidence, whether a disease which is epidemic, is to be considered contagious or infectious, or neither, this circumstance may be deserving of being kept in recollection, and of being employed as a test.

The influence of age (the next particular noticed in this return) is strongly marked in the numbers attacked, and how (taking the numbers as a criterion) the tendency to the disease diminishes with advancing age ; and, what is very remarkable, how, after 28, almost a complete exemption appears to have been afforded. I regret that I cannot give the numbers attacked of different ages, from one year upwards. farther on a return of deaths on this plan, will be furnished, from which it may be inferred as probable that the diminution of tendency to contract the disease, at least after a certain period of life, is not in the exact ratio of augmentation of age.

It is hardly necessary to point out that the strong disposition to infection in infancy, especially in the first year, is deserving of being impressed on the minds of parents; it may be brought forward as a powerful argument for early vaccination.

The columns under the head of vaccination in the return show what a large number had the disease after supposed vaccination, and also what a considerable number, who had small-pox before, were attacked by it a second time. Farther on I shall have some remarks to offer on this subject.

RETURN of those who died of Small-pox included in the general Table of Deaths, specifying Sex, Age, &c.

Months.	Sex.		Age.				Vaccination, &c.			
	Males.	Females.	Infants to 7 years.	8 Years to 14.	15 Years to 28.	Beyond 28 years.	Not vaccinated.	Supposed to have been vaccinated.	Well vaccinated.	Had before Small-pox.
March,	...	2	1	1	...	...	2	...	...	...
April,	10	6	8	2	6	...	11	5	...	...
May,	17	12	16	6	7	...	22	7	...	...
June,	57	38	47	20	28	...	32	8	1	4
July,	103	82	125	27	32	1	159	25	1	...
August,	102	88	127	27	35	1	168	18	2	2
September,	98	75	126	24	23	...	143	20	8	2
October,	88	73	98	22	41	...	133	19	9	...
November,	71	65	87	17	29	3	125	6	4	1
December,	39	25	44	4	14	2	62	2	...	...
January,	28	18	34	2	10	...	45	1	...	...
February,	16	16	22	2	8	...	32	...	...	...
March,	6	12	11	5	2	...	17	1	...	..
April,	6	9	6	3	6	...	11	4	...	...
May,	5	2	6	1	...	...	7	...	...	...
June,	...	1	1	...	...	...	1	...	...	...
July,	...	1	1	...	...	...	1	...	...	...
August,	1	...	1	...	...	...	1	...	...	...
Total,	647	525	761	163	241	7	1022	116	25	9
Sex of each Age. { Males,			409	86	146	6				
{ Females,			352	77	95	1				
			761	163	241	7				

Comparing, in this Table, the mortality of the two sexes, the males are found to have suffered in a somewhat higher ratio than the females; the total number of females carried off was 525, but had it been in the same proportion as the males, for the number attacked, it would have amounted instead to 576: this difference, perhaps, is not more than might be expected, taking into account the greater proportional mortality in the male sex than in the female, which is commonly found to occur, whether owing to their different habits and manner of life, or to these combined with peculiarities of constitution.

The influence of age on the mortality, as might be anticipated, is well marked, especially of tender age: thus, whilst the general mortality, including all ages, has been 1 in 6.8 of those attacked, in infancy it has been in the proportion of 1 in 3.7; in the next period, viz. between 8 years and 14, as 1 in 15.2; in the next, between 15 and 28, as 1 in 11.2; and in the last, those above 28 years of age, as 1 in 9.7.

For the farther illustration of the relation of age to small-pox, I shall insert here a Table of the ages of all those who died of small-pox from March to December, beyond which month it was not continued; and also one of those who experienced a second attack of small-pox.

RETURN, showing the respective Age and Sex of the persons who died of Small-pox from the 16th March to December 31, 1830

Years.	Males.	Females.	Years.	Males.	Females.	Years.	Males.	Females.
1	151	154	19	20	7	37	...	...
2	87	57	20	25	12	38	1	...
3	43	31	21	6	5	39	...	...
4	31	25	22	11	12	40	...	...
5	24	22	23	3	4	...	...	...
6	22	11	24	4	1	...	...	...
7	11	10	25	1	...	...	...	...
8	9	8	26	2	2	...	...	...
9	18	16	27	2	1	...	...	...
10	8	8	28	1	...	...	...	...
11	7	5	29	1	1	...	...	...
12	11	10	30	...	...	...	...	...
13	11	8	31	...	...	...	...	...
14	17	14	32	1	...	...	...	...
15	15	12	33	1	...	...	...	...
16	10	8	34	1	...	...	...	...
17	13	8	35	...	...	...	...	...
18	16	14	36	1	...	...	...	...
								...

Males,	585	
Females,	466	
Total,	1051	

RETURN of the Age and Sex of 91 individuals reported to have had Small-pox a second time.

Sex.	Attacked.					Died.	
	Infants to 7.	8 to 14 years.	15 to 28.	Above 28.	Total.	15 to 28.	Above 28.
Males, . .	...	...	43	3	46	..	...
Females, .	...	...	42	3	45	...	...
Total,	...	...	85	6	91	9	...

Calculating on the results contained in the Table, under the head of vaccination, it appears that the mortality amongst those not vaccinated was 1 in 4.7 ; amongst those supposed to have been vaccinated, 1 in 23.4 ; amongst the well vaccinated, 1 in 15.6 ; and lastly, amongst those attacked a second time by small-pox, 1 in 10.8.

Why the proportion amongst the well vaccinated should be greater than amongst those supposed to have been vaccinated, I am not able to explain. Perhaps the apparent anomaly may be connected with the circumstance, that the majority of the former may have belonged to the infantile age.

As regards the general effect of vaccination, in its influence both as affording protection from small-pox to a considerable extent, and mitigating its severity when not preventing the attack, the facts given are clear and satisfactory. It is a curious circumstance, that the proportion of those who died after a second attack of small-pox, was, as has been already pointed out, greater than in the instances of those who had the disease after vaccination. The strongest confirmation, however, of the beneficial effect of vaccination, was afforded by the comparative exemption of the troops serving in Malta, as shown in the following returns :—

RETURN of the Men, Women, and Children belonging to the Troops serving in Malta, who had been previously Vaccinated, or had had Small-Pox.

Sex.	Strength.	Previously Vaccinated.	Had Small-Pox previously.
Men, ...	2219	706	1513
Women, . . .	196	49	147
Children, . . .	315	305	3
Total,	2730	1060 7*	1663

RETURN of Cases of Small-Pox amongst the Troops.

Sex.	Attacked.	Of these, previously Vaccinated.	Had Small-Pox before.	Died	
				After Vaccination.	After Small-Pox.
Men, . .	10	7	4	1	1
Women, .	1	1	...	...	...
Children, .	3	3	...	2	...
Total,	14	11	4	3	1

The native population, in 1830, was estimated at 100,839 persons; amongst whom it appears, from preceding returns, 1 in every 12.1 was attacked with the disease, and 1 in every 85 died; but amongst the military, including their wives and children, the proportion attacked, as shown above, was 1 in 188, and the mortality was only 1 in 682.

These results, demonstrative of the protecting and

* Requiring to be vaccinated, and were immediately.

mitigating power of vaccination, are the more remarkable, and the more to be depended on, as no
precautions whatever were taken to prevent intercourse between the military and the inhabitants. It
is true that the majority of the soldiers lived in barracks, but they were not confined to barracks; during
the whole time the epidemic prevailed, they had the
usual liberty of going at certain times into town, free
from all restriction. And, as regards their families,
many of them lived in the close streets adjoining the
barracks, and the children mixed freely with the
other children of the place; notwithstanding, one
woman only became infected, and three children—a
remarkable fact.

Reasoning from the facts contained in the preceding returns, the influence of vaccination in preventing
small-pox, appears to have been less than that of
small-pox itself in preventing a second attack,—
whilst the mitigating power of the former, compared
with that of the latter, seems to have been greater:
thus, of those attacked by small-pox, after having
been vaccinated, as it was supposed, the mortality
was only 4.2 per cent.; but amongst those who had
the disease a second time, the mortality was as high
as 9.3 per cent.,—a result which, I believe, is in
accordance with common experience, if I may so
express myself respecting an event (a second attack
of small-pox), which is held to be a rare occurrence.
The recurrence of the disease shows a peculiar susceptibility to it,—and on this ground, the severity of

its effects have been attempted to be explained. But in such matters, I fear it must be confessed that explanation commonly is unsatisfactory, and that our knowledge is limited by the facts. An instance has been related to me of a lady, the mother of ten children, who had small-pox eleven different times; first in infancy, and subsequently on the occasion of each of her children having it, and, what is very remarkable, the latter attacks of the disease were not less severe than the first; no mitigating influence appeared to have been imparted to the constitution even by frequent repetitions of the specific morbid actions peculiar to variola. This information I received from one of the sons of the lady,—an accurate observer himself, and a man of unquestionable veracity.

In consequence of the comparatively large number of persons who were attacked with small-pox, after vaccination and after small-pox, an opinion prevailed in Malta at the time, and was spread abroad, that the disease in question was not true small-pox—that it was peculiar in its nature, and somewhat different from genuine small-pox. This opinion, I believe, was rather popular than medical, and was founded on a very superficial knowledge of the history of small-pox, and of the varieties to which it is subject. All that I saw and heard of the disease, relative to its origin, diffusion, and symptoms, satisfied me that it was ordinary small-pox, nowise peculiar in its nature, and of a comparatively mild kind.

As in every endemic, some peculiarities were observed. In the worst cases, especially in the summer months, a hæmorrhagic tendency was prevalent, as bleeding of the gums, bloody stools, and petechiæ. The individuals thus affected generally died before the eighth day; and, in some instances, without any other eruption appearing excepting the petechial ; so that a superficial observer might have considered the disease petechial-fever. Some cases occurred, in which the premonitory fever was smart and distinct, accompanied with all its usual symptoms, but followed by very few pustules; in one case, which was under the observation of an attentive and accurate medical man, one pustule only appeared. In two cases not a single pustule succeeded the fever, and the patients were convalescent on the fourth or fifth day. As the individuals were exposed to the contagion of small-pox, persons in the same families, then labouring under the disease, the natural inference is, that the fever was that of small-pox, though not followed by the eruption.

In most instances that the disease occurred, after vaccination had been previously successful, it was mild, and ran its course in an unusually short time; often more resembling chicken-pox than small-pox.

I endeavoured to collect information on the important problem of the nature of chicken-pox, whether it is a distinct disease, or merely a variety of small-pox, as has been so ably maintained by Dr John

Thomson. But I could learn nothing decisive. After the appearance of small-pox, and during its prevalency, chicken-pox also was common—ninety-one cases were reported to the police physician; and he told me, that he believed that many more occurred which were not reported to him. So far this is in favour of the identity of small-pox and chicken-pox. But, in opposition to this opinion, chicken-pox has been known to prevail in Malta when small-pox did not exist; Dr Gravagna, the intelligent police physician, has assured me that he has witnessed this himself, and in more instances than one. However, even if admitted to be correct, the fact is not conclusive. The advocates of the new doctrine may say, the state of atmosphere constituting atmospheric constitution, using the term in its medical sense, may have been favourable only to the production of the mild variety. In December 1831, three months after the termination of the last case of small-pox, some cases of chicken-pox occurred, and amongst them was one, at first of a doubtful character, in the person of the daughter of an advocate, aged thirteen, who had been previously vaccinated. I saw her when the pustules were well formed; and from their appearance, and the after progress of the disease, was obliged to come to the conclusion, that it was an example of genuine small-pox, though of a very mild kind. Her father supposed that she had contracted it at school, from children there who had chicken-pox. The disease spread no farther. Now, in this instance, unless

particular attention had been paid to the case, it
would have passed as one of chicken-pox. Where
quarantine restrictions hang over a people *in terrorem*,
the tendency always is to conceal solitary examples
of diseases which subject the individuals to be taken
from their homes and shut up in a lazaretto—exposed
to discomfort and annoyance, which the sick are ill
fitted to contend with. This may be deserving of being
kept in recollection in weighing evidence on such a
point as that in question.

Before concluding, it may be right to say a few
words relative to the returns which have been inserted. I have already mentioned how they were
furnished. I may add that they were drawn up, at
my request, under the direction of the police physician, and agreeably to my suggestions, as nearly as
possible. They were framed from the daily reports
made to his office by persons employed to collect the
information, and the deaths were certified by the
medical men who attended the sick. That all of
them are not deserving of the same degree of confidence must be admitted ; some of them are necessarily more exposed to error than others.

1*st*, There can be little doubt that more cases of
the disease occurred than were reported ; and those
kept back, it may be inferred, were chiefly of the
mildest kind.

2*dly*, In relation to vaccination, confidence may
be placed in the numbers reported " not vaccinated,"
and tolerable confidence in the numbers " supposed

to have been vaccinated;" that is, the numbers on whom the operation of vaccination had been performed ; but a much less degree of confidence is due to the numbers reported " well vaccinated," owing to vaccination in Malta having previously been conducted in a very unsatisfactory manner, it being seldom ascertained at the time whether it had taken effect, the individual rarely returning to the vaccinators after the operation, though urged so to do by them. It may farther be stated, that the column of " well vaccinated" was filled up very much on a supposition till the month of December, when, at my suggestion, the inference was made from the appearance of the cicatrix ; and, consequently, it is only for the latter months that this column is deserving of attention.

3dly, In the numbers reported to have had the disease a second time, tolerable confidence, I believe, may be placed ; as in the determining of them there does not appear to have been any material source of fallacy.

4thly, As regards age and sex, I apprehend the numbers given may be considered as tolerably accurate; the age and sex of each case reported to the police physician having been specified.

I have not thought it necessary to describe the manner in which the disease was medically treated, because I am not aware of any peculiarities in the method employed ; the antiphlogistic plan, including the cooling regimen, whenever a medical man was called in, was, 1 believe, exclusively used; and the habits of the natives, and their mode of diet, and the poverty of the major part of the population, must have conduced greatly to the proper observance of it.

CHAPTER XV.

ON THE CLIMATE OF CONSTANTINOPLE, AND ON SOME OF THE HABITS OF THE PEOPLE IN CONNEXION WITH CLIMATE AND HEALTH.

Climate of Constantinople different from what might be expected *a priori*. Its chief Peculiarities. Observations in Illustration. Some Errors and Exaggerations pointed out. Meteorological Tables for the Years 1839 and 1840 kept in Pera. Comments on them. Observations and Remarks in Connexion with Climate. On the Temperature of the Bosphorus and Black Sea at different Seasons. A Peculiarity in the Temperature of the Bosphorus pointed out. Brief Notices of the Dress, Dwelling-Houses, Manner of Living, &c., of the Turks, in Connexion with Climate and Health. Notices of the Principal Diseases to which they are subject in the Capital, and of those to which they are either little Liable, or are Exempt from. Remarks on the Climate in Relation to the Inquiries of Invalids and Travellers.

LYING nearly in the same latitude as Naples, situated on the shore of the Sea of Marmora and the banks of the Bosphorus, at no considerable distance from the Mediterranean, and close to the Black Sea, it might be expected that the climate of Constantinople would differ but little from that of southern Italy ; that it would be characterized by hot summers and mild winters; and would be distinguished by equability of temperature. Such, however, is only very partially

the case.   Its summer season is commonly hot, but
its winters are often irregularly severe and protracted.
The circumstances most peculiar in the character of
its climate are, irregularity—variability, the sudden
changes of temperature, with changes of wind and
weather to which it is liable, and the wide range of the
thermometer.   When I arrived in Constantinople the
year before last (1840), on the 24th of November,
nothing indicated, excepting the falling leaf, and the
russet foliage, the approach of winter.   No fires—no
warm clothing were required—people were sitting with
open windows, or in the open air,—the temperature
very agreeable, between 60° and 70°.   This pleasant
state of air lasted till the 1st of December, when it was
suddenly interrupted by a violent snow-storm from the
north of about three days' duration, accompanied by
a fall of the thermometer below the freezing point.
On the 3d of the month, at nine o'clock in the morning, I find, by my notes, that it was as low as 29° in
my bed-room, and that in the open air it was two
degrees lower.   Thus was winter rudely ushered in.
And great was the change in the habits of the people.
The   mangal, tandour, and stoves, were hurriedly
brought into use—the windows, at their openings,
were made as tight as might be with the aid of paste
and paper, as I witnessed in one of the best lodging-
houses in Pera; the windows in the houses of the
opulent Turks were fortified with double sashes;
the plants which had hitherto ornamented their gardens, the orange, the lemon, the oliander, and other

exotics, were taken from the open air, and deposited for safety in their large, tile-roofed conservatories. Nor was the change of dress less striking: the snow or mud-boot was pulled on; the warm fur pelisse, and the padded winter coat, one or other was brought into general use; and, amongst the troops, the sentinel on duty appeared in his watch-coat well lined with fur.

This violent setting-in of winter was soon again interrupted by change of temperature, from cold to mild, and the latter, before the end of the month, by a recurrence of cold,—marking the vicissitudes for which, as I have observed, the seasons are distinguished, especially the winter. On the 16th of December it is set down in my note-book that the weather was delightful, the thermometer, at three o'clock in the afternoon, at 60°. A week after, viz. on the 23d, it was as low as 22°, and the ground was again covered with snow, which fell the preceding night, when it was reported that two persons had been frozen to death, and were found so in the morning, on the wooden bridge across the Golden Horn, connecting Pera with Constantinople.

Other instances, hardly less remarkable, might be given, of sudden and great changes of temperature in the other seasons. A fall of snow is not considered remarkable in April; a shower of snow has suddenly masked the bright verdure of the early May; even in summer, the most equable season, the range of the thermometer is considerable, and the fluctuations of temperature are often great. In July last it was often so low as 70° before sunrise, and as high as 90°, or above that, in the afternoon in the shade.

The variability of climate is well exemplified in the usages, as regard dress, of the opulent natives, or rather was, when their dress was strictly oriental. A few years ago, it is said, that a Turk of rank, when going to take a walk, was followed by attendants bearing pelisses of different degrees of warmth, in preparation for changes of temperature, whether depending on change of wind, or on going from the sunshine into the shade—from a sheltered to an exposed situation—or to other circumstances of situation or state of atmosphere likely to render one description of cloak too heating, or another description not a sufficient guard against cold.

Probably erroneous ideas of the climate of Constantinople have been derived from the incidental notices of it contained in Lady Mary Wortley Montague's Letters. This charming writer appears to have viewed every thing that came under her notice in the most favourable light. Occupying the ambassadorial residence; having about her every comfort and luxury; under no necessity to quit her well-aired and well-warmed apartments to encounter the occasional inclemencies of winter, it is not surprising that she rather dwells on the mild days of that season, when the soft south wind wafted warmth from the Mediterranean, and in the middle of January she could sit writing, with her windows open, exposed, with the jonquil and rose that perfumed her room, to the influence of the atmosphere. It may be that, during the time she was in Turkey, the winters were unusually mild; but this is not probable—hardly more so than that they were more severe when the disconsolate Ovid wrote his " Tristia" on the shore of the Euxine. The feelings of each, doubtless, tinged their descriptions. In most things there is a tendency to exaggeration, and, the simple truth is, of difficult attainment. It is remarkably so in regard to the weather and the seasons, as the home experience of every one may testify. Amongst other exaggerations in regard to the climate of Constantinople, I have heard it said that there there is no spring—that it is passed over, so rapid is the transition from winter to summer. It is true that the spring is backward, that the transition is rapid, but yet there is a transition, well marked by the gradual rise of the mean temperature of the atmosphere in March and April, and still more, by the state of vegetation, and by the appearance of certain birds. April, in its general character, is almost as much a spring month on the banks of the Bosphorus as of the Thames. In this month the stork, the dove, the nightingale arrive. Early in last April doves crowded the burying-grounds, pleasantly cooing in the cypress-trees; and before its end, the nightingales were in full song in the sheltered valleys. Early, too, in the month, wild flowers were brought to market in Pera in plenty—the leaf-buds of many trees were opening

—the leaf of the weeping willow was almost fully expanded—and the rose-bushes were little less advanced.

In England, spring is, as it were, a struggle between winter and summer—this having the upper hand to-day, that to-morrow. Such contention is even more remarkable at Constantinople, where the mean annual temperature of the ground is higher—the sun, when unclouded, more powerful—and the northern influences, when the wind blows strong from that quarter, more severely felt. This is well exemplified in the different degree of progress of low plants and of lofty trees, or even of large shrubs, and in the lingering stay of certain birds. The white-thorn was not in full bloom till the middle of May; the wheat harvest was commenced towards the end of June; the woodcock was to be had in the market in the middle of April.

Since Constantinople has been occupied by the Turks, the sciences and literature have been almost utterly neglected there—that is to say, the modern sciences and European literature,—what is strictly national of each hardly deserving the name. This neglect has not been confined to the Turks; it has appeared almost equally in the Frank portion of the population. Science and literature amongst them is nowise respected; as merchants, traders, or dragomans, they are mainly intent either on money-making or the study of languages. In the whole of Pera there is no public library—no museum of any kind

—no collection of philosophical instruments—no maker of such instruments;—it is not, therefore, surprising that meteorology has had little attention paid to it, and that we are less minutely acquainted with the climate of this celebrated capital than with that of almost any other town of note in the world. Individuals, probably, have made observations on the weather, aided by instruments; but they have been lost to science. Nor is this more than might be expected, considering the difficulties that have existed till recently in the way of communication,—the want of aid and encouragement, through the medium of societies,—and the indifference of the public there to such observations. Up to the present time the dark middle age has been protracted in Constantinople. Now, it is to be hoped, that the dawn of a better time is appearing, and that there will be a reflux of know-ledge to that city to which Europe generally has been under no small obligation on account of letters. This hope is founded chiefly on the increased facilities of intercourse recently afforded by means of steam navigation; and the greater interest taken in the affairs of Turkey by the powers of Europe, and on the necessity for introducing European science into the country in aid of its resources, if the Turkish empire is to be preserved, and not doomed to perish, as has been recently so often and so confidently foreboded.

Whilst I was in Constantinople I was fortunate in becoming acquainted with one gentleman, Mr Redhouse, who had lately begun to pay attention to the subject of meteorology. The results of his observations for two years are contained in the following Table. It may be premised that they were made in Pera, at an elevation of about two hundred feet above the level of the sea; that the barometer was placed in an open hall; that the rain-gauge stood about twenty feet from the ground; that the thermometer was in the open air, with a north-westerly aspect, and was observed at eight A.M., two and twelve P.M.

GENERAL RESULTS OF METEOROLOGICAL OBSERVATIONS AT CONSTANTINOPLE FOR THE YEARS 1839 AND 1840.

Year and Months.	Barometer.					Rain. Inches.			Thermom. Fahrenht.					Days Wind blew.				
	Highest.	Lowest.	Mean.	Greatest daily Variation. Rise.	Fall.	Monthly.	Greatest daily.	Rainy Days.	Highest.	Lowest.	Mean.	Greatest daily Variation. Rise.	Fall.	N.E.	N.W.	S.E.	S.W.	N.
1839.																		
Jan.,								14	52 30	36		9	12	23	0	2	6	0
Feb.,								10	52 29	42		5	10	9	4	1	14	0
March,								13	59 30	40		7	13	7	0	13	11	0
April,		Not observed.						11	54 34	43		5	6	16	0	5	8	1
May,								6	70 47	52		15	12	13	0	0	18	0
June,								5	89 60	70		16	16	21	0	0	9	0
July,								7	88 64	72		18	19	19	0	8	4	0
Aug.,								1	89 64	80		13	14	20	0	4	7	0
Sept.,								4	84 61	68		13	14	28	0	0	2	0
Oct.,	30.03	29.80	29.90	0.13	0.10	0.00		8	72 57	63		7	9	28	0	2	1	0
Nov.,	30.02	29.64	29.81	0.21	0.23	1.71	1.34	9	67 51	57		7	7	19	0	0	11	0
Dec.,	30.18	29.37	29.81	0.29	0.39	2.14	0.72	14	58 36	46		18	12	12	8	0	8	3
	30.18	29.37	29.84	0.29	0 39	3.85	1.34	102	89 29	56		18	19	215	12	35	99	4
1840.																		
Jan.,	30.28	29.50	29.875	0.44	0.25	6.20	1.15	14	54 24	40.7		17	12	7	10	0	14	0
Feb.,	30.21	29.48	29.873	0.37	0.33	2.68	0.49	15	58 26	39.4		12	6	1	10	2	7	9
March.	30.18	29.26	29.719	0.40	0.31	4.91	1.16	19	55 25	40.4		15	10	13	1	0	13	4
April.	30.01	29.42	29.754	0.41	0.28	2.61	0.57	11	63 36	46.0		16	11	19	1	0	9	1
May,	30.06	29.50	29.807	0.41	0.42	0.83	0.50	6	85 47	59.9		20	23	14	2	0	15	0
June,	29.95	29.64	29.696	0.15	0.19	0.37	0.20	3	82 51	69.0		22	21	25	0	0	5	0
July,	29.82	29.53	29.742	0.08	0.12	0.07	0.05	2	91 62	76.1		13	14	26	0	0	5	0
Aug.,	29.90	29.49	29.712	0.17	0.16	0.97	0.50	5	87 62	73.3		17	17	23	0	0	8	0
Sept.,	29.90	29.58	29.770	0.20	0.21	3.28	1.75	6	89 59	69.6		17	17	24	2	0	4	0
Oct.,	30.00	29.33	29.802	0. 0.25		3.27	1.00	12	82 44	60.1		14	16	18	2	0	11	0
Nov.,	30.10	29.53	29.807	0.21	0.24	1.69	0.32	11	70 32	54.8		14	18	14	0	1	15	0
Dec.,	30.38	29.55	29.946	0.48	0.42	4.77	0.80	18	60 24	37.8		20	17	15	9	0	7	0
	30.38	29.26	29.793	0.48	0.45	31.65	1.75	122	91 24	58.6		22	23	199	37	3	113	14

Limited as these observations are to the short space of two years, yet they are valuable, and give a better idea of the climate of the place than can be conveyed by mere description, unaided by numerical results regularly taken.

The range of the barometer, it would appear, has been inconsiderable—especially during the summer season—when, as might be expected, the climate, like that of the Mediterranean generally, approaches in its character to a tropical climate.

The quantity of rain which fell in 1840 is comparatively small for the latitude, and may be considered below the average quantity; for that year, and the year before, and the following, were more than usually dry, as was attested by the state of the crops. The number of rainy days—or rather, it should be said, of days in which rain or snow fell—was considerable, but very unequally divided, comparing the winter and spring, with the summer and autumn.

The thermometrical observations demonstrate fully the vicissitudes of temperature on which I have commented, as one of the principal features of the climate; and this would have been shown by them even more strongly, had the morning observation been made at an earlier hour, just before sunrise; and had the thermometer, which was attached to a wall, fronted by another wall, at the distance only of a few feet, been freely exposed to the open sky. The same observations are also in accordance with the preceding remarks on the spring months,—the backward-

ness of that season, and the contention it exhibits
between winter and summer.   It is observed by Mr
Redhouse, that snow fell in each year in the middle
of April.*

The columns in the Table denoting the direction
of the winds, show a well-known peculiarity respecting them,—I allude to the great prevalence of the
north-east wind—the Etesian wind of the ancients;
one year blowing 215 days; the other, 199 days.
The opposite wind, the south-west, is next remarkable in point of prevalency.   These two winds are
essentially different in character, as might be expected
from the regions from whence they proceed.   The
one, coming from countries and over a sea in winter,
and spring subject to cold more or less severe, and
in summer to drought and a high temperature; the
other, coming from the Mediterranean, over the
Archipelago and Sea of Marmora, subject, indeed, to
variation of temperature, but, compared with the
other, comprised in narrow limits.

In Vol. I., Chap. VII., the variation of temperature
of the Mediterranean, through the greater part of the
year, has been given, so far as my observations permitted, showing that, when highest at the surface, it

* The observations referred to in the text having been made at a
certain elevation, and in a constantly shaded place with a north-
westerly aspect, express atmospheric temperature little affected by
the earth: this requires to be kept in mind; if neglected, an exaggerated idea will be formed of the cold of spring, and the absence of
genial warmth in lower sheltered situations, open to the sun, and
defended from the bleak winds of the north.

did not exceed 82°, excepting once during a calm, and that, when lowest, it was not below 55°. A series of like observations on the varying temperature of the Black Sea could hardly fail to be interesting and instructive. I apprehend they would be strongly illustrative of some of the peculiarities of this remarkable sea, and might throw some light on its varied influences on the climate of its shores, which, as regards temperature, and consequently rigour and mildness, differs very much more than could be expected, considering merely differences of latitude. Compare, in this respect, for instance, Trebizond and Odessa; the one in about 41°, the other little more than five degrees farther north; the one washed by a sea always open, enjoying a mild winter climate, suitable to the olive-tree, which is extensively grown in the neighbourhood of the town;—the other, having its port closed every winter by ice extending many miles, and experiencing a severity of winter cold comparable almost to that of the arctic regions.*

As a contribution to this inquiry, I shall give such

---

* Great as is the contrast between the winter of Odessa and Trebizond, that between the winter weather of Odessa and the almost adjoining eastern coast of the Crimea is even more remarkable. The sheltered valleys along this coast, screened by lofty hills from the north, skirted by a deep sea, are peculiarly mild, rivalling in mildness the most favoured spots in the south of Europe. The olive and even the palm, we are told, are there met with, accompanied by other plants of a warm climate, seeming to justify the lavish praise bestowed by an accomplished writer on the climate of this region.— *Vide* Mrs Guthrie's interesting account of the Crimea.

observations as I was able to make, whilst in Turkey, on the temperature of the Black Sea at its surface, and on the current of the Bosphorus, which is strictly a river flowing out of that sea, and a fair specimen of its water,—hardly perceptibly differing from the nearest part of it in degree of saltness.*

* The following are the results of the trials I have made on the specific gravity of the water of the Black Sea and of the Bosphorus:—

No.		Sp. Gr.
1.	Taken up about two miles off Trebizond, and where the sea is about 125 feet deep, . . .	10127
2.	From off Cape Sinopè, about 200 or 300 yards, water about 275 feet deep, ...	10115
3.	About a mile from Penderaclea, . . .	10115
4.	From the entrance of the Bosphorus, taken up with the preceding early in July, ...	10115
5.	Taken up September 22, about twenty miles from Costangi, on the western shore of the Black Sea, .	10090
1.	From middle of Golden Horn, taken up December 16,	10110
2.	From mid-channel, off Therapia, March 8, . .	10120
3.	From the same situation, March 20, . .	10120
4.	From the same situation, July 13, . .	10124
5.	From the same situation, August 30, . .	10124
6.	Off Genoese Castle, September 22, . .	10110

Many fishes are common to the Mediterranean, the Black Sea, and the Bosphorus; many of them are migratory from one to the other, passing into the fresher water, like the salmon, for the purpose of breeding; some well known in the Mediterranean are never caught in the Bosphorus or Black Sea; the torpedo is one of these. A strict comparison of the fishes of these seas might reward the naturalist by some interesting results.

TEMPERATURE OF BOSPHORUS AND BLACK SEA, AS OBSERVED AT
THE SURFACE, AT DIFFERENT TIMES, IN 1840-41.

Time.	Situation.	Temp. of Water.		Temp. of Air.	
1840.					
Nov. 24,	Between Constantinople and Therapia,	59°	57°	60°	58°
Dec. 5,	Between Topana and Scutari, . .	54	53	48	44
7,	Between Topana and the Lazaretto of Kulili,	54	52	44	
21,	In Golden Horn, opposite the arsenal or dockyard, ...	49		56	
25,	Golden Horn ; off Galata, . . .	46		33	
1841.					
Jan. 3,	Ditto ; opposite the arsenal, . . .	45		50	
Feb. 14,	Ditto ; between Galata and Constantinople,	40	39	39	
18,	Ditto ; off Galata, ...	43		54	
Mar. 4,	Ditto ; between Galata and Constantinople,	44	43	48	
5,	Between Topana and Therapia, . .	39	37	44	43
20,	Golden Horn ; off Galata, . . .	46		50	
April 5,	Ditto, ditto, ...	44		55	
May 9,	Between Topana and Bebek, . .	51	50	60	58
14,	Golden Horn ; off the arsenal, . .	57		62	
18,	Ditto ; off Topana, ...	51		56	
23,	Between Topana and Therapia, . .	61	58	68	65
June 4,	Golden Horn ; off the arsenal, . .	65		70	
6,	Between Topano and Scutari, . .	64	60	75	
10,	Between Topana and the Lazaretto, .	67	61	77	75
15,	Between Topana and Therapia, . .	68	62	75	70
16,	Between Therapia and Black Sea, .	69	67	64	
23,	Between Topana and Chalcedon, .	68	62	70	
27,	Between Topana and Therapia, . .	74	64	80	78
29,	Between Topana and Princes Islands, in the sea of Marmora, . . .	73	64	64	
July 2,	Between Topana and the Black Sea, .	72	63	78	75
11, 13,	Between the entrance of the Bosphorus from the Black Sea and Topana, .	75	68	72	
	Between Galata and Constantinople, .	75	71	87	
20,	Between Galata and Becktictash, .	73	71	77	
Aug. 9,	Golden Horn ; off Galata, . . .	71		80	
10,	Between Topana and Buyukdere, .	77	68	80	77
13,	Between Topana and Therapia, .	77	69	78	72
19,	Between Topana and Emirguen Oglou,	75	71	80	
30,	Between Topana and Therapia, .	77	71	80	75
Sept. 10,	Between Galata and Constantinople, .	77	76	74	
13,	Between Topana and Therapia, . .	77	74	76	74
15,	Between Topana and Therapia, .	78	74	75	73
22,	Between Topana and the Black Sea, .	74	70	66	64

TABLE OF TEMPERATURE—*(continued.)*

Time.	Situation.	Temp. of Water.		Temp. of Air.	
1841. Jan.	Off Trebizond, in the Black Sea, in about five fathoms water,* . . .	46.7°		60°	50°
July 2,	At entrance of Black Sea from the Bosphorus,	74		72	
3,	Off Penderaclia, about five miles, .	72		73	
...	Off Penderaclia, about three miles,	71		72	
	Close to the port of Penderaclia, . .	72		75	
...	Between this port and the coal-mine of Kossiagisi, ...	76	71	75	74
4,	Between Penderaclea and the coal-mine of Tchaousagsi, ...	73	70	75	71
10,	Between Penderaclea and the Bosphorus, about one mile from port, 6½ A.M., .	73		69	
...	About ten miles off the coast, 8¾ A.M.,	77		75	
...	About one mile off the small island of Kefkene, close to shore, 1 P.M., .	78		76	
...	About six miles off shore, 2 P.M.,	79		75	
...	About four miles off Kilva, 4 P.M., .	77		76	
...	About eight miles from mouth of the Bosphorus, 6 P.M., . . .	78		74	
...	About a mile off shore, a little to the eastward of the lighthouse at entrance of Bosphorus, 6½ P.M.. . . .	75		74	
...	About one-fourth mile off the lighthouse, at entrance of Bosphorus, 6¾ P.M.,	74		74	
Sept. 22,	At mouth of Bosphorus, 3¾ P.M., .	73		62	
...	In Black Sea, 4 P.M., ...	71		61	
...	Ditto, 5½ P.M., ...	72		61	
...	Ditto, 6½	72		55	
23,	Ditto, 6 A.M., ...	68		58	
...	Ditto, 9	70		58	
...	Ditto 10	70		60	
...	Ditto, 11	69		65	
...	Ditto, 12	68		64	
...	Ditto, 1 P.M., ...	67		65	
...	Ditto 2, ...	68		65	
...	Ditto, 3, ...	67		65	
...	Ditto, 4, ...	68		65	
...	Ditto, 5, ...	...		...	
	About one-fourth mile from Constangie,†	65		60	

On these observations I shall offer a few com-

* For this observation I am indebted to Dr Bell.

† The voyage to Penderaclia and Constangie, in the Black Sea,

ments. Those on the Bosphorus show two circumstances worthy of notice—the wide range of temperature to which its waters are subject, and the difference of temperature of the stream on the same day.

The range of temperature observed throughout the year was so high as 39°; in February and March being only 5° above the freezing point; in August as high as 77°, and in September one degree higher. In some years, it cannot be doubted that the variation of temperature has even been greater. In the memory of man the Golden Horn has been known to have been frozen over; and it has been handed down traditionally, and, I believe, recorded in history, that the greater part of the Bosphorus between Topana and Scutari has been covered with ice.

The difference of temperature exhibited on the same day in the stream of the Bosphorus is remarkable; when greatest, as in the month of June, amounting to 10°. This may require a few words in explanation. The difference is of two kinds : one is a trifling one, depending on the time of the day. In

was made in a steam-packet, going at the rate of about eight miles an hour.

I have been particular in giving the temperature of this sea, especially on approaching the Bosphorus, with the hope that, were a series of observations of the like kind made for every month in the year, the result might be of importance in navigation,—might afford the means of finding the mouth of the Bosphorus in the dense fogs to which the Black Sea is subject,—in which, in the attempt alluded to, innumerable vessels have been lost.

the afternoon, under the influence of sunshine, I found the temperature of the same place, and of the Bosphorus generally, one degree higher than at an early hour,—a result that might be expected from all previous experience of the influence of the sun's rays on water at the surface. The other, the greater difference, is connected with situation and the course of the current. It may be right to give some observations in illustration.

On the 27th of June, between the hours of twelve and five in the afternoon, in going and returning from Therapia, the following differences were noticed :—

Just outside the Golden Horn, where the current ascends along
    the European shore, the temperature of the water was   64°
In the three rapids, which occur on the same side of the Bosphorus, between the villages of Arnaudkoi and Emirguen
    Oglou, in which the descending current is very powerful,*
    it was   70
In the main stream, outside the bay of Therapia, it was   .   74
In mid-channel, a little above the Castles, it was   .   .   71
The greater part of the way down, in mid-channel, after passing the Castles, it was about   .   .   .   67
Near the entrance of the Golden Horn, in the counter-ascending
    current, it was   65

On the 29th of June, the following observations

---

* The strength of the great current of the Bosphorus depends a good deal on the wind,—being greatest with a strong north-easterly wind, and least with the opposite : when the wind is in favour of the currents, the ascent of the rapids, particularly of that called the Devil's Rapid—*Scheitan* Akindissi, is not easy; the oars of the dexterous and powerful Turkish boatmen are of little avail, and accordingly they are put aside, and the tow-rope is substituted, drawn commonly by one man, but sometimes requiring two.

were made in going to the Princes Islands, situated
in the upper part of the Sea of Marmora:—

4 15 P.M. in Golden Horn, temperature of water, . .	.	64°
4 30 ... Off the Seraglio, ...	.	64
4 35 ... Off the Seraglio Point, where the descending current		
is strong, ...	.	66
4 45 ... Off Scutari Barracks, . . .	.	67
4 50 ... Off Kadikoi or Chalcedon, . . .	.	68
5 0 ... Off the Point of Chalcedon, . .	.	69.5
5 25 ... Ditto, . . .	.	70
5 55 ... Ditto, . . .	.	71
6 5 ... About a mile off Kalki, . . .	.	72
6 20 ... About a quarter of a mile from Prinkipo, .	.	72
6 35 ... Close to shore, ...	.	72

It will be seen, by referring back to the observations made at different times of the year, that the
greatest variation of temperature was noticed in the
beginning of summer, and that in winter it was very
inconsiderable. The general idea that I am disposed
to form, from all the facts I could collect, is, that
the reduction of temperature in certain parts of the
Bosphorus is owing to deep water being brought
to the surface, in consequence, it may be conjectured,
of the deep current meeting with obstacles which
impede its free downward course and throw it back,
producing those counter-currents for which the Bosphorus is so remarkable, and which, well known to
the boatmen, are of essential service in enabling them
to make good their way in proceeding upwards towards the Black Sea. That the ascending counter-
current is cooler than the descending main stream
and the rapids, and greatly cooler in the beginning

of summer (when the difference is most remarkable) than either the Black Sea at one end of the Bosphorus, or the sea of Marmora at its other extremity, are the circumstances chiefly in favour of this view, and which, I apprehend, it would be difficult to explain in any other manner.   Be this as it may, the facts are curious and deserving of attention; and it is to be hoped that they will be further investigated.

The influence of the great range of temperature of the waters of the Bosphorus on the climate of its shores, cannot be questioned,—tempering the summer heat, tempering the severity of cold of the early winter, and chilling the air of the advanced spring and early summer.   Even the colder ascending currents have a perceptible influence; the portions of shore nearest to them, in several instances washed by them, seem to be considered by the natives as favourite spots; they are the sites of the principal palaces of the Sultan, and of the villas and charming gardens of the most opulent of his subjects.   The effect of the climate generally, along the banks of the Bosphorus, is manifested in the vegetation.   The olive is cultivated in the Princes Islands, where the cold of winter is moderated by the warmth afforded by the sea of Marmora, and this within sight of Constantinople.   I have met with the myrtle growing wild luxuriantly, close to the shore of the Black Sea, near Penderaclea, in sheltered situations, having the advantage, in winter, of a source of warmth in the contiguous deep water. But neither the olive nor myrtle is to be seen on the shores of the Bosphorus excepting, perhaps, in some villa garden, reared with care, and protected from the cold winds.

The few observations made on the temperature of the Black Sea, indicate a range of temperature somewhat less than that of the Bosphorus. This may be true, for the southern part of that sea to which the observations were limited, that part being generally deep, fed by few rivers, and those generally pouring into it water little less warm, or even warmer than its own. But it is far from the truth for the Black Sea generally. I have already contrasted the mild winter of Trebizond with the almost arctic winter of Odessa. That season is little less severe all along the western shore. At Constangie, considerably to the westward of the mouth of the Danube, I was assured that the sea is every winter frozen in the month of January, and to a considerable distance from the shore. The shallowness of the Black Sea, in its western portion, and its comparative freshness, are favourable to its freezing. And the great rivers which flow into this part of it, of northern origin, promote equally its freshness and the reduction of its temperature,—the latter effect, after they have lost their summer heat, and are pouring in water either reduced nearly to the freezing point, or quite to that point, and are discharging into it floating ice. The range of temperature of the two extremities of the Black Sea, or of the western extremity throughout

the year, must be very great, probably not less than
65°.   In summer and the beginning of autumn, it is
likely to rise to nearly 60°, and in winter to fall to
25°, or even lower.   Horace, at Tomos, lamented
the freezing of the wine; at Constangie, the severity
of the winter cold is now similarly marked.*

When the character of the two seas is considered,
between which Constantinople is situated, and also
the character of the connecting stream of the Bosphorus, there seems to be but little difficulty in
accounting for most of the peculiarities of its climate,
and especially for those great vicissitudes, as regards
temperature, to which it is subject,—the comparatively high temperature of its autumnal months,—
the comparatively low temperature of its spring, and
its hot summers.   The nature, too, of the adjoining
country—of the high naked moorland, which stretches
northwards immediately from the outskirts of the

* Ovid's notice of the place of his exile is still strictly applicable
to the adjoining country :—a country still without a tree, without
the vine, without the apple; where the rivers and sea are frozen in
winter; where creaking waggons, of rude construction, drawn by
oxen, are still in use, and constitute, as of old, the chief possession of
the poor natives; who, now as then, are bearded, and, excepting the
face, completely covered with a dress formed principally of sheep-
skin; and who still leave the earth unploughed, unsown, partly, it
may be, in dread of an invading enemy.—(*Vide* Tristium, lib. iii.,
10, el *et passim*).   From Constangie to the Danube, a distance of
about forty miles, the whole way, as far as the eye can reach, excepting very near the Danube, the low, almost flat, country, is such
as that alluded to ; and poor and naked as it is, it is not without
marks of hostile invasion, viz., that of the Russians, in 1827.

city, presenting an extraordinary contrast with the beautiful and highly cultivated shores of the Bosphorus, is not less favourable, in a limited way, to the peculiarities alluded to. There, the snow lies in winter; from thence, damp fogs, proceeding from the Black Sea, pour down in the spring months, chilling the air of the warmer valleys; and in summer, when parched and heated, this desert surface by day rather increases than mitigates the heat and dryness of the passing wind.

Before offering any remarks on the climate of Constantinople, in relation to health, it may not be amiss to notice some of the habits of the people, especially as regards dress, habitations, and way of living, which, on account of their peculiarities, can hardly fail to have a considerable effect on health.

The old national oriental dress of the Turkish people is still in common use, excepting amongst the military and those employed in the public service, who, in obedience to the orders of the late Sultan, enforced by the present, have substituted the fez— the cylindrical high red cap with a blue tassel—for the skull-cap and the turban; the frock-coat of the Franks for the caftán or loose Turkish gown; the close fitting trowsers, suspended by bracers, for the ample loose shalwár or Turkish drawers, drawn by a running string in its waist-band round the loins; and lastly, the tight European boot, to which the foot is made to conform, for the easy natural-shaped shoe or boot and its slipper.

The oriental dress may well be advocated against the western, as founded on principle and reason, and approved by experience—not the production of caprice or fashion. The intent of it appears to be, to defend the head, for which the turban is so well adapted ; to keep the feet dry and moderately warm ; the loins well girded and warm ; the chest free and cool ; and the neck free, without any pressure on its blood-vessels, depending for warmth on the beard. All who have made trial of the Turkish costume have, I believe, expressed approval of it—regarding merely their comfort, its suitableness to the climate, the ease with which it is worn—independent of its beauty and picturesqueness of effect. As regards the feet, it secures from corns and bunions, which, until the introduction of the tight boot, were unknown amongst the Turks. As regards the loins, the folds of the shalwár, and the pressure there applied by the waistband, are a good protection from lumbago and dysentery. The turban is equally a defence from the sabre, the sun's rays, and the cold blast.

The change of dress has been ill received, and probably will not be permanent. All who have it in their power, on going home, resume, more or less, the costume of their ancestors. The aversion to the new costume is shown in the negligent adoption of it. The stock is little worn by the Turkish soldier, and a slipper very generally—preserving the shuffling gait in the march of the infantry.*

* The sandal has been proposed to be substituted for the boot

The dress of the Turkish women continues unaltered ; indeed, whilst I was in Constantinople, a suspected disposition to expose more of the charms of the face was opposed by an edict expressly on the subject, requiring a strict observance of the ancient rule of propriety. In principle, the female costume is similar to the male ;—avoiding ligature, excepting about the loins; allowing the limbs to be free in their movements, and affording a graceful drapery, not designed to display the form of the individual limbs, and well suited to decorum and a modest nature. The yashmac—the veil of the women—holds the place of the manly turban ; it covers the head, the neck, and the whole of the face, excepting the eyes and nose ; and the feridjee, or loose cloak or mantle, performs the same service for the rest of the body, excepting the hands and feet. The under-clothing of both sexes is very similar ; and, whether shirt or waistcoat, boddice or drawers, is on the same plan of easy looseness.*

amongst the Turkish troops. As regards service, no doubt, it would prove an excellent substitute ; but it is questionable that it would be approved by the Mussulman, accustomed to the convenient slipper. It is this which he takes off in going into a mosque, or even into a barrack-room : it is not necessary, as it is commonly supposed, on entering the former, to bare the feet—the object being merely cleanliness, which the removal of the slipper insures.

* The form of Turkish drawers is well fitted for the dressing-room ; having no opening in front, and of ample dimensions, it is easily slipped on on rising ; and confining a large quantity of air, it is well fitted to prevent the lower part of the body from being chilled, on which account it is not undeserving of the attention of persons of

The Turkish houses in Constantinople, as it is well known, are commonly of wood. The best of them, of ample dimensions, gaily painted, are pleasing to the eye; and all of them, however poor, are, from their form, invariably picturesque. Even the most splendid of the palaces of the sultan are of the same destructible material. The preference is given to wood by the Turks, not chiefly on account of economy, but from the persuasion that it is more wholesome than stone ; and also, it is said, from a feeling of humility, it being considered by them presumptuous to dwell in buildings like their mosques, made, as it were, for eternity, and keeping no measure with the frailty of the occupants. The idea of the unwholesomeness of stone buildings is not, perhaps, without foundation in such a climate. The stone houses in Galata, built by the Genoese, with walls of extraordinary thickness, are of bad repute. Unless the rooms are kept warm in winter, they must be damp in the spring and early summer; so long as the walls are cold, on the occurrence of a southerly wind, they will act as refrigeratories, and occasion a precipitation of moisture from the humid warm air. The thin walls of wood, on the contrary, conform more to the temperature of the atmosphere. None of the sitting-rooms of the houses

delicate constitutions and of invalids, especially when travelling. It answers very well even when made of muslin, so as to occupy very little space in a carpet-bag or portmanteau. The Turkish shirt may be mentioned with commendation as an excellent night-shirt—without collar—nicely fitted to the shoulders, with ample sleeves.

have fixed fire-places or chimneys, they are heated in winter chiefly by a charcoal-fire, contained in the open mangal, or covered tandour.* The mode of warming their rooms is also suitable to the manner in which they are constructed. The crevices in the wooden work allow of a certain admixture of common air and escape of carbonic acid gas, sufficient to prevent any dangerous accumulation of the gas, so that the rooms are easily warmed, and kept warm and dry, without risk of life.†

Their manner of living—their habits of life—require little remark, they are so well and generally known. Fashion is as little concerned in them as in their dress, and they are equally oriental and primi-

* The mangal is a brazier (one copper vessel within another—the latter, it may be, gilded or plated), of graceful form, and often high price—its size and value being, in some measure, in proportion to the rank and wealth of the individual using it. The tandour is a brazier, covered with a wadded coverlet, sustained by a wooden frame. In the latter, there being little circulation of air, the consumption of fuel is very slow, and the fire is long retained; it will keep-in twenty-four hours, affording a mild warmth. The tandour is often the gathering-place of the family party amongst the Franks of the Levant; sitting round it as a table, their feet and legs, beneath the coverlet, are kept of an agreeable warmth, more agreeable, it is probable, than wholesome.

† I never heard of any fatal accident from the use of charcoal fires in Constantinople, although no precautions are taken to prevent them. Headach, however, is a common effect of breathing an atmosphere containing an undue proportion of carbonic acid gas. Were the doors and windows of Turkish rooms suddenly made air-tight, and the fissures in the wood-work closed, there being no chimney to give vent to the fixed air, half the population of Constantinople might be suffocated any winter night between sunset and sunrise.

tive, and domestic. Their household furniture consists chiefly of cushions. They are independent of
chairs, and tables, and bedsteads. A low couch is
their ordinary seat; a mattress spread on the floor,
on a mat, or carpet, their bed, provided with pillows,
sheets, and coverlet. Neither forks or knives, or
plates, are used at their meals. Sitting round the
circular tray, raised on a low stool, with washed
hands, using the fingers of the right hand, each helps
himself from the well-dressed dish, or with a horn or
wooden spoon, if liquid or of soft consistence. Their
best cookery is elaborate—their dishes various and
excellent. Dinner is their principal meal, which is
served after sunset, after the termination of the
labours of the day. Coffee and sherbet are their
principal drinks ;* these, at all hours, with pipes, are
presented to visitors. They rise early, and early
retire to rest. After the last call to prayer the streets
are deserted. The vapour-bath is used by them re-

---

* People of all classes in Constantinople use these drinks. A good
cup of strong coffee may be had for a farthing, and a glass of sherbet
for little more. Their coffee is made in a simple, easy manner—and
most expeditiously. When a single cup is called for, the attendant
in the coffee-house pours hot water into a little copper pan, or rather
pot; puts it over a charcoal fire for an instant to make it boil; then
adds a proportion of well ground or pounded coffee, either alone or
mixed with sugar : returns it again to the fire, to boil for an instant,
and the coffee is made. It is poured, boiling hot, into a small porcelain cup, and handed to the customer ; the coarser grounds quickly
subside, in a few seconds, whilst cooling down to the drinking point.
Disagreeable at first, a taste for this strong unclarified coffee is soon
acquired. It is an excellent and safe substitute for a dram.

gularly, and commonly at least once a-week. Wealthy persons have a bath-establishment in their own houses. The public baths are numerous, and of prices suited to all ranks.* The baths, the mosques, the bazaars, and pleasant shaded spots on the banks of the Bosphorus are the principal places of resort;—the last mentioned in the fine season, when they delight to live in the open air, and form pic-nic parties—the women and men, as at home, always eating apart. As their manner of living is as suitable to the camp as the city, they adopt with great ease the military life. Last year in the spring, when the sultan resided for a

* The Turkish baths, as it is well known, are vapour-baths. The temperature of the inner room or Sudatorium, I have never found to exceed 98° F., though, judging from the sensation experienced, it might be inferred to be very much higher. The effects of the bath are two-fold,—one connected with the perspiration excited; the other with the perfect cleansing of the skin. The former is not without danger to persons of a full habit, disposed to apoplexy. The latter may be considered always salutary. It is effected by friction, by means of a glove, made of the silky hair or wool of the Angora goat. The form of the glove is that of a bag, just large enough to hold the hand. It is an article which might be introduced into this country with advantage, as a substitute for the coarse, harsh horse-hair glove at present in use for the purpose of friction, better fitted (as was remarked to me by a distinguished physician), for the hide of the rhinoceros than for the human skin. So cheap is the bath-glove in Constantinople, that it is within the reach of the poorest people; one costs half a piastre, little more than a penny. If imported, it might be sold with a large profit, at fourpence or sixpence a-pair. It is equally fitted for the purpose of ablution with soap and water, supplying the place of a sponge, and for dry-rubbing, in place of the flesh-brush.

Their tooth-brushes, as well as their bath-gloves, are deserving of notice. They are not of hogs'-bristles, like ours (the Mussulman ab-

short time in a small palace at the " Sweet Waters,"
his court was encamped around him, and the ground,
including a circuit of several miles, was kept and carefully guarded by a cordon of troops stationed on the
adjoining hills.

As regards health, the climate of Constantinople
appears to be good, not productive of more disease
than might be expected from the vicissitudes of temperature to which we have seen it is liable.   The diseases most common are inflammations, especially of
the lungs and its investing membrane, and bowel complaints.   The latter, probably, are as much connected
with irregularities of diet and the use of crude fruits,
to which the Turks are partial, as with the sudden

horring every thing belonging to this animal as impure), but of wood
—the branch or root of a tree that grows in Syria, of a fibrous structure, with a tough, strong, reticulated envelope of bark.   The fibrous
wood is impregnated with a bitter gummy matter.   For use, a portion of the bark, about an inch, is removed, and the decorticated end,
after having been soaked in water, is beaten with a mallet; thus a
brush is produced.   The daily use of it appears to be equally serviceable to the gums and teeth, cleaning the one, and rendering firm the
other.   The bitter gummy substance probably has a beneficial effect.
Another kind of wood is also used, which is even more esteemed.   Its
wood has a pungent aromatic flavour.   The estimation in which both
are held by the Turks is very great.   I have heard a learned mufti
descant on their virtues, attributing to them no less than forty good
qualities.   He ended his discourse by a caution, that the brushes
should never be placed horizontally, but always inclined, or, what is
best, perpendicularly—the objection to the horizontal position being
the very serious one of turning the owner mad.   This is one of the
many instances that have come to my knowledge of the extreme superstition of these people, arising, no doubt, from their ignorance of
the physical sciences.

changes in the temperature of the atmosphere. Typhus fever, too, may be mentioned as a prevalent disease in winter amongst the lower classes and the troops; * and fever with gastric and intestinal derangement during the summer and autumn. On the score of exemption, or little liability, several important diseases may be enumerated, as intermittent and remittent fevers,† insanity, gout, scrofula, and pulmonary consumption. The little tendency to insanity amongst the Turks is very remarkable. For the whole of Constantinople there are only two receptacles for lunatics—one for men, one for women ; and the total number of patients, when I saw them, did not exceed forty.‡ Their

* In the winter of last year, typhus-fever proved very destructive amongst the troops in Constantinople and its neighbourhood. It was considered, and probably justly, contagious. Its origin was obscure ; it was most generally attributed to the bad quality of meat supplied to them, and to undue exposure to the weather on sentinel duty during the cold season.

† Spots in the neighbourhood, it is reported, are not exempt, as the beautiful suburb Eyoub and the adjoining valley of " Sweet Waters," in the beginning of summer ; and the village of Therapia, on the Bosphorus, in autumn.

‡ The miserable state in which these wretched lunatics are kept, calls for severe reprehension ;—it is disgraceful to the Turkish government—an opprobrium on Turkish humanity. In cold cells, in the winter season (there was snow on the ground when I saw them), with barred unglazed windows, the poor men are chained by the neck to the wall by a heavy iron chain, about six feet in length,—a space to which their exercise is limited. No medical aid is afforded them. They are open to the public gaze, and subject to irritation of an aggravated kind from mischievous boys and lads, who, as I witnessed, seemed to take a pleasure in tormenting them, making, even by blows, the violent doubly furious. In consistency with their treatment, the insane establishment is contiguous to a menagerie ; one has

little liability to this sad malady is probably, in a great measure, connected with their temperance, especially their abstinence from ardent spirits. The greater the abuse of ardent spirits, so in proportion, it would appear, is the prevalence of mental disease. Thus it exists in no small degree in England, in a greater in Ireland, and in a still greater degree in Scotland. Other circumstances may promote a healthy state of brain amongst the Turks and comparative exemption from its worst class of maladies—such as the mental faculties not being overwrought, the ordinary tranquillity and regularity of their lives, and their resignation under misfortune to the dispensations of Providence. Perhaps, too, their being little subject to scrofulous disease may be another cause of exemption, it being now generally admitted that scrofula and insanity are often connected,—the changes produced by the one in the intellectual organ being, it may be inferred, productive of the symptoms constituting the other.

The exemption of the Turks from gout is probably also in part dependent on their abstinence from fermented liquors, and in part on the regular use of the vapour-bath. That it is not owing to temperance in eating (a virtue they do not lay claim to) is marked by the obesity commonly prevalent amongst the inhabitants of the capital in easy circumstances. Whe-

to pass through the yard containing the cages, in which a few wild beasts are exhibited, to enter that in which are the cells of the lunatics; and the payment for both is the same.

ther the composition of their dishes, their common fare, is concerned in the exemption in question, it is not easy to determine; vegetables enter largely into them, and butter and *grasso*, to our taste, in excessive proportion.

I have mentioned pulmonary consumption amongst the diseases to which the inhabitants of Constantinople are little liable. This I do not consider as proved in so satisfactory a manner as the exemption of the Turks from gout, and their comparative exemption from insanity. Where *post-mortem* examinations are never instituted,—where no statistical returns are made of diseases and of mortality,—and where the number of enlightened physicians is small, it is not surprising that the conclusion relative to the rareness of this disease should be matter of conjectural, rather than of certain, knowledge. Supposing the conjecture to be well-founded, as, after collecting the best available information on the subject, I believe it is, there are circumstances in the habits of the people and their manner of living, which may conduce to prevent the formation of tubercles, the organic cause of this deplorable, and amongst us, most fatal malady. I shall enumerate what may perhaps be considered the principal, and merely enumerate them, as to discuss them would almost require a volume. They are, as it appears to me, early marriages; early hours; little exposure to the night air; warm clothing; the use of the yasmac by the women when they go into the open air, by which

the air-passages are in a measure protected as by the
respirator; and the wearing of the moustache and
beard by the men, which has a somewhat similar
effect; the manner in which their rooms, without
chimneys, are warmed, incompatible with currents of
cold air, and productive of a dry state of air; and
lastly, their indulgence in the open air when the
weather is favourable,—as it is during the hot season
of summer and the warm autumnal season,—and
their disposition to relax and amuse themselves, in a
quiet way, without dissipation,—to which the use of
the bath may also conduce,—and their fondness for
and constant use of the pipe and coffee.

I have sometimes been asked, Is the climate of
Constantinople a fit one for invalids? From the
particulars already given, it may be conjectured, that
the answer I have felt it right to give, has been
negative. Not only is the climate, during the greater
part of the year, unfavourable to those who are in
delicate or precarious health, but likewise other circumstances,—especially the want of comfort in the
inns and lodging-houses of Pera,—the difficulty
that attends taking exercise, owing to the wretched
state of the streets and roads, with the bad description of carriages in use,—and the want of agreeable
society and all rational amusement. For a short
time, as between the middle of May and the middle
of June, the weather is generally delightful, the perfection of fine weather; the temperature between
60° and 70°; the shores of the Bosphorus in full

beauty. This is the time to see Constantinople to advantage, and to feel its attractions. To the traveller in good health, the enjoyment will be of a very high kind. But the invalid should not be seduced by the temptation. To him the difficulty will be in arriving there without suffering, at the enjoyable season, and in retiring from it, without risk of mischief. If he come by the Mediterranean, he will suffer from heat,—if by the route of the Danube, he is likely to suffer from cold; and in going away he exposes himself to greater annoyances,—to still hotter weather by sea,—and to heat and the torment of insects on the Danube,*—and to danger of malaria-fever whilst performing quaran-

---

* From May to August insects, particularly musquitoes, are extremely numerous on the Danube, and excessively troublesome, forming a serious objection to proceeding by this route. After August they almost entirely disappear. Whether the whole course of the river is infested by them, or only the lower part of it, I do not know. At Orsova, they are spoken of as a plague, and also in the adjoining lazaretto of Schupanack. This lazaretto, at the same season, is considered unwholesome; persons performing quarantine there, are liable to attacks of ague, and occasionally of severe remittent fever. The situation is close, surrounded by hills, and excessively hot in summer,—singularly contrasted with the cool, salubrious, delightful Miadia, about twelve miles distant in the interior,— the resort, during the hot season, of the gentry of the surrounding provinces,—some attracted by its sulphureous waters, others by the natural beauty of the spot, its excellent accommodations, and agreeable society. Its remarkable coolness it probably owes chiefly to being in the shade of enormous precipices of limestone, and on the bank of a clear, cold mountain stream (in which the trout is described as being always in good condition), and also to the profusion of wood on the adjoining hills.

tine.   Another short period of pleasant weather is
the latter part of autumn, viz., the greater part of
October and the early part of November.   Then the
active traveller can again derive enjoyment from
Constantinople and its environs ; but the objections
which ought to weigh against the visit of the invalid
are not lessened ; the weather is hardly so certain as
in the early summer, and the risk from travelling is
rather increased than diminished.

CHAPTER XVI.

NOTICE OF SOME OF THE PUBLIC INSTITUTIONS IN CON-
STANTINOPLE, IN CONNEXION WITH THE PRESENT
STATE OF TURKEY.

Opposite Hypotheses respecting the Present Condition of the Turkish
Empire. Opinion of their Futility. Military Hospitals in Constantinople and its Neighbourhood, Described. Naval Academy.
Military College. Medical School. How defective. Notice of
the great Barracks belonging to the Capital. Of the Quarantine
Establishment. Of some of the Government Manufactories.
Contrast between them and the Native Work-Shops—between
the New and the Old Schools—as demonstrative of different
Periods. Prospect of Improvement, founded on the Capacity of
the Turkish Youth. Observations on the Vices of the Government, connected with the Training of Official Men. Conjectures
respecting Reform, and Revival of Power, on the Supposition that
the People are little changed, and that existing Abuses may be
Swept away by a Master-mind. Farther Conjectures on the
same Subject. Remarks on the Rayah-Christian Population.

Two hypotheses are at present entertained relative
to the existing condition of Turkey. According to
one, the Turkish people are in their infant state, full
of life and susceptibility, but uninformed, uneducated,
weak ; and, if their existence as a nation be precarious, it is so in consequence of infirmities analogous

to those of infancy.   According to the other hypothesis, the empire is in its old age, worn out, exhausted, tottering, unable to stand unaided, from sheer and
unreclaimable debility.   Neither of these hypotheses
I apprehend to be just, because both are founded on
analogies, which, however specious, are not applicable,
with any strictness, to races of men or empires,—the
rise, decline, and fall of which seem to depend on a
complication of circumstances of difficult analysis.

One hundred and fifty years ago, equally extreme
views were taken of the political condition of Turkey.
Then it was considered, too, in its exhausted old age,
and its empire about to expire.   The visible tokens
of decline were not less conspicuous and in favour of
the worst prognostics.   A Kiuprili appeared,* and in
a few short years effected a revival—imparted strength
and energy, where before there was only debility and
languor.   And I imagine, if such a man were to
appear now and to guide the helm of government,
like results might follow, and the Turkish power
might again be formidable.

But I am anticipating a conclusion which existing
circumstances hardly seem to warrant; most of them,
indeed, are apparently more in favour of the old age
and worn-out hypothesis.

These circumstances are tolerably apparent in all
the public institutions of the capital which I had an
opportunity of examining, chiefly military hospitals,

* Kiuprili Mustafa Pasha was appointed Vizier in 1689.

schools, and colleges. Of these I propose now to give
a brief account; partly with a view to the recording
of their condition, at, it may be, a critical time, and
to the inferences deducible from them as marks of
the government; and partly with a hope, far, indeed,
from sanguine, that the notice of these defects may
meet the eye of some individual interested in their
improvement, with influence to promote it, and effect
more than oral exhortation on the spot could accomplish.

The military and naval hospitals which I visited
were five in number, all of them situated in the
suburbs or vicinity of the capital. I shall enumerate
them in the order of their size and importance. 1*st*,
The hospital of Maltepeh, calculated for 1200 patients,
situated about four miles from Eyoub, on the rising
ground between the two great barracks of Daoud
Pasha and Ramistchiftlik, from each about a mile
apart; 2*d*, The hospital of the imperial guard at
Scutari, calculated for 500 patients; 3*d*, The arsenal
or naval hospital of Sakiz Aghateh, built on a height
a little above the arsenal, calculated for the same
number; 4*th*, The military hospital in Tophana, capable of holding about two hundred patients, which
was crowded with three hundred; and, 5*th*, The
small naval hospital of Epleckcanai, or that of the
rope-walk, on the shore of the Golden Horn, a little
below Eyoub, calculated for one hundred and fifty
patients.

As regards the buildings—their equipment in the

important articles of bedding and dresses, the number of servants in attendance, the number of medical officers attached, the state of the wards as to cleanliness and order—there was little occasion for finding fault ; indeed, in some particulars, especially the bedding and dresses, one was rather disposed to praise. The bedding * was generally superior to that in use in our military hospitals, and the dresses† of much better description.   The faulty parts were a bad system of administration—no subordination—a want of method and carelessness in the conducting of the medical duties—and a culpable neglect in supplying many articles of medicine and diet required.

These establishments are under the orders of the Seraskier, the commander-in-chief of the army ; or of the Capitan-pasha, the commander-in-chief of the navy ; and all of them are under the nominal superintendence of the Hakem-bashi, the chief physician of

---

* The beds were invariably raised from the ground, supported by boards and trestles, the latter commonly of iron.   The bedding consisted of two mattresses—the upper of wool or cotton, the lower of hair or hay—of one or two pillows, of cotton sheets, and a coverlet ; the sheets not loose, but tacked to the coverlet and mattress as a lining.   Even itch-patients had the comfort of beds of this description —a treatment singularly contrasted with that in use in the British military hospitals, the itch-ward of which is an abomination (the men in it lying on boards, naked, excepting the covering of a single blanket), worthy only of the hold of a slaver.

† The hospital-dresses consist of a warm padded cap, nicely fitting to the head ; a cotton shirt and drawers, and a warm cotton gown or great-coat, with a pair of slippers.   The hospital utensils, the plates, bowls, and drinking cups, are of a good description, and very durable, being of tinned copper.

the sultan—a Turk—the head of the medical profession, in its various departments throughout the empire. Belonging to the ulemah, holding a distinguished rank in that order, invested with high judicial powers, he is as little qualified as inclined to inspect hospitals, and inquire into the care of the sick. He was expected, it was said, at all the hospitals at the time of our visit, it having been an official one, by the desire of the government—but he never appeared. At one of them, there is reason to believe, that he was expected in reality—for it was newly washed and decked with flowers—a compliment to him.

Each hospital is under the immediate charge of an officer, a Turk, in the joint capacity of commandant and commissary, who has the control of the establishment and the management of its supplies, aided by a clerk, or clerks, and ward-masters, according to the extent of 'duties.   He draws supplies by requisitions —unchecked, and liable to great abuse ; his accounts are unaudited, as is the case generally in Turkey in the government departments—all public accounts being kept in such an imperfect and irregular way as to defy satisfactory examination.

The medical officers are of three classes—physicians, surgeons, and apothecaries; most of them are Franks and adventurers, appointed without examination as to qualification ; owing their appointment to favour, and insecure of holding it.   Ill paid as most of them are,*—not respected, without rank in regu-

* The pay of medical officers in the Turkish service varies from

lar gradation, without a commission, without half-pay, liable to be dismissed without inquiry, even without warning,—is it surprising that they spare themselves as much as possible, perform their duties as easily as possible (if the term be applicable to such performance), and make, as far as they can, a convenience of the service? Their regular visit is restricted to once a-day in the morning, and it may occupy about an hour. It is not repeated in the evening; one of each class remaining, in succession, as orderly officer, in case of emergencies. Each physician and assistant-physician is attended at the bed-side of the sick by an apothecary, who writes on a scroll of paper the medicine prescribed from dictation, and marks the diet. No returns are required from them, no registers are kept by them, no reports are made by them.* The duties of the surgeons are confined chiefly to the dressing of wounds and sores, and the minor operations of surgery,—as blood-letting, the opening of boils, &c. An important or delicate operation is rarely attempted; instruments are deficient,†—the skill and requisite knowledge are com-

---

3000 piastres a month to 200, *i. e.* from twenty-seven to two pounds sterling. Few, however, have more than 2000 piastres monthly, the majority about 1000. The rate of pay is very much a matter of favour.

* The only return made is one (of admissions, discharges, and deaths), by the commandant of the hospital to the seraskier, or in the instance of the imperial guard, to the high officer commanding that body, to be submitted to the Sultan.

† In the large hospital of Maltepeh, in which, at the time of our visit, 390 patients were under the charge of fifteen medical officers, five of each class, there were no surgical instruments, excepting a few

monly wanting. In the hospital of the Imperial Guard, containing, on an average, above three hundred patients, an amputation even had not been performed for many years. The instruments belonging to its surgical department were comprised in an old case,—judging from its appearance more than a century old,—and out of repair and unfit for use. The medicines are obtained on requisition from a central pharmacy, which has to furnish supplies for the whole of the army and navy, but is so scantily provided as to be quite inadequate to meet the wants of either service. The medical officers are required and are obliged to exercise a miserable economy in prescribing, and to limit themselves very much to the ordering of simples, such as infusion of camomile flowers, gum-water, infusion of Iceland moss, and the like, in place of more expensive and energetic drugs. A like wretched parsimony is followed in the dieting of the sick.* The regular diets are of the simplest

scarificators for cupping,—not even a catheter or turniquet; if required, they could be procured only from the central depôt, several miles distant.

* The following is the scale of diets in use in the arsenal hospital, from which that followed in the other hospitals differs but little :—

1. Rice in water, thirty drachms per diem.
2. Rice in water, thirty drachms; bread, one-fourth.
3. Rice in water, thirty drachms; bread, one-half.
4. (Quarter diet). Rice in broth, thirty drachms; bread, three-fourths.
5. (Half diet). Rice in broth, thirty drachms; bread, four-fourths; meat, fifty drachms.
6. (Three-quarter diet). Rice in broth, thirty drachms; bread, five-fourths; meat, fifty drachms.

kind: the lowest, rice-water; the highest, rice, bread, and meat. Extra articles of diet are said to be allowed, but are not actually permitted. I have heard a humane physician lamenting the restrictions he was under: he could not procure milk for patients labouring under dysentery or phthisis; neither an egg, or an orange, or a lemon was permitted. I have seen a poor lad thrusting out his emaciated arm, with a small coin in his hand, begging his medical attendant to allow a lemon to be bought, for which, with parched lips and tongue, he had a longing.

As might be expected, the mortality amongst the patients is occasionally very great. In the hospital of the Imperial Guard, during six months, viz., from November 1840 to the end of the following May, it amounted to 16 per cent. of those admitted, which, considering the class of patients, chiefly young soldiers, is enormous;* and at the Maltepeh Hospital, during the same period, I was informed the loss of

7. (Full diet). Rice, thirty drachms; bread, six-fourths; meat, a hundred drachms.

The loaf of bread, portioned as above, weighs from ninety-eight to a hundred drachms. The quality of it varies; in the hospital of the Imperial Guard, it is of one quality—good white bread; in the other hospitals, this description of bread is restricted to the fever cases; the other patients have brown bread, similar to that supplied to the troops.

* The following return, for which I was indebted to the colonel-commandant of the hospital of the Imperial Guard, shows the mortality amongst the soldiers treated there, during twelve consecutive months, in 1840–41, amounting, on the whole, to the high number of 11.4 per cent. The document, probably, is not much to be

life was even greater; during the three last months of it, when the severity of sickness had abated, it amounted to 12.4 per cent.

In these brief notices, I have understated the evils of the existing system, under which the military and naval hospitals in the neighbourhood of the capital are conducted,—a system of much expense,*—of idle forms, without a just guiding principle, and without efficacy,—the shadow of a substance rather than the thing itself.

If such be the state of the hospitals about the capital, under ordinary circumstances, what can be expected of them in the remote provinces, and during the existence of an epidemic such as cholera or

depended on for accuracy, judging from the want of accordance, in several instances, between the figures in the respective columns.

Months.	Sick re-maining.	Admitted.	Dis-charged.	Died.	Remain-ing.
May, ...	204	135	217	25	97
June, ...	97	233	295	13	122
July, ...	122	261	264	8	111
August, ...	111	275	217	12	157
September, . . .	157	777	632	20	282
October, ...	282	234	278	43	195
November, . . .	195	245	251	62	327
December, . . .	327	493	471	96	393
January, ...	293	652	475	86	344
February, . . .	244	598	507	86	349
March, ...	349	394	427	58	248
April, ...	248	301	264	52	233

* No stoppage is made from the pay of the Turkish soldier, whilst in hospital, as in our service: his small pay of twenty piastres a-month is allowed to accumulate.

Amongst the hospital expenses, the pay of servants is considerable. In the hospital of the Imperial Guard, the number of servants altogether was sixty (the patients 223), with a pay to each of thirty piastres a-month, besides rations and clothes. In this number washermen are included, and others occupied in repairing dresses and bedding.

the plague, or after the storming of a town or a great
battle.   Under such circumstances, I have reason to
believe that their state baffles description; the sick
are left to die neglected; the wounded are left to
die neglected; the loss of life is terrible; the effect
on the minds of the survivors appalling.   What has
come to my knowledge during the recent campaign
in Syria, after the taking of Acre, and subsequently,
whilst plague prevailed in that province,—in brief,
during the whole period that our troops were stationed in the country, fully bears me out in the
above remarks.   The inefficiency of the medical
branch of the service there was deplorable :—hospitals sometimes without medical officers; medical
officers without medicines; surgeons without instruments; and the majority of the so-called medical
officers mere pretenders, uneducated, taken from ser-
vile situations ;—as a whole, such a system of inefficiency, blunder, and ignorance, exceeds the ordinary
powers of imagination.

The Turks have the reputation of being charitable
and humane.   I believe the feeling exists amongst
them; it is a feeling belonging to human nature; it
is strongly inculcated by their religion.   But there
is little public proof of it; not a single Turkish hospital for the reception of the sick-poor exists in Constantinople; not a single dispensary.   Their charity
has not yet gone beyond the distribution of food—
the establishment of alms-houses.   And it probably
has been so limited, in consequence of the low state

of medical science in the country, in common with the East generally, and the ignorance of the people on the subject of medical relief, ably and judiciously administered. It would be unreasonable to expect that a people unacquainted with mechanics, totally uninstructed in the physical sciences, should form a railway or construct a steam-boat. Two things are required as preliminaries—knowledge to originate the attempt, and skill to execute it. The public mind in Turkey, in a similar manner, in relation to medical institutions, requires to be enlightened, to become conscious of the need and advantage of such establishments ; and when enlightened, medical men will be required, who are not at present to be found amongst the natives, competent to take charge of them and conduct them successfully.

In connexion with the hospitals, it may not be amiss to notice briefly the barracks belonging to the capital, for the accommodation of the troops. They are so many and so large as to be capable of holding sixty thousand men ; three of them alone are calculated for twenty-five thousand men. These are—the magnificent barrack of the Imperial Guard, at Scutari, with complete accommodations for three regiments, each of three thousand men ; and the two great barracks of Daoud Pasha and Ramistchiftlik, outside the walls of Constantinople, in the situation already alluded to when noticing the hospital of Maltepeh, each capable of holding about eight thousand men. These and the barracks of Constantinople

generally, are superior, in many respects, to any barracks which I have seen at home. They chiefly
excel in the loftiness of the rooms, in the judicious
means of ventilation, and in the conveniences attached
to them. Most of them are built in the form of a
hollow square, including a considerable extent of
parade-ground. Their entrance is generally a handsome gateway, within a portico, surmounted by apartments for the reception of the Sultan, elegantly furnished. They are commonly of two stories, each
consisting of a spacious well-lighted gallery or passage, and of rooms opening into it, lighted by numerous windows in the outer wall, and admitting of
ventilation by a window looking into the passage,
over each door. In the smaller barracks, as in the
Cavalry Barrack, close to the English burying-ground,
above Pera, and in the Infantry Barrack, adjoining
the official residence of the Seraskier in Constantinople, a different construction is observed, well fitted
also for ventilation. The building is surrounded by
a double gallery, the upper one supported by columns,
not unlike a gallery in an English church, open
within, without partitions, making one uninterrupted
large room. The rooms in the great barracks are of
different sizes, some calculated for fifty men, some for a
hundred. The men sleep on a platform raised about a
foot, on a short mattress, with a coverlet. The rooms
I visited were in excellent order. In the gallery or
corridor of the barrack of the Imperial Guard, there
are marble fountains, where the men are required to

wash their feet before entering their rooms. The kitchens in this barrack, the wash-houses, the store-rooms are excellent, as is also its pharmacy. An air of grandeur and of splendour pervades the whole, which is very striking. In the great kitchens (one for each regiment), the boilers are fixed in a platform of marble ; they communicate with each other and with the open air by a tube, attached to the covers of each pair, preventing the unpleasant and unwholesome effect arising from the escape of steam into the room. The wash-houses, where the men wash their own linen, are furnished with troughs or basins for the purpose, of white marble, and are amply supplied with hot water by pipes. They are sufficiently large to permit of fifty men being occupied in them at the same time. The store-rooms for the clothing of the troops are furnished with presses, with glass fronts, in which, in summer, the winter clothing of the men is laid up in safety, and in a very neat and orderly manner ; and, in winter, their summer dresses. There are no barracks apart for the officers ; men and officers are all under the same roof ; and the subaltern officers are little better accommodated than the private soldiers. Even captains have not each a separate apartment ; a room is allotted to four.

It might be expected that, in such good quarters, apparently so well taken care of, and with an ample allowance of food, exempt as the Turkish soldier is from the temptation of the canteen, and of drunkenness, the Turkish troops would be distinguishedly

healthy.   But I believe this is far from the case, and
that they suffer from disease in a high ratio, and especially from typhus fever and nostalgia (home sickness).   I have already alluded to the supposed causes
of the former.   The latter is connected, no doubt,
with the manner in which the army is recruited, on
a severe conscription-plan, and the listless life to
which the young soldier is subjected, when not actively engaged in the field, without the resources
which our men find, as I once heard a facetious person observe, in making love, and in getting drunk,—
the one being as strictly prohibited by the Sultan, as
the other is by their prophet.   A circumstance leading
to severity of disease amongst the troops, is the
neglect of it in its early stage, owing to the careless
manner in which health-inspections are made, if
made at all, by the regimental medical efficers *, commonly incompetent, and the want of regimental
hospitals.   The barrack establishments, like the hospital ones, afford a striking example of the little
advantage of forms, unless regulated by principle, and
of the abuses to which they are liable, under a bad
system.

The principal schools or colleges instituted by the
government, for the ostensible purpose of supplying

---

* Each regiment has nominally a certain number of medical officers
attached to it, sometimes only one, sometimes more, of the same
description as the individuals employed in the general hospitals;—
under no system, without medicines and instruments, as is commonly
the case, they may be considered altogether useless.

well-educated and efficient officers to the army and navy, are the naval and military academies, and the medical school of Galata Serai.

All three are entirely supported by the government. The students are not only taught without entailing expense on their parents, but are also lodged and fed and clothed, and each has an allowance of pocket-money.

The naval school has been long established; I was informed eighty years: and, notwithstanding, the Sultan has not a sufficient number of officers to command a fleet; I believe it may be stated, without any exaggeration, he has not a sufficient number to take charge even of a frigate. When the fleet, detained by the Pasha of Egypt, returned from Alexandria, it was said that there were only three or four of the captains who could read and write, and were acquainted with the use of the mariner's compass.

The building belonging to the naval school is finely situated on the summit of a hill, within the precincts of the arsenal. It is a handsome substantial edifice, constructed chiefly of marble, white-washed. The number of students in it, nominally in process of education, when I visited it in the spring of 1841, was 260, of different ages, from eight years old to twenty. Three masters had charge of them, with a superintendent. Their teaching was entirely oral; strange to say, no books were used. It was limited to Arabic, a smattering of French, and a little navigation, with the addition of naval architecture, re-

stricted to a limited number. Though books are
dispensed with in the teaching, a printing-press is
attached to the establishment, in the business of
which students are unprofitably employed. The work
in hand, at the time of our visit, was a code of instructions for the regulation of the navy A library,
as it was called, was also attached to it; the collection of books consisted of about fifty volumes, a few
Turkish, a few French, and a few German works. In
the same room were a pair of globes, and a very few
mathematical instruments. In the yard of the building, the fore-half of a vessel was exhibited, with fore-
masts and bowsprit, rigged, and provided with cannon,
for the purpose of exercising the students in gunnery,
teaching them to climb, &c. It was in bad order,
requiring repair, which led to the remark, that there
was not a man in the fleet sufficiently acquainted with
the ropes and sails of a ship, to rig it correctly. It
might be supposed that, close to the Bosphorus, and
within a few hours sail of the two seas, the Black Sea
and the Archipelago, well fitted for a nursery of sailors,
with numerous ships lying at anchor unemployed, a
different and more natural method would be taken
of teaching the students practical navigation.

The military academy or college, the fruits of which
hitherto have been no better than those of the naval,
as has been sadly proved in all the recent campaigns,
is situated on the side of a hill, at a considerable
elevation above Dolmabagdsche, the winter palace
of the Sultan, skirting the Bosphorus. It is a struc-

ture of wood, of two stories, in the form of a hollow square, inclosing a garden; and, though built only a few years (five, as I was informed), it was in want of repair, decaying, and called old. The number of students it contained, when I visited it, was 256, varying in age from twelve to twenty-one. From what I could collect, the system of instruction in use was almost as limited, and as little efficient, as that followed in the naval school, being confined chiefly to languages, Arabic, Persian, and French. The class-rooms, the dormitories, the eating-room, at least showed attention to the comfort of the youth; they were spacious, and well warmed and ventilated. A mosque is attached, and forms a part of the establishment, which every morning the students are required to attend. A library, too, is attached to it; but, from its appearance, it was of little use; never used. The collection of books was larger than that belonging to the naval academy; perhaps twice or thrice as large, consisting chiefly of French works, with which a few English and German were mixed, and a small number of Turkish. There was in the same apartment a small collection of philosophical instruments, many of them of a very antiquated structure, and some plans and drawings of fortified places.

The medical school of Galata Serai is situated in Pera, in a building, or rather a group of buildings, which had been an imperial palace. It was established by the late Sultan, by whom the palace, from which it derives its name, was assigned to it. The number of students belonging to it in 1841 was 260, of various ages from eight to twenty.   Their studies are of two kinds, preparatory and medical, and the teachers are similarly divided.   The preparatory studies,—necessary in consequence of the ignorance of the lads, in many instances, even in the most elementary acquirements,* comprise, the Turkish, Arabic, and French languages, with writing and arithmetic, the first principles of geometry, geography, the elements of zoology and Turkish history.   The course of preparatory instruction occupies three years.   After its completion, if found fit on examination, they enter on their medical studies, also of three years' duration. These are directed by five professors: one who lectures on chemistry and pharmacy; one on anatomy; one on physiology; one on surgery, botany, and materia medica; and one on natural philosophy.   Two of these professors are Germans, two Greeks, and one a Periote.   The German professors, in lecturing, use the French language: each has an assistant, who repeats the discourse in Turkish.

This college as at present organized has been established four years.   Besides its professors, it has a president, an inspector of the classes, and a director. The first is the Hakim Bashi, the chief physician to the Sultan, already alluded to; the last, a well-in-

* According to the regulations of the college no student is admissible who cannot read and write; but, owing to the influence exercised by pashas, many are received who have made little progress in either.

formed German physician, Dr Barnard, who is also professor of surgery, of botany and materia medica, or, at least, gave lectures on these subjects. The inspector of the classes is, or was, a Turk; the appointment, I believe, a sinecure. It was enjoyed by the son of the Hakim Bashi.

As in the other two colleges, the students in this appear to be well taken care of. Their dormitories are two large rooms, with an upper gallery extending the whole length on each side, on the construction of the smaller barracks, in which their beds (one for each student) are arranged, resting on boards and tressels. In each room a guardian is placed to keep order. They take their meals at a common table, at which they sit, using a plate, knife, and fork, and provided with a napkin. They have three meals a-day—an early breakfast, dinner at noon, and supper in the evening. Bread and broth for breakfast; bread and meat, with a portion of vegetables, for dinner; and bread and meat again for supper. Water is their only drink. The diet of the students in the other schools is very similar. It is ample in quantity, the allowance of meat being a pound, and that of the bread rather more, and appears to be favourable to health; for, from what I could collect, the students in each school were generally healthy. In common with the other students they wear a uniform, of a neat description and good material, of the same form as that of officers of the army and navy, with a distinctive mark on the green velvet collar of the coat. From the information which I obtained, it would appear that they were generally well conducted, studious, with good capacities, especially for the acquisition of languages, and that they were making respectable progress. Their advance is yearly tested by public examinations, at which hitherto the Sultan has been present, with his principal ministers, and reward is then given to merit by the distribution of prizes.

Within the precincts of Galata Serai is a botanical garden, yet in a very imperfect state; a library-room, in which, at the time of my visit, there were only a very few books;* an anatomical theatre of a large size, well fitted for the pursuit and study of practical anatomy, hitherto hardly used; a pharmacy, with a depôt of medicines, called the central pharmacy for furnishing supplies of these articles to the army and navy, of a description, as already observed, very inadequate to the wants of either service; an infirmary for sick students, neatly fitted up as an hospital; and a mosque for daily worship. Moreover, in the range of building containing the class-rooms, there are other apartments for various uses. In one was a respectable collection of minerals and of rock speci-

* They were almost entirely French and elementary; there was only one modern professional work in Turkish,—a treatise on anatomy,—said to be an indifferent compilation. This was in the winter of 1841, since which time probably an addition has been made to the collection of a considerable number of standard French works on medicine and the collateral sciences, a list of which had been submitted by the director to the Hakim Bashi, and approved by him.

mens, procured from Germany; in another a variety of philosophical apparatus, many of them of a useful kind, for the purpose of teaching; and, in a third, some anatomical models in wax, and anatomical plates, and two moist preparations, the commencement, it was said, of a pathological museum.

The notice which I have just given of this institution may probably have raised a favourable idea respecting it in the mind of the reader, which, I fear, is not well founded in reality, considering the many defects of the establishment, and its precarious existence—defects owing to want of support on the part of the government, and that want of support owing to ignorance or mistaken views regarding its usefulness.*

Chemistry, of so much importance in connexion with medical science and all the useful arts, is attempted to be taught—without a laboratory, without apparatus, and, consequently, without experiments. The teaching of pharmacy is not better conducted ; nor is the teaching of anatomy. The excellent anatomical theatre has hardly yet been used for the purposes of practical anatomy. And of a piece with this —the teaching of practical medicine and surgery, have been undertaken without an hospital. The defects in the system of teaching have been often and strongly pointed out, in conjunction with the advantages

* The present state of the medical school in Egypt appears to be very similar to that of Galata Serai, and owing to the same causes. In the Appendix will be found an account of it, in a letter addressed to me, written by Dr Robertson, already referred to.

which may be fairly expected from the college, were it liberally maintained and ably conducted—advantages of no ordinary kind, and which ought to make an impression even on uninstructed minds (if uninstructed minds can take in such subjects), if alive to the public good, and to the interests of a great empire. The more important of the advantages enumerated were, the introduction of sound medical knowledge into the country,—the forming of an efficient class of practitioners amongst the natives,—the supplying of the army and navy with good medical officers,—and the rendering both services and the people generally, independent of foreigners for medical aid.

I have noticed the good abilities and disposition to study exhibited by the Turkish youth, on the report of a competent judge. It is these abilities—it is this disposition, which justify the favourable view just taken. It can hardly be doubted that, had the young Turks the same means of education as are available in the schools and universities of Europe, they would prove themselves worthy of them, and that many would be distinguished. It is difficult, if I may judge from my own feelings, to see Turkish boys at play even, without forming a favourable opinion of them—they are so active, bold, and energetic. It would be extraordinary were they without curiosity and a thirst for knowledge. I apprehend they have both, in a degree not inferior to our own youth. The very little that has hitherto been done in practical anatomy at Galata Serai has already been alluded to. The winter before last, only two bodies could be obtained, (and those were of Christians), to make a commencement of the study.   I was present at the first dissection conducted in the anatomical theatre—the first in Constantinople in modern times—and perhaps even the first ever attempted there.   I never saw young students more intent, more interested, as if they fully appreciated the benefit of obtaining valuable knowledge in so direct and impressive a manner, instead of in the dilute, feeble, third-rate way of elementary manuals and barren epitomes.   It was at night that the dissection or demonstration was made; the scene offered a fine subject for the pencil of the artist.   There was no apprehension expressed by the young Mohammedans of being defiled by touching a corpse,—there were no marks of fear—none of disgust—all seemed to be overpowered by the stronger feeling of curiosity and desire of knowledge.

The Turkish government, in most of its measures, has found either defenders or apologists.   The low state of the treasury I have heard assigned as a reason for its not giving that support and assistance to the medical school which it absolutely requires to become efficient.   The same apology has been made for the wretched state of its medical department, including the hospital establishments.   The apology is little else than a subterfuge; the neglect, as I shall endeavour to show further on, is the result of other circumstances connected with vicious administration and selfish views on the part of the governors—the influential few—who, under the sanction of the name of the Sultan, constitute the executive. Low as the treasury is at present, funds do not appear to be wanting to pay the exorbitant salaries of ministers* and other high officers of state, or to show the bounty of the Sultan, even to individuals dismissed from office,† or to preserve an idle form, and add to an almost useless navy. Other public establishments, which may be mentioned, especially the quarantine department and certain manufactories, are most of them hardly less demonstrative of profusion than the preceding are of parsimony.

The quarantine system, which has existed now about four years, dating from the period of its organization, is extensive and costly. The number of distinct stations are, at least, fifty, and these, it is certain, are far from adequate to the wants of the empire, on the principle, that every part of the country is to be under observation, and an account to be rendered regularly to a central board, or superior council of health, of all such occurrences as are liable to affect the public health, and more especially the

* The principal ministers and high officers of state have salaries, varying from about ten thousand to eighteen thousand pounds sterling a-year.

† Just before the late Minister for Foreign Affairs, Reschid Pasha, was dismissed, a present was made to him by the Sultan of a sum of about ten thousand pounds, with a rich decoration—a mark, it was said at the time, by those conversant in the habits of the people—that his influence was on the wane, and his downfall at hand.

breaking out or appearance of any contagious disease, and, above all, of plague.

At each station there is a medical officer and a director of quarantine,—the former, in almost every instance, a Frank,—the latter invariably a Turk. They are reponsible to the government for carrying into effect the quarantine regulations; and the former has to report every fifteenth day, or oftener, to the superior council of health, on every thing of importance connected with the health of the district in which he is placed, and also to the consuls or vice-consuls of the European powers residing there, should a case of plague or of any other contagious disease occur.

The superior council of health is composed of a president, a Turk of high rank,—of a director-general of quarantine, a Frenchman,—of delegates from the respective embassies of the principal European powers, and of other individuals, chiefly medical men, appointed by the government, some of whom receive pay, others not. The duties of this council are to form regulations; to meet in consultation on all matters of importance connected with the public health; and to give their sanction to all sanatory measures issued for the preservation of the same, according to the subjoined form, in the French language, in which their proceedings are conducted, and their regulations drawn up.*

This council is the most important and vital part

* Discuté et approuvé par le Conseil Supérieur de Santé à Constantinople, le   , 184 .

Le Directeur-Général des Quarantaines.

of the system; and it is so in consequence of the members belonging to it, being independent of the Porte, free to offer their opinions conscientiously, and sure of the support and protection of the ambassadors, under whom they act, and to whom they have to report proceedings. It is generally understood that, were it not for their presence and exertions, quarantine, very shortly after its institution, would have been abolished, the Turks generally having an aversion to it, and especially certain influential individuals, who regard it with an eye of jealousy on account of the manner in which the council is constituted.

Of the directors of quarantine, and of the health officers, little can be said in commendation—they are the weak part of the system. The former, being natives, are very ignorant of all that relates to the subject; and, on entering into office, are necessarily totally destitute of experience. Absurd stories are related of the proceedings of some of them on points of quarantine very characteristic of such ignorance, as well as of extreme carelessness and indifference. The health-officers are commonly medical men, imperfectly educated, chiefly French, Italians, and Germans, who, like those employed in the other branches of the public service, have come to Turkey as adventurers. The reports of many of them can be of little value, owing to their very limited knowledge and professional incompetency.

At each station there is or should be a lazaretto.

Most of the lazarettoes are of a bad description, totally unfit for the purpose for which they are designed. A very small number, perhaps, may be excepted, and even these, I believe, at present, are worse than useless, owing to the ill manner in which they are conducted.

Taking into account the comparatively short time that the attempt has been made to establish quarantine in the Turkish dominions, and the many and great difficulties that have been encountered and are still in the way;—difficulties connected with the government, either lukewarm or averse to the measure; the directors little satisfied of the necessity of it; both they and the health officers such as have been described; and lastly, the guardianoes, if possible worse than the directors, with public opinion decidedly and strongly hostile,—it is not surprising that more has not been done to improve the system,—it is rather surprising that it has been tolerated.

The regulations which have hitherto been issued are such as might be expected from the respectable source from whence they have proceeded, viz., the Superior Council of Health. And they have been formed evidently mainly to be in harmony with the regulations of the old sanità establishments of the Mediterranean, and of the countries bordering on Turkey on the European side, with a view, by their improvement, to establish, in the absence of plague, a free intercourse between Turkey and these countries, to the very great advantage of both.*

* Hitherto this advantage has not been enjoyed by Turkey, except-

The principal manufactories belonging to the government are three,—one of gunpowder, one of small arms, and one of cannon.

The gunpowder manufactory is on the shore of the Sea of Marmora, a few miles from the capital, conducted without the aid of any foreigner, by a very able and intelligent Armenian, who has had the advantage of foreign travel through most parts of Europe, engaged in expressly for the purpose of studying the best methods of making gunpowder. About fifteen hundred-weight of powder are made annually, of a quality said to be equal to the English government powder. All the processes are carried on with much skill, and in a very scientific manner. The machinery used is of the best kind: the steam-engine and the air-pump apparatus were imported from England. The mill-stones are of marble. The sulphur used is Sicilian, purified on the spot; the nitre also is purified there: it is entirely the produce of the country, collected in different parts of Roumelia. The charcoal, also, is prepared on the spot, made of the branches of the willow. The neatness and order of the establishment, with the intelligence

ing, indeed, a few weeks' intercourse with the Danube. Probably, even Turkish patience will be exhausted, before the advantage will be experienced to any profitable extent. It is very questionable if the governments of Europe will ever be satisfied with the manner of conducting quarantine in Turkey; or that it is even practicable to conduct it there in such a manner as to give satisfaction to those who are guided by the old sanatory rules, and consider them efficient and necessary.

displayed in all the operations, are very pleasing, and reflect credit on the conductor; whilst the expensive style of the buildings, and the profusion of marble, sufficiently indicate that they are government works.

The small-arms manufactory, and the cannon foundry and manufactory,—one at Dolmabagdsche, the other in Tophana,—are both conducted with considerable skill, and in great part on the improved European plan.   Both are under the superintendence of Turkish officers, who have been in England for instruction, and who, it is said, made whilst there considerable attainments in mechanical science.

In the small-arms manufactory, muskets, complete in all their parts, bayonets, pistols, and lances are made, of a good description, but, it would appear, at a cost much exceeding that at which they could be imported from England.   The steam-engine in use for boring the barrels is of fifty-horse power.   About sixty native workmen were employed, at the time of my visit, under two English engineers.

In the other manufactory, that of cannon, the business of casting is entirely managed by natives,—an operation with which they have been long familiar, and in which they have considerable skill, limited, however, hitherto to brass.   The boring of the cannon and the completion of them is now effected by the steam-engine, one of twenty-horse power; which, with that of larger size in the small-arms manufactory, was procured from England, and has, till very lately, with the beautiful machinery attached to it, been under the direction of an English engineer. The building in which the operation of boring is conducted is a large and substantial one, planned by an English architect, and erected at the enormous cost of L.200,000 sterling. This I learned from the intelligent English engineer, who also gave some curious particulars of the superstitious usages observed on first opening the manufactory ; how a lucky day, hour and minute, was calculated ; and how,— on the very minute determined on, every preparation having been previously made, the Sultan present with the great officers of state,—the operation of boring not one, but many cannon of various sizes, was simultaneously begun,—a complicated train of machinery starting into action in an instant as if by magic,—the moving power,—the steam-engine being in an adjoining room, and hid from the sight of the astonished spectators. Before I left Constantinople, the Englishmen in both manufactories were discharged, from views of economy. But whether the machinery can be used without such aid, is very questionable. The engineers were decidedly of opinion, that no native was competent to the management of it,—not even of the steam-engine alone,—and that, consequently, the Turks would be under the necessity either of resuming their old rude processes of manufacture, or of calling in further foreign assistance, begrudging the payment.

A striking difference exists between these manufactories so recently introduced into the country, that

they can hardly be said to be established, and those
of the old standing, which may be considered as indigenous. Nor is the difference less strongly marked
between the new schools and mode of instruction (I
speak of the design and not of the execution) commenced by the government on the modern European
plan, and the old schools and manner of teaching,
and the subjects taught. The new manufactories,
the new system of education, belong to the present
period of advance in art and science,—the period of
the connexion of the two. The old belong to past
times, have been continued from generation to generation unaltered; the schools under the influence of
the ancient philosophy, if any; and the arts, unconnected with, and unimproved by, science. Turkish
learning and the state of the arts in Turkey are both
of them much the same now as they were two or three
hundred years ago, or as learning and the arts were
in the East two or three thousand years ago. In the
higher colleges, where the men of the law receive
their education, a ten years' study, independent of
that of the Koran, which is the main subject, is
confined chiefly to the barren and wordy logic and
metaphysics of the Arabs, derived from the Greeks,
extended, perhaps, to astrology and Galenical medicine. In the minor schools, one of which is attached
to every mosque throughout the empire, and in
which a large proportion of the Turkish youth receive instruction, it is believed seldom to go beyond
lessons in reading and writing, and the committing

to memory verses of the Koran, in Arabic, without a knowledge of the language.

The unadvanced state of the arts is most obvious to every one who walks through the streets and bazaars of Constantinople, in which they are carried on with little or no combination of labour, with little capital, with a few and cheap implements; the work-man commonly his own shopman,—when not engaged in selling to the passing customer, occupied in mak-ing the article. There we see the unimproved hand-loom still in use; the small spinning-wheel; the hand-mill; with a variety of other implements and simple pieces of machinery, indicative of the stage adverted to. It would be vain to inquire amongst the people, or to seek in their workshops for any articles that may not be found in the bazaars of India, requiring more than individual dexterity, aided by a few simple tools. I never heard of a clock, or watch, or a telescope, or indeed of any complicated piece of machinery, made in the workshops of the capital. Constantinople is even without a glass-house, except-ing one hardly deserving the name, managed by Jews, of a very rude kind, in which vials and a few other articles, requiring little skill, are made from broken glass, remelted. Constantinople, too, is without a printing-press, excepting that which belongs to the government, and that on a small scale, and employed chiefly in printing official papers.

This backward, or unadvanced state, is not, I ap-prehend, owing to want of capacity of mind on the part of the people, any more than in the middle ages the rudeness which then prevailed amongst the nations of Europe, was attributable to this cause.   I have alluded to the aptness for learning, and the good abilities displayed amongst the students in the medical school of Galata Serai.   Even in the useful and ornamental arts, simple as most of them are, ingenuity of contrivance and some invention may often be witnessed, as well as much dexterity.   The works of the loom in Turkey are many of them beautiful and excellent.   The art of dyeing, in a limited way, has attained very great excellence.   Some articles of cutlery, of native manufacture, are also very excellent. In architecture, in ship-building,—arts more depending on individual talent than on scientific knowledge, resting on a few simple principles,—native Turks have distinguished themselves.   In the construction of their great mosques, their aqueducts,* and ships

* No country probably is better supplied with water than Turkey, and no city in Europe better than Constantinople.   This is not surprising, considering its climate and religion ; the latter restricting the inhabitants, in a great measure, to water as a drink, and requiring its almost constant use for the purposes of purifying ablution.   The Turkish plan of procuring water is simple, economical, and easy, and deserving of being generally known.   It is well exemplified in the great works constructed in the neighbourhood of the capital, on which the population is almost entirely dependent for this most necessary article.   They may be described as consisting of three parts—1st, Of " Bendts," or tanks, great reservoirs, vallies dammed up, in which rivulet and rain-water is collected ; 2d, Conduits, by which the water so collected is conducted to any distance, made in part of solid masonry, grand arched structures, in part of earthen-ware tubes, and in part of leaden pipes ; and, 3dly, Of " Sootcrays," or towers of

of war, proof has been given not less convincing than that afforded in the cathedrals of Europe, in the dark ages, of intellectual capacity, requiring only culture and encouragement, under favourable circumstances, to make progress in the arts and sciences generally, and attain excellence comparable with that attained by the western nations in the short space of a very few centuries.

I have alluded, in the opening of this chapter, to the two opposite views that have been taken of the present condition of the Turkish empire,—one that it is in the weakness and decline of old age, the other, that it is in its infancy, and has not yet put forth its strength, pointing out, at the same time, the little value of such speculations, founded on fanciful analogies, and offering a conjecture relative to the restorative influence of even one great man, were the re-

various use, communicating with the conduits, the summit of the sooterays being an elevated, little, open cistern, into which one pipe, ascending its side, terminates, and another pipe, descending, commences—a grating dividing the well. The uses of these structures, which commonly mark the line of a Turkish aqueduct, standing apart at certain distances, seem to be principally fourfold, viz. to determine practically the height to which the water will rise ; to render easy the finding out any accident that may befall the aqueduct; the purifying the water ; and, *lastly*, the escape of air. Of the many agreeable excursions which may be made in the neighbourhood of Constantinople in the fine season, as in the beginning of June, I know no one that will so well repay the traveller as a ride to Belgrade, affording him an opportunity of seeing the different artificial lakes, or bendts alluded to, surrounded by noble forest scenery, and the great and magnificent aqueducts by which the water is carried over vallies in its distant way to the city.

sources of the country placed at his disposal,—that is, if he held the reins of government.

Let us consider for a moment the description of men who, at present, conduct the government, and the system on which they act.

A Turkish minister is a man apart from the people. He may have started in life as a waiter in a coffee-house, as a boatman, even as a slave. His good looks may have attracted the attention of the Sultan, or of some influential person at court. He is made a page; he ascends from one grade to another amongst the ranks of courtiers till he has attained the highest rank. If it be the will of the Sultan, he may become Seraskier, Capitan-Pasha, or Grand Vizier. The only art he need cultivate is that of pleasing his superiors, and gaining their favour; the only knowledge, that of court forms and court intrigue. No knowledge of political economy,—no truly statesman-like knowledge is required;* it is not even necessary that he should be able to read or write; with a secretary and

---

* The above remarks apply to the system, not to individuals. Some of the high functionaries are the sons of men who have enjoyed high official rank; some have inherited wealth; some may be individually honest; but, it seems to be understood, that bribery, and corruption, and flattery, constitute the channel to favour and power, as the rule, —directed either to the principal in office in each department, or to his subordinates. The late Capitan-Pasha was considered a man of great integrity; yet, medical officers, to obtain an appointment whilst he was in office, had to pay, in advance, to some one influential under him,—a month's pay as a douceur,—without which he had no chance of success in his application: merit and professional qualification were entirely disregarded.

signet-ring,* he can dispense with both. The consequences of such a training are of the worst kind,
marked by disregard of honour and honesty, by indifference to the interests of the state,—in brief, by
intense selfishness. Power, with low sensual enjoy-
ments for its end and reward, is the aim of the regularly trained courtier. With an uncultivated mind,
what other enjoyment can he have? What I state,
I have been assured, is true, not only by Europeans,
well conversant with the Turkish people, acquired
during a residence of many years in Pera, but also
from Turks themselves. I remember once sitting in
a garden close to the Bosphorus, in the most charming season of the year, in the beginning of June,
when the air was in a manner vocal with the singing
of the nightingale, surrounded with flowers, and
orange and lemon-trees in fruit and flower, and hearing a confession of the kind from the luxurious owner,
himself, I fear, a striking example of the prevailing
character, which he pretended to deplore and depre-
cate—the sensual egotist, without regard for pos-
terity, satisfied if secure of his palace and gardens,
his houses and harem,—satisfied if the empire should
last his time,—totally indifferent as to its future

* The signet-ring is often used in Turkey by official persons of
high rank, and even by those who can write. The secretary, who
prepares a document, on presenting it for signature, has ready a kind
of printer's ink to apply to the signet, which he receives from and
returns to his chief, by whom the impression is made. The signet is
carefully kept in a little chain purse, made of fine gold or silver wire,
and is suspended from the neck.

condition. It is consistent with such a character that bribes should be offered and accepted,—that right and justice should be overlooked,—that merit should be put aside, and vice rather than virtue encouraged as that by which it can expect most to profit.

I have said that the Turkish minister is apart from the people. He appears to be so in a remarkable manner, owing to the vicious mode of his training. The people are commonly considered honest and truthful—influenced in a high degree by their religion—the forms of which are commonly strictly observed. They, too, are equally apart from the government. As Mohammedans, possessed of a good deal of personal freedom—all on an equality as to civil rank, under the Sultan—they can hardly be said to have any political rights. To express opinion, they must almost rebel. Indeed, without newspapers, without festivals bringing them together in large numbers, it can hardly be said that there is any public opinion—that it can be either formed or declared. The different provinces of the widely-spread empire— the different districts of each—their towns and villages—may be considered as so many separate families, and liable to fluctuations—such as we witness in families—this prospering, that decaying—owing to peculiar circumstances, without sensibly affecting the whole.

It is often asserted, in accordance with the hypothesis of the old age of the people, that the Turks have greatly degenerated : that they have lost their military ardour and their religious zeal. This, I apprehend, is very doubtful. The character of the government is changed, but, probably, not the character of the people. In the prosperous days of the empire the sultans were men of talent and energy— trained young to war and to business—in the command of provinces, and who had an eye to merit and fitness for office in the choice of their ministers. This palmy time terminated with a change of measures, especially the manner of bringing up the sons of the Sultan—when, debarred from manly exercises, deprived of all opportunities of acquiring a knowledge of mankind and of public affairs, they were, in consequence of jealous fear, confined in the seraglio, to the company of uneducated women and slaves. Such a training necessarily fitted them for sensual life rather than for command, whether in peace or war—fitted them to choose the adroit, flattering courtier, rather than the upright, talented man, and rendered them, more or less, dependent on ministers, and the tools of favourites.

The Turkish people seem little liable to change ; with the same climate—the same habits, and manners, and institutions—no cause is obvious which is likely to produce any material change. A similar remark applies to their religious feeling. They are attached to their religion by its forms—the daily uses required of them, as well as by the simplicity of its doctrines. When we see the Mohammedan, at the hours of prayer—whether in the bazaars of Constantinople, in a barrack-room, or the deck of a steamer in the Danube, surrounded by Franks— turn his face to Mecca, and perform the requisite prostrations, with an earnestness and abstraction, which may be a habit, but can hardly be affected, it is not easy to believe that his religion can be a matter of indifference—that he can be lukewarm about that to which he owes distinction—to which he has been taught to attach the greatest importance—his law and constitution, as well as his faith.   The little tendency to change in the Turkish people is very strongly exhibited in Constantinople.   Though for several centuries in daily communication with Pera and its Frank population, the Turks of the capital are as much an oriental people, are as little altered in their ways and habits, and modes of thinking, as if separated by a wide sea, instead of the Golden Horn. Their religion and language act more effectually than such a sea.   The distinctness of races in Constantinople, and the little tendency to amalgamate, presents a curious phenomenon.   Jews, Greeks, and Armenians, as well as Turks, equally keep apart, having the same great causes of separation—religion and language.

If the views which I have taken of the Turkish government and people be correct, it is easy to imagine a restoration of power to the empire—a widely spread improvement in the condition of the population—the introduction of science and useful know-

ledge, could honour, integrity, and patriotism be
infused into the administration. This is the very,
very great difficulty. Where low intrigue, bribery,
and corruption are the rule of conduct ; where the
majority entrusted with power are corrupt and intriguers, men of ordinary abilities and ordinary honesty are little inclined to seek office, and, if thrust
into it, have no chance of success in opposition,
if they have the desire to attempt it; they will
be carried away by the strength of the stream,
or thrown out and stranded. A master-mind seems
to be the one thing needful to perform the more
than Herculean task of effecting a regeneration
of the country through its government. Had the
Sultan such a mind, or any minister such a mind,
with supreme controlling influence, so that he could
act the part of a dictator, it is not difficult to imagine that, in a very short time, a complete reform
might be effected, and a new order of things established to a certain extent, even with existing institutions, under the Mohammedan religion and law,
which no more now than in the best times of the
Arabs seem to be incompatible with the study of
the sciences and with intellectual culture. The late
Sultan appears to have had some of the qualities of
the kind of mind requisite—fixed resolve—freedom,
in a great degree, from prejudice—no undue attach-
ment to usages. He destroyed the power that threatened and coerced him in the janissaries. He attempted to remodel the army, and place it on a footing

with the armies of Europe; he founded schools for instruction in modern science; and encouraged innovation generally.   Had his reign been prolonged, he might have effected much; but, it would appear, that he accomplished little in the way of radical reform.

Almost with the opening of the new reign of his son the Hatti Scheriff of Gulhane was published.*

* The ceremony of its publication was an unusual and impressive one.   It took place in the neighbourhood of the capital at Gulhane, " the Plain of Roses," on the 3d of November 1839.   Reschid Pasha, then Minister for Foreign Affairs, and the reputed author of it, read it aloud, in the presence of the Sultan and others of most weight in the empire, as appears from the heading of the document, of which the following is a translation, taken from the Globe newspaper of the 27th of November of the same year :—

   " Hatti Scheriff, read by Reshid Pasha on November 3, 1839, in
       presence of all the Ministers, Ulemas, Pashas, and Deputations
       of Nations, Sects, and Races subject to the Sultan.
   " All the world knows, that in the first times of the Ottoman monarchy, the precepts of the Koran, and the laws of the empire were a rule ever honoured, in consequence of which the empire increased in force and grandeur, and all its subjects, without exception, acquired a greater degree of ease and prosperity.   But, since a century and a half, a succession of accidents and different causes have led to the people's ceasing to conform to the sacred code of laws, and to the rules which flow from it.   Thus, the internal prosperity and force became changed to weakness and poverty.   An empire loses its stability in ceasing to observe its laws.
   " These considerations are always present to our mind ; and, since the day of our accession to the throne, the thoughts of the public good, of the amelioration of the provinces, and the alleviation of the people's burdens, have occupied me solely.   If one consider the geographical position of the Ottoman provinces, the fertility of their soil, the aptitude and intelligence of their inhabitants, one remains convinced that, by seeking out efficacious remedies, these may be obtained and put in practice within the space of a few years.   So that, full

Two views have been taken of this measure. By some it was considered as the consummation of the

of confidence in the succour of the Most High, and relying on the intercession of the Prophet, we judge fit to seek, by new institutions, to procure for the provinces of the empire the benefits of a good administration.

" These institutions relate principally to three things, which are—1st, Guarantees which insure to our subjects the security of honour and fortune ; 2d, A regular mode of levying imposts; 3d, A regular mode of levying soldiers, and fixing the duration of their service.

" Are not, in fact, life and honour the most precious benefits which exist ? What man, no matter how averse to violence be his character, could refrain from recurring to violence, if his life and honour be threatened ? If, on the contrary, these be secured, a man will not quit the paths of loyalty and fidelity. If such security be absent, every man remains cold to the voice of either prince or country. No one thinks of the public fortune, being too anxious about his own.

" It is most important to fix the rate of taxes. The state is obliged to have recourse to them for the defence of its territories. Fortunately for the people, some time back, they have been delivered from the vexatious system of monopolies, those bad sources of revenue. As bad a source of revenue still exists, in the venal concession of offices. By this system, the civil and local administration of each region is delivered up to the arbitrary will of one man; that is, to the most violent and greedy passions ; for, if such farmer of the revenue be not super-excellent, he can have no guide but his interest. It is henceforth requisite that each Ottoman subject should pay a certain sum of taxes proportioned to his fortune and faculties. It is also requisite that special laws should fix and limit the expenses of the military and naval force.

" Although the defence of the country is an important and universal duty, and although all classes of the population must furnish soldiers for the purpose, still there ought to be laws to fix the contingent of each locality, and limit to four or five years the term of military service. It is dealing a mortal blow to agriculture, as well as an injustice in itself, to take more hands from districts than they can fairly spare ; and it is to reduce soldiers to despair, and to depopulate the country, to retain them all their life in service.

reform commenced by his father—a magna charta of rights, including the Christian Rayah population

" Without such laws as these, of which the necessity is felt, there can be neither empire, nor force, nor riches, nor happiness, nor tranquillity. All these blessings may be expected from new laws. Henceforth, moreover, every accused person shall be publicly tried, according to the Divine law, after act and examination ; and no power shall secretly, or otherwise, cause any one to perish by poison, or by any other means, until a regular judgment has been passed. No one shall hurt another's honour, and each shall possess his property with liberty and in fear of no one. The innocent heirs of a condemned person shall inherit his property, nor shall the goods of the criminal be confiscated.

" These imperial concessions extend to all our subjects, of every religion without exception. Perfect security is accorded to all the inhabitants of the empire in life, honour, and fortune, as wills the text of our law.

" With regard to the other points, which must be regulated by enlightened opinions, our Council of Justice, augmented by new members, and by the adjunction of the ministers and nobility of the empire, shall assemble, in order to prepare laws for the security of life and fortune, and the regulation of imposts. Each person in these assemblies will state freely his ideas, and offer his advice.

" The laws respecting military service shall be debated, in a military council at the palace of the Seraskier. When the law is prepared, we will give it our sanction, and write with the imperial hand a heading.

" These institutions being to cause religion and government to flourish, we will permit nothing contrary to our promise.

" We will have these laws placed in the Chamber of the Prophet's Mantle, and will then swear to them in the presence of the ulemas and the grandees, making grandees and ulemas also swear. Whoever shall infringe these laws shall be punished with the legal penalty, and a penal code shall be drawn up for the purpose.

" All venality and traffic of offices shall be abolished, as the great cause of the decadence of the empire.

' These dispositions, being a revocation of old usages, shall be pub-

within the pale of equal justice, and defence from oppression. By others, it was viewed merely as a *coup d'etat*—a proclamation of words—a fiction to conciliate, on the threatening emergency (the Pasha of Egypt then almost threatening the capital), the good-will of the people, and the support of foreign powers, without intention of ever carrying the measure into effect. The result, it must be confessed, hitherto is rather in favour of the latter hypothesis than the former. The little that has been done in accordance with the Hatti Scheriff has been a failure —it has been so imperfectly done and so ill supported; the greater part has been passed over as a dead-letter; and the government now, constituted as before, seems to have fallen back on its old practices —its Conservative system, as it is sometimes called, —meaning, in Turkey, the perpetuation of abuses— that most corrupt system, acting on which no regard is paid to the public good—every thing good is sacrificed to ambition and lucre working by intrigue.*

lished at Constantinople and throughout our empire, and communicated officially to the ambassadors resident there.

" May the High God keep you in his guard ; and malediction on those who shall act contrary to these institutions."

* Already, probably, this Hatti Scheriff has been formally set aside. In an article in the Times of the 7th of February, under the head of private correspondence, bearing the date of Constantinople, January 12, it is stated,—" The Sultan on that day presided at a grand council, in which the proposal of issuing a *tauzeemat jedeedy*, or new organization, was solely mooted ;" which, adds the writer, " will have the effect of entirely upsetting it (the ordinance of Gulhane) in its main objects." And, in another article, of the 17th of the same

Had the Pasha by whom the Hatti Scheriff was promulgated (supposing him to have been sincere, as is commonly believed, in his liberal views and good intentions), had he been a wiser and abler man, grave in character, determined of purpose, sound of judgment,—securing him from being duped by foreign adventurers,—he might, perhaps, have made head, and triumphed over the party that opposed, and finally overthrew him. The time, in many respects, was propitious;—a young Sultan of unformed views, not, it was supposed, averse from change, owing to the instructions of his father; the empire in difficulty and extreme danger, from the machinations of the Pasha of Egypt; foreign powers tendering their aid to ward off the danger; and the British government affording varied and ample assistance in furtherance of the best interests of the country at this critical

month, a story is related of the proceedings of the new prime vizier quite in accordance with the olden usage—of his going in disguise, and punishing in the most summary manner, at the cost of life, a saucy pastry-cook, for refusing to sell him, under the disguise of a mendicant, a half a piastre worth of a delicate kind of pastry. . . . "Disdaining to make pennyworths, he told him to go about his business; and upon the seeming beggar importuning him still further, and stating his particular longing to eat a small piece of cadaif, he answered, he might eat a piece of his posteriors, if he liked. ' Well,' rejoined the beggar, throwing off the hood and cloak, and displaying the grand vizier in all his terrors—' Well, sirrah, if I must eat a piece of what you say, I will at least have it roasted. Ho there !' he continued, addressing four stout cavasses, who now rushed from their hiding-places, ' take the caitiff, and roast him in his own oven. The order was no sooner given than executed, and the consequences, I lament to say, were terrible."

period. It seemed a magnificent opening for a genuine reformer such as the country requires for its regeneration, if not doomed to perish,—a magnificent opening for such a man as Kiuprili,—one who, by the energies of a great mind directed to the public good, could overcome even intrigue and master abuses. Under the enlightened rule of such a man, acting as dictator, it is not difficult to imagine that a new character might be given to the empire, even without any material alteration in its framework, and that it might be made to assimilate to the kingdoms of Europe, which are not governed by free institutions. Colleges might be established; the sciences taught; good masters might be attached to the mosques; a system of education might be immediately commenced, and soon spread throughout the country; the provinces might be ruled with justice; the revenue, unoppressed as it is by a national debt, rendered productive and adequate to the wants of the state;* agriculture, and commerce, and the arts might be

* The Turkish revenue, if justly managed, it is supposed, would be more than adequate to the wants of the state. Its sources are few, and chiefly direct, of a kind not to be oppressive to any class; they are, chiefly, a land-tax, one-tenth of the produce; a capitation-tax, the haratch, confined to the Rayah population, of small amount (varying from about seventy to thirty piastres a-head, according to the means of the families); a trifling tax on houses in towns; and a three per cent. *ad valorem* duty on exports and imports. So reduced is the revenue at present,—so exhausted the treasury,—so low government credit,—that a paper currency lately issued to the extent only of a few hundred thousand pounds sterling, has been ill received; and though bearing an interest of twelve per cent., is at discount.

encouraged and improved; the army might be reorganized; the navy rendered efficient; posts for letters might be established; lines of road of easy communication opened; and various other ameliorations effected, calculated, as experience has universally taught, to benefit the people and strengthen the state.

Great as such a reform would be, a greater still may be conceived, founded on a change of religious views and of domestic manners; substituting, in the one, the humane and meek spirit of Christianity for the fierce and persecuting spirit of Mohammedanism; abolishing polygamy, and allowing woman her due influence and place in society. These are things merely to hint at; it would be idle to speculate on them in detail, and perhaps presumptuous.

Whatever measure of reform may take effect,— whether small or great,—it cannot be expected to originate in the people; the government must be looked to for it, and in the government it will be easy to witness its manifestations.

By a distinguished individual intimately acquainted with the condition of the country, thinking favourably of its innate vigour and resources, and considering that those persons labour under a great mistake who suppose that it is falling to pieces and about to perish, I have heard the empire compared to a Turkish dwelling-house, which has been patched and mended with wood and clay; ricketty to look at, and yet serviceable, and which, with patching and mending, may last a long while, he did not know how long. It may be compared, also, to a fine property neglected and abused,—its spendthrift owner having entrusted its management to a rapacious unprincipled agent, intent only on enriching himself, equally regardless of the interest of the proprietor and the tenantry.

Amongst those who speculate on the destinies of Turkey, and draw unfavourable auguries respecting the future, there are some who express their belief that the Rayah population, especially the Greeks and Armenians, are rising in importance, in wealth and intelligence, in activity and enterprise, as rapidly as they consider the Turks declining; and that the time is not very far distant, when they will form the dominant party. That the Greeks and Armenians have shown an increased desire, of late years, to have their children educated, seems universally admitted; and also that education amongst them is making progress. But it appears to be slow, for want of good schools; and for the same reason, of a very indifferent kind. Neither the Greeks or Armenians, with a joint population, estimated at about 400,000 in the capital and its suburbs, have a single college in Constantinople, nor I believe in the Turkish empire, in which the modern sciences are taught, and not a single school even, of any distinction.*   The

* The only good school belonging to the Greeks that came to my knowledge, is that in Kalki, one of the group of the Princes Islands, in the upper part of the sea of Marmora. It owed its establishment to the exertions of an enlightened Greek, sensible of the real wants of the people. Whilst presided over by him, its condition was flourish-

clergy of both people are generally very ignorant, and the Greek clergy especially opposed to the introduction of knowledge ; believing, with the hierarchy of their church, that knowledge and infidelity are intimately associated, having witnessed the production of the latter from superstition and bigotry. The moral condition of both people is, I fear, even less in advance than their intellectual, and at present so low as to render them totally unfitted to exercise, with success, a commanding control over others, or even to conduct a government of their own, supposing it possible that each people could be insulated and rendered independent. The vices peculiar to the Turkish government are considered as common amongst the Rayah population. They have not credit for honesty, straightforwardness, and that regard for truth, supposed to mark the Turkish character. Disunited amongst themselves, each sect of nominal Christians, hating the other, even with a greater hatred than they feel for their masters, it is highly improbable that they will be able to combine to act with effect against the government, even if they pos-

ing ; now it is less so. The number of students, when I visited it, in July 1841, was about sixty, from the age of eight upwards to twenty, the majority of them from Constantinople ; a few from Odessa. Under a principal, a Greek priest, and three professors, they are instructed in ancient and modern Greek, in writing, arithmetic, mathematics, and French. A small select collection of philosophical instruments belonged to the establishment, which bore no marks of use. The charge for board and education of each boy is about L.25 sterling a-year, paid by the parents.

sessed the courage requisite to attempt it. Mixing more with Europeans, some of the most respectable of them, having had the advantage of a liberal education in France, Switzerland, or Germany, they are more European than the Turks in their habits, tastes, and pursuits, and more inclined to assimilate with the great European family, with which they are united by religion, and the Greeks by blood.* This

* The Greeks of Constantinople have shown their disposition to imitate the institutions of Europe, by the establishment of a civil hospital outside the walls of the city, about five miles from Pera, into which are admitted all applicants of the Greek religion, including Russians. The building is of stone, new, good and ample, capable of accommodating about five hundred patients, and liberally supported by subscription. When I visited it, in August 1841, it contained about 125 patients, a small number of lunatics, and some infirm paupers, being used in the triple capacity of hospital, lunatic-asylum, and poor-house. Its expenditure then was as high as 33,000 piastres a-month, or about L.330 sterling. Under the management of a committee of some of the principal Greeks of Constantinople, its state was nowise creditable to them. So bad, indeed, was it, that we could not avoid coming to the conclusion that more lives were lost in it than saved, and that it would be a charity to close it. It was difficult also to avoid the conclusion that it was jobbed, and the funds abused. The wards were dirty and ill-ventilated; the walls begrimed with spittle; an attendant, bearing a brazier, into which, on the live-coals, he threw in, every now and then, sprigs of juniper, for fumigation, to overpower the bad smell, accompanied the surgeon from bed to bed, occupied in dressing sores. Such filth, such bad air, was accompanied, as might be expected, by hospital gangrene; the smallest sore, the slightest wound, often became gangrenous, and proved fatal; and gangrene, as a sequela of fever, was common. I need hardly observe, that no medical registers were kept, no cases recorded, no *post-mortem* examinations instituted; nothing, in fact, was discernible, indicative of a more scientific manner of conducting the business of the establishment, than that followed in the military hospitals of the Turks, to which

disposition, under favouring circumstances, may have an excellent effect, especially if it should induce them to cultivate the virtues of the west, its literature and science. It would be a glorious triumph for them, could they take the lead in what is good, be an example, in these respects, and earn an independence in civil rights by the force of merit, proving themselves deserving of it. The Sultan, by the Hatti Scheriff of Gulhane, has promised his Rayah subjects justice. If the great powers of Europe see to the performance of this promise, and exert their influence over the Porte accordingly, the opportunity will be given for that improvement so much required, so much to be desired, and which may be so important in its consequences. The breaking out of the Greek revolution was marked by dreadful atrocities. Similar scenes are likely to occur, unless the Rayahs estimate their weakness more justly, and are content, if not oppressed (which the powers of Europe may prevent),

this was much inferior in point of order and cleanliness. And the portion of it used as a lunatic-asylum, was only a grade better than that in the city already alluded to, adjoining the menagerie. The lunatics in this also, were all secured by heavy chains attached to the neck; had to sleep on the floor, in their clothes, on a rug, and were under no medical treatment ; and, horrible to be related, a poor lad, subject to epilepsy, was chained in the same manner, and his malady equally neglected. These horrors I notice, with the hope of drawing attention to them. It is extraordinary the abuses which are fallen into and tolerated, when there is an indifference to public opinion, or rather a want of means of forming and expressing it. In all institutions the constant tendency is to abuse, requiring to be perpetually checked by inspection and exposure.

to work out their " good estate" by self-improve-
ment.　Last winter, when there were risings in Bul-
garia and Candia, rumour was loud and frequent of
conspiracies amongst the Greeks, even in the capital.
How disastrous would the consequences have been,
had there been any demonstration!　Insurrection on
foot, the massacre of the christian population would
be almost inevitable.　Even the best disciplined
troops cannot act, on such occasions, with moderation ; and what chance of success for the insurgents,
ignorant even of the use of arms.　They have much
to answer for, who talk lightly of the weakness of the
Turks ; of the strength and union of the Christians in
Turkey ; of the decline of the one, and the advance-
ment of the other,—if with a view, as has too often
been the case, to spirit up the latter to resistance,
which must end, if attempted, in their ruin.

APPENDIX.

APPENDIX.

APPENDIX.

LETTER from Dr ROBERTSON, Deputy Inspector-General of Hospitals, to the Author, on the Present State of the Medical School at Cairo ; with some Remarks on Turkish Military Hospitals ; the Treatment of Medical Men by the Turks ; the Question of the Contagion of Plague ; and the System of Quarantine, as observed in Egypt.*

London, March 18, 1842.

MY DEAR SIR,—I promised to give you some account of the much talked of medical school of Egypt, so far as it came under my notice during my late visit to that country. The idea of forming such an institution among a nation of barbarians, unprepared by preliminary education for scientific studies, originated, as you are, no doubt aware, with Clot Bey, the principal medical officer attached to the army. The scheme, however, was only a part of that system which Mehemet Ali was induced to adopt, by the advice of designing and flattering foreign adventurers.

He was persuaded that the manufactures, and even the learned institutions of the civilized nations of Europe, could at once be introduced among the ignorant and prejudiced Egyptians.

* Dr Robertson, at my request, having obligingly permitted me to make any use I may think proper of this private letter, I am induced to insert it, believing that, though hastily written, as he informed me was the case, under the pressure of business, it is accurate as to information, and well fitted to enlighten the public on several points.

Some of these, while supported by an immense expenditure of money, had an appearance of success, but of late, the finances being exhausted, and having no inherent vigour, are now rapidly going to decay.

The medical school was established in 1827, at a place called Abouzabel, on the border of the Desert. This site was selected as there was a large military hospital, and the camp of military instruction at Kanka was in the neighbourhood.

Medical men, all foreigners of course, and I believe for the most part previously employed in the army, were appointed as *professors*.

A more difficult task was to find pupils ; and it was found necessary to receive children, taken almost by force from their parents : these, of course, required to be put under a course of preliminary instruction, which I believe, however, was very imperfect.

These pupils were perfectly ignorant of the language of their professors, who are said to have written their lectures in French, which were afterwards translated into Arabic by persons perfectly ignorant of any science.

Whatever may have been the talents of the teachers, no one, acquainted with the difficulties which even well prepared pupils experience when commencing the study of the medical profession, could expect any other result than failure from such a mode of instruction. So unsatisfactory were the services of the persons sent from the school for medical duty in the army, that Ibrahim Pacha sent many of them back.

I believe Clot Bey contradicts this ; but I am free to declare that I never heard any other than an unfavourable opinion of the acquirements of those persons from those competent to form a judgment. The camp for military instruction no longer exists, and the military hospital and the school of medicine have been transferred to Cairo. The hospital and school form one establishment, the medical duties of the hospital being performed by the professors, as they are called. The building is excellent, and the site well chosen, about two miles from the town, on the banks of the Nile. The hospital could accommodate a thousand patients or more ; the wards are spacious, a double row on each story, with a fine corridor in the centre.

The apartments for the school are at one end of the hospital, and form a square ; on one side, the library, lecture-rooms, &c. ; on the other, the dormitories, kitchen, stores, &c.

I may now mention that, since the late political changes in Egypt, foreign *employés* are being dismissed from all the public establishments, partly for retrenchment, and partly from the vanity of some of the natives, who think they can stand alone. The only foreigner now employed in the school of medicine is the director, Monsieur Perron ; all the other officers are natives, who have been, in some degree, educated in Europe, chiefly at Paris.

Supposing these gentlemen properly qualified, they would have great advantages over the foreign professors, in being able to communicate directly with the pupils in their own language.

Here we have a splendid display—a fine hospital—a school for medical science, conducted by native professors ! Is not Mehemet Ali a great man ; and have not the Egyptians made rapid progress in civilization ? will exclaim the superficial observer.

I regret to say, that the impression left on my mind, from personal inspection of the details, was, that it is a mere display—a splendid exhibition—which deceives Mehemet Ali and strangers, who either examine superficially, or are incompetent to judge of the matter.

I first examined the library ; it is a small room, with a collection of books, chiefly French, and a few elementary compilations from Broussais and others, translated into Arabic by Mons. Perron, who, every one reports, is a good linguist. Here also are some wax figures for anatomical illustration, and a few commonplace philosophical instruments—the last carefully locked up, and apparently never used. The library has no appearance of being frequented.

The next apartment I visited was a small pharmacy containing the medicines required for the use of the hospital. I observed that the nomenclature used was without system.

From the pharmacy I was introduced into the museum. It contains only a tolerable collection of the birds of the country. Some of the specimens are splendid. The anatomical theatre and operating room is well constructed, lighted from the top, and arranged much as one sees in Europe. It was the winter season, the time for dissection ; and I at least expected to see some signs of practical anatomy being carried on. I was told it was; but not a sign could

I observe of such being the case. No part of the human body, not even a bone, no tables, no instruments, not a vestige of work. Not a single preparation of either morbid or natural anatomy could I observe in any part of the institution. I cannot, therefore, think otherwise than that although a knife may occasionally be applied to a dead body, yet that anatomy is not taught practically, and that prejudice against dissection is not overcome, or that the professors are incompetent or careless. Disappointed with the anatomical department, I asked to see the chemical one; the same disappointment followed. No furnaces; only a few of the most common kind of apparatus. It was quite evident that no proper course of chemical instruction was being carried on.

The Native Professors were not visible; and, although I expressed a wish to be present at some of the lectures, it was evaded. I have already stated, that the hospital is an excellent building; the wards are good; the bedding also is superior for the class of patients. It is a military hospital; and when I saw it, it contained about 200 patients only, nearly all chronic cases. No medical records are kept. The ophthalmic and venereal patients are kept separate. There are also surgical and medical wards. I did not see any medicine in any of the wards. Of 100 ophthalmic cases, not twenty had escaped the loss of either one or both eyes. The treatment, as far as I could ascertain, was inert. There existed no marks of local blood-letting, or of counter-irritation ; the more strange as these are very generally used even by the Arabs. It was the director who accompanied me during my visit; he was, I believe, not a medical man originally, but a chemist, and did not seem to understand the stimulating mode of treatment, at least by nitras argenti.

It must be allowed that the establishment of hospitals has been of great advantage to the Egyptian soldier. He is at least well lodged, and tolerably well fed; but my experience both in Syria and Egypt, convince me that he has rarely the benefit of proper medical treatment. The medical school, I am of opinion, will ere long cease to exist, from the inefficiency of its conductors, and the little encouragement that exists for medical men among the natives. An intelligent and well-educated Egyptian would find it much more advantageous to follow commercial pursuits, than to study medicine. Turks and Egyptians have no respect for a physician, unless he boasts of knowing *specifics* for every disease. If a particular mode of living, and attention to the natural functions be recommended for the cure of a disease, it only excites their contempt for your ignorance. They are also extremely illiberal in the remuneration of medical men; indeed often I have been told, they will not pay at all.

As an instance of the preference for quacks, I may mention what I heard from a medical man, who was attending a Pacha, and also one of his harem. Both were doing well under a system of treatment, when one day he sent his secretary to ask the doctor if he could promise to cure them in a fortnight? who replied that he neither could nor would; that the cure was going on well; and that, by pursuing the same treatment, they would certainly recover. The secretary then said, I am, in that case, desired to tell you that an Arab has promised to perform a cure in a fortnight, and the Pacha will employ him unless you will promise to do so in as short a period.

No encouragement exists for a school of medicine among the people; such an institution is far beyond the general state of civilization. The government, also, have less motives to support it, and very diminished resources. The army is now reduced to 18,000 regulars, and there is less demand for medical men in the service.

The position of medical men in the service of the Pacha is far from being what it has been represented. The pay is perhaps sufficient for a native, but not such as would induce a respectable and well-educated European to serve. The medical officers are treated with little consideration; it is true they have comparative army rank; but any rank in the Turkish or Egyptian army, under that of a colonel, obtains little respect.

During the time I was in Egypt, plague was not prevalent; an occasional case was reported by the officers of the quarantine establishment at Alexandria; at Cairo it was said not to exist. It is probable, however, that had there existed a quarantine establishment at Cairo, cases would have been found equally deserving the name of plague as those at Alexandria.

From all I could learn from the best sources of information, plague is an endemic disease in Egypt, and at all times, although *rarely* in the extreme heat of summer,—sporadic cases may be met with.

At some periods, from causes that escape the most scrutinizing observation, the disease rages in an epidemic form ; such was the case in 1835. During the periods when the disease is only of occasional occurrence, the symptoms are comparatively mild. When prevalent in an epidemic form, a large proportion of the cases are fatal.

All the medical men I met with were decidedly of opinion that the disease arises from local causes (not known), and that contagion is neither necessary for its production or propagation. Some, however, appear to believe that, under particular circumstances, it may be communicated from the sick to the healthy. All evidence, however, goes to prove, that this is at least very rarely the case.*

I was informed by Mons. Perron that he has known the disease to be prevalent in a village, while a neighbouring one, not more than a mile or two distant, was free, the inhabitants all the time communicating without restriction ; and the next year circumstances were completely reversed, the disease altogether leaving the unhealthy village, and attacking the other.

The wonderful stories that are told, to show the extreme contagious nature of plague, in my opinion prove exactly the contrary. Europeans, when plague is epidemic, shut themselves up,—observe the most rigid seclusion. Notwithstanding all their precautions, the disease attacks them. Having previously convinced themselves that the plague is never produced except by contagion, they begin to inquire how it could have been introduced ; in vain they endeavour to find that there has been some breach of the system of seclusion that had been established. At length, however, they find that a *dog*, a *bird*, or a *feather*—above all, some unfortunate cat, has made an entry, and communicated the disease. Now, would it not be much more rational, in these cases, to doubt at least the justice of the preconceived notice of contagion. It does not appear that those

---

* Before Dr Robertson visited Syria and Egypt, in common with most of his professional brethren at home, he considered plague a virulently contagious disease : this he authorises me to state. And further, that as he gained experience, his faith in this doctrine has diminished and is now much shaken.

persons, who adopt a system of seclusion during the prevalence of plague, more frequently escape than those who take no precautions ; but this is easily accounted for, from their being generally lodged in the most healthy locality, and avoiding all the predisposing causes to disease.

Taking for granted that the principles on which quarantine regulations are formed are just, the system pursued in Egypt is absurd. Quarantine is enforced at the sea-ports, while communication by land with places where plague may be prevalent is left free.

Political reasons alone, I am convinced, induce Mehemet Ali to keep up quarantine establishments. I believe also a revenue is derived from them.

The annoyance, and even real suffering and danger incurred by travellers is great. At Damietta, for example, there is no lazaretto, and it has often occurred that travellers from Syria (perhaps that country at the time free from plague) have been obliged to live in an open shed on the sands for ten days. From my own knowledge, this lately occurred to some English gentlemen.

I do sincerely hope that our government may be induced to take up seriously the question of quarantine. Our own rules in England are bad enough ; the system adopted with the Alexandrian steam-vessels is a perfect farce.

I am, my dear sir, most truly yours,

J. ROBERTSON.

INDEX.

INDEX.

	Vol.	Page
Ænos, Mount, in Cephalonia, climate of,	i.,	240
Agriculture, state of, in the Ionian Islands,	i.,	318
... in Malta,	i.,	274
Antiquity, remains of, in the Ionian Islands and Malta,	i.,	19
Aqueduct in Corfu, ceremony of opening,	i.,	133
... Malta,	i.,	170
Aristotle, his opinion respecting the cause of earthquakes in Greece,	i.,	192
Arts, state of, in the Ionian Islands,	ii.,	32–42
... Constantinople,	ii.,	458
Asphaltum of Antipaxo,	i.,	88
Assembly, Legislative, of Ionian Islands,	ii.,	4
Asylum, Lunatic, in Corfu,	ii.,	118
... Constantinople,	ii.,	421
Bacile, measure of land in Malta,	i.,	388
Bank, Ionian, lately established,	ii.,	74
... Island Savings,	ii.,	78
Barometer, observations on, in the Ionian Islands,	i.,	234
... ... Malta,	i.,	308
... ... Constantinople,	ii.,	400
Baths, Turkish,	ii.,	419
Births, in Gozo, return of,	i.,	433
Bituminous matter in mountain limestone of the Ionian Islands,	i.,	49
Black Sea, climate of,	ii.,	403
Bleaching, experiments on,	i.,	295
Bosphorus, temperature of,	ii.,	405
... specific gravity of water of	ii.,	404
Bowring's, Dr, observations on quarantine,	ii.,	329

	Vol.	Page
Breakwater, floating, suggestion respecting	i.,	163
Bread, in Malta, return of price of,	i.,	409
Breccia-bone, in the Ionian Islands,	i.,	55
Campi artificiali, in Malta, how formed,	i.,	392
Caprification, particulars respecting,	i.,	367
Catacombs,	i.,	20
Cattle, neglect of, in Ionian Islands,	i.,	381
... attention to in Malta,	i.	411
Calamo, district of, in Cerigo,	i.,	387
Catastari, a village in Zante,	ii.,	157
Carriages, in Malta, return of,	ii.,	388
Caverns, remarkable ones in Ionian Islands,	i.,	62
Cemetery in Corfu, recently opened,	ii.,	144
Cisterns in Malta, manner of forming,	i.,	168
Chicken-pox, remarks on,	ii.,	388
Climate of Ionian Islands in general,	i.,	244
... mountainous and hilly region,	i.,	239-244
... Malta,	i.,	251
... ... of town and country,	i.,	259-263
... Constantinople,	ii.,	393
Church, Greek, effect of its ordinances on the state of agriculture,	i.,	325
Coolness, suggestions for procuring, in sleeping apartments in hot climates,	i.,	289
Colonia-system in Ionian Islands, effects of on agriculture,	i.,	322
Corn-lands and crop in Ionian Islands,	i.,	329
... ... Malta,	i.,	408
... kinds of, grown in Malta,	i.,	407
Commerce, capabilities of Ionian Islands for,	ii.,	57
Conglomerate rock, now forming in Santa Maura,	i.,	55
Commissioner, Lord High, of Ionian Islands,	ii.,	1-12
Consumption, Pulmonary, remarks on in the Mediterranean,	ii.,	280, 322
... ... proportional mortality from,	ii.,	312
... ... suggestions for prevention of,	ii.,	318
... ... remarks on, in Constantinople,	ii.,	422
Council, primary, of Ionian Islands,	ii.,	4
... municipal,	ii.,	5
Constantinople, observations on climate of,	ii.,	393
... meteorological table for,	ii.,	400
... diseases of,	ii.,	420
... public institutions,	ii.,	427

	Vol.	Page
Constantinople, schools and colleges of,	ii.,	440
... manufactories,	ii.,	454
... aqueducts,	ii.,	459
... barracks,	ii.,	437
Cotton-plant in Malta,	i.,	402–407
Consultation, Greek Medical,	ii.,	197
Crimes, prevailing, in Ionian Islands,	i.,	321
Crops in Ionian Islands, return of,	i.,	327
... Malta and Gozo,	i.,	396
... ... rotation of,	i.,	398
Currant-plantations of Ionian Islands,	i.,	339
... trade, particulars of,	ii.,	64–90
Cummin, its exhausting effects on the land,	i.,	399
Currents, sea, flowing into land,	i.,	165
Decoy for doves,	ii.,	55
Dew, observations on, in Ionian Islands,	i.,	237
... ... Malta,	i.,	292
... composition of,	i.,	293
Dimecks, their workshops and sculpture in Malta,	i.,	120
Douglas, Sir Howard, his description of the earthquake of 1840,	i.,	187
... remarks on deficiency of timber-trees in the Ionian Islands,	i.,	382
Drakea, islet of, on coast of Corfu,	i.,	84
Dress of Ionian people,	ii.,	136
... Turks,	ii.,	415
Drought, effects of, in Malta,	i.,	296
Dust, shower of, in the Mediterranean,	i.,	301
Dyeing, in Ionian Islands, methods of,	ii.,	51
Earthquakes in Ionian Islands,	i.,	176
... some remarkable ones described,	i.,	185
... conjectures respecting their cause,	i.,	193
Ecclesiastical establishments in Ionian Islands,	ii.,	9
Education, state of in the Ionian Islands,	ii.,	102
... ... in Santa Maura,	i.,	323
Elphinstone, Sir Howard, his meteorological tables in Malta,	i.,	259, 263–278
Egypt, medical school and military hospitals in, notice of,	ii.,	482
Exports, Ionian Islands, return of,	ii.,	60
Fano, islet of,	ii.,	206
Farmer, in Malta and Gozo, condition of,	i.,	415–430

Vol. Page

Fishing, modes of, in Ionian Islands, . . . ii., 54
Fevers of Ionian Islands, ... ii., 218-240
   ... Malta, ... ii., 262-273
Ferrara, M., analysis of dust of a shower, . . i., 306
Flocks of Ionian Islands, ... i., 372
Fog, observations on, ... i., 248
Foundlings, hospital for, in Ionian Islands, . . . ii., 119
Forest of Black Mountain, conflagration of, . . . i., 75
Freestone of Malta, ... i., 105
Frere, Right Hon. J. H., his account of a remarkable funnel-shaped
   cavity in Malta, ... i., 312
Fruits of Ionian Islands, ... i., 362
   ... Malta and Gozo, ... i., 422-430
Funeral ceremony in Ionian Islands, ... ii., 144

Gales, observations on, in Malta, ... i., 278
Galland, Dr C., his tables of average life in Gozo, . . i., 432
Garden-ground in Ionian Islands, ... i., 360
   ... Malta and Gozo, . . . i., 422-429
Georgio, St. monastery of, in Zante, ... ii., 165
Giant's Tower in Gozo, ... i., 20
Gilliamano in Zante, village of, ... ii., 180
Government of Ionian Islands, form of, ... ii., 1
   ... character, ... ii., 11
   ... Turkish, ... ii., 461
Gozo, climate of, ... i., 311
Goats, mischief from, ... i., 384
Grease spring, erroneously so called, ... i., 147
Grain in Malta, return of, ... i., 409
Granite in Cerigo, ... i., 48
Grafting in Ionian Islands, methods of, ... i., 364
Gypsum, its abundance in Ionian Islands, . . . i., 86

Hail in Malta, ... i., 310
Handcock, Mr, his remarks on the currant-trade, . . ii., 91
Harmattan wind, ... i., 270
History of Ionian Islands, sketch of, . . . i., 22-33
   ... Malta, ... i., 34-46
Hoe, different forms of, used in Ionian Islands and Malta, . i., 330-417
Homeric notices of Ionian Islands, ... i., 21
Horticulture in Ionian Islands, ... i., 362

	Vol. Page
Horticulture in Malta and Gozo,	i., 423–430
Houses, Ionian,	ii., 132
... in Constantinople,	ii., 416
Hospitals, Turkish military,	ii., 429
... Egyptian,	ii., 484
Ice, its artificial production,	i., 291
Implements, agricultural, of Ionian Islands,	i., 329
... ... Malta,	i., 417
Instruments, musical, of Ionian Islands,	i., 374
Imports, return of, for Ionian Islands,	ii., 59
Insanity in Turkey, remarks on,	ii., 422
Institutions, charitable, of Ionian Islands,	ii., 117
... public, in Constantinople,	ii., 449
Ionian Islands, enumeration of,	i., 33
Irrigation in Ionian Islands,	i., 344–363
... Malta,	i., 420
Jameson, Mr R., observations by,	i., 58, 65, 93
Judicial establishments of Ionian Islands,	ii, 7
Justice, defective administration of, in Ionian Islands,	i., 380
Kieri, village in Zante,	ii., 189
Knights of Malta, form of oath that was taken by, on entering the order,	i., 40
Knife, pruning, forms of in use in Ionian Islands,	i., 344
Knowledge, state of, in the Ionian Islands,	ii. 96
Lamps in use in Ionian Islands,	ii., 46
Labour-field, particulars of,	i., 376
... ... in Malta and Gozo,	i., 416–430
Land tenures in Ionian Islands,	i., 378
... Malta,	i., 395
... waste in Ionian Islands, return of,	i., 386
... ... Malta and Gozo,	i., 412, 429
... rent and selling-price in Malta,	i., 413
Laws, new codes of, for Ionian Islands,	ii., 15
Leo, St., in Zante, mountain village,	ii., 175
Lazarettoes, remarks on their insecurity,	ii., 243
Life in Gozo, low average duration of,	i., 431
Lignite, localities of, in Ionian Islands,	i., 88

Vol. Page

Leftimo, in Corfu, district of, ... ii., 201
Lime, carbonate of, enamel-like deposit of, on shores of Ionian
    Islands, ... : . i., 90
Lightning, a particular effect of, ... i., 96
Longevity, instances of, ... ii., 176–181

Maklouba, a singular pit in Malta, ... i., 109
Malta, its state before occupied by the knights, . . . i., 37
   ... when most flourishing, under the rule of the order, . i., 39
   ... its commercial prosperity, ... i., 43
Malaria considered, ... ii., 241–273
   ... precautions against, ... ii., 258
Maize, its culture in Ionian Islands, ... i., 333
Manure, neglect of, ... i., 379
   ... valued and used in Malta, ... i., 419
Marriage ceremony in Ionian Islands, ... i., 433
Marriages in Gozo, return of, ... i., 433
Maries in Zante, village of, ... ii., 171
Manganese, its localities in Ionian Islands, . . . i., 93
Marble statuary of Cerigo, ... i., 48
Marl deposit of, in Ionian Islands, ... i., 53
Mediterranean Sea, peculiarities of, ... i., 195
   ... ... density of its water, ... i., 199
   ... ... its temperature, . . . i., 205–215
   ... ... comparative moisture of its air, . i., 217–219
   ... ... conjectures respecting its saltness, . . i., 222
   ... ... its currents, ... i., 223
Medals Prize, founded by Sir H. Douglas, . . . ii., 104
Metairie system, effects of, in agriculture, . . i., 321–324
Meganisi, islet of, ... ii., 199
Meschiato, ... i., 409
Merlera, islet of, ... ii., 207
Mill, notice of a very primitive one, ... ii., 44
Mist, on the formation of, ... i., 248
Mortality, return of for Gozo, ... i., 431
Mountains, Ionian Islands, summer climate of, . . . i., 242
   ... as masses of matter, their tendency to equalize tempera-
      ture, ... i., 258
Monuments, ancient, destruction of, in Ionian Islands, . . i., 25
   ... ... in Malta, . . . i., 36

Vol. Page

Mummy cloth, its composition, ... i., 402

Napier, Sir C., observations on the summer climate of the Black
mountain, ... i., 240
... ... account of Seraglia—impositions in Cephalonia, i., 347
... ... of the mischief from goats, . . i., 384
Nile, mud, composition of, ... i., 53
Nitre, observations on its formation, . . . i., 121

Ocean, specific gravity of, between Ceylon and England, . . i., 202
Olive plantations in Ionian Islands, . . . i., 350
... process of extracting the oil, . . . i., 353
Oven in use in Ionian Islands, ... ii., 45

Patarella, rude boat of rushes, ... ii., 53
Pasture lands in Ionian Islands, ... i., 369
Paxo, island of, ... ii., 212
Parliament, Ionian, particulars of, ... ii., 4
... examples of acts of, ... ii., 22
Pegada (Perapapigada) in Ithaca, ... i., 77
Perjury, prevalence of in Ionian Islands, . . . i., 322
People, Ionian, character of, by different authors, . ii., 148–154
... Turkish remarks on, ... ii., 464
Pieta Monte de, ... ii., 117
Pitch Wells in Zante, ... i., 153
Plague, oriental, remarks on, ... ii., 330
... in Malta in 1813, ... i., 44
Porter, Mr, his Tables on the trade of the Ionian Islands, . ii., 80
Pluviometer, observations on, at Gibraltar, . . . i., 253
Plough, notices of, ... i., 330–417
Pottery, antique, examination of varnish, . . . ii., 71
... of Ionian Islands, ... ii., 72
Population of Ionian Islands, return of, ... ii., 58
... particulars respecting, ... ii., 124
... of Malta, ... ii., 372
Poor, destitute in Ionian Islands, ... ii., 120
Pronos in Cephalonia, ... i., 163
Produce, agricultural return of, for Ionian Islands, . . i., 327
... ... for Malta and Gozo, . . i., 396
Press, remarks on, in Ionian Islands and Malta, . . ii., 392

	Vol. Page
Quarry, ancient one of sandstone in Cerigo, . . .	i., 84
Quartz in mountain limestone of Ionian Islands, . .	i., 49
Quarantine, remarks on, ...	ii., 323
... objections to classification of substances, . .	ii., 337
... inconsistencies, ...	ii., 347
... connexion with police restrictions, . . .	ii., 349
... necessity for further inquiry, . . .	ii., 352
... facts in favour of a milder and more efficient system,	ii., 357
... notice of, in Turkey, ...	ii., 450
... remarks on, in Egypt, ...	ii., 487
Rain in Ionian Islands, observations on, . . .	i., 232
... in Malta, ...	i., 297
... in Gibraltar, ...	i., 252
... disastrous effects of, . . .	i., 256, 186, 298
... shower of, with dust, ...	i., 300
Radiation of heat in Ionian Islands, . . .	i., 237
... ... in Malta, ...	i., 281
Rice, suggestions for its cultivation in the Ionian Islands, .	i., 358
... upland of Ceylon and Sumatra, note respecting, .	i., 359
... grounds, injurious effects of on climate doubtful, .	i., 360
Revenue of Malta, ...	i., 409
Roads of Ionian Islands, ...	ii., 76
Robertson, Dr, his remarks on quarantine, and medical school and hospitals in Egypt, ...	ii., 481
Rocks of Ionian Islands, ...	i., 47
... Malta, ...	i., 102
... action of plants on, ...	i., 118
Salines, ...	ii., 71
Salm, Maltese measure, ...	ii., 3
Samitraki, islet of, ...	ii., 207
Samos, ancient tombs at, ...	i., 19
Sandal in use in Ionian Islands, . . .	ii., 51
Scopo, mount, in Zante, ...	i., 79
Seasons in Ionian Islands, peculiarities of, . .	i., 226
... Malta, ...	i., 257
... Constantinople, ...	ii., 394
Schools of Ionian Islands, . . .	ii., 102, 112
Senate, Ionian, ...	ii., 3

	Vol. Page
Sincliti, qualifications of,	ii., 2
Shepherd in Ionian Islands, habits of,	i., 371
Seraglie, notice of,	i., 347
Shipping of Ionian Islands,	ii., 58
Schupanack, lazaretto of,	ii., 425
Spiliotissa, monastery in Zante,	ii., 159
Slate, calcareous, of Ionian Islands,	i., 51
Sirocco wind, observations on,	i., 268
... its peculiarities,	i, 271
... conjectures on its origin,	i., 277
Spenser, Sir Robert, his notice of a shower of dust,	i., 303
Small-pox in Malta, account of.	ii., 368
Smuggling, remarks on, in connexion with quarantine,	ii., 344
Springs, situation of, in Ionian Islands and Malta,	i., 122–167
... temperature of, in Ionian Islands,	i., 227
... ... in Malta,	i., 265
... varieties of,	i., 129
... mineral,	i., 143
... sulphuretted,	i., 144
... bituminous,	i, 153
... saline,	i., 143–172
... anomalous peculiarities of,	i., 160
Spring of Alexandria Troas,	i., 141
Soils of Ionian Islands,	i., 313
... Malta and Gozo,	i., 389
Society, agricultural, in Malta,	i., 427
Still in use in Ionian Islands,	ii., 47
Stock in Ionian Islands, return of,	i., 327
... in Malta and Gozo,	i., 397
Strofades, islets,	i., 141
Sulphur, its localities in Ionian Islands,	i., 87
Sulla, manner of its cultivation,	i., 410
Superstitions of Ionian people,	ii., 100
Tar, mineral of Zante,	i., 157
Temperature, atmospheric, of Ionian Islands,	i., 229
... ... Malta,	i., 259
... peculiarity of in hollows,	i., 250
Thunder storms in Malta,	i., 310
Tombs, ancient Greek, at Samos,	i., 19

	Vol.	Page
Towns of Ionian Islands, ...	ii.,	131
Tufa, notice of a fact in illustration of its formation, . .	i.,	138
Tulloch, Major, his conclusions respecting pulmonary diseases in the Mediterranean, ...	ii.	281
Turks of Constantinople, particulars respecting, . .	ii.,	418–463
University, Ionian, notice of, ...	ii.,	102
Valetta, town of, ceremony of its foundation, . . .	i.,	38
Vallies, basin-like, in Ionian Islands, . . .	i.,	71
Vaccination in Malta, proof of its efficacy, . .	ii.,	383
Valonea oak, its valuable produce, . . .	ii.,	383
Venetian government of Ionian Islands, . .	i.,	28
Verdea, a wine of Zante, ...	i.,	338
Vestis melitensis, conjecture respecting, . . .	i.,	401
Village life in Zante, ...	ii.,	182
Vineyards in Ionian Islands, particulars of, . .	i.,	334
Vrachiona, ascent of, a mountain in Zante, . .	ii.,	161
Vromi, bay of, in Zante, ...	ii.,	169
Wages of labourers in Ionian Islands, . . .	i.,	376
... ... in Malta, . . .	i.,	416
... remarks on, in connexion with price of food, .	i.,	427
Water cistern, particulars respecting, . .	i.,	142, 171
... rain, composition of, ...	i.,	299
Watering of ground, methods of in Ionian Islands, .	ii.,	48
Washing, manner of conducting, . . .	ii.,	49
Wines of Ionian Islands, ...	i.,	336
Winds prevailing, ...	i.,	238, 247
... ... of Malta, ...	i.,	265
... ... at the Dardanelles, . . .	i.,	240

FINIS.

MURRAY AND GIBB, PRINTERS, GEORGE STREET, EDINBURGH.